Health Counseling

Health Counseling

Judith A. Lewis
Governors State University

Len Sperry
Medical College of Wisconsin

Jon Carlson
Governors State University

Brooks/Cole Publishing Company
Pacific Grove, California

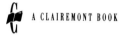 A CLAIREMONT BOOK

Brooks/Cole Publishing Company
A Division of Wadsworth, Inc.

Printed in the United States of America
10   9   8   7   6   5   4   3   2   1

Library of Congress Cataloging-in-Publication Data
Lewis, Judith A., [date]
    Health counseling / Judith A. Lewis, Len Sperry, Jon Carlson.
      p.   cm.
    Includes bibliographical references and index.
    ISBN 0-534-13446-7 :
    1. Health counseling.   I. Sperry, Len.   II. Carlson, Jon.
III. Title.
R727.4.L48   1993
362.1'04256—dc20   92-37322
                                      CIP

Sponsoring Editor: Claire Verduin
Marketing Representative: Thomas L. Braden
Editorial Associate: Gay C. Bond
Production Coordinator: Fiorella Ljunggren
Manuscript Editor: Barbara Kimmel
Permissions Editor: Karen Wootten
Interior Design: Katherine Minerva
Cover Design: Susan Haberkorn
Typesetting: Kachina Typesetting
Cover Printing: Phoenix Color Corporation
Printing and Binding: Arcata Graphics/Fairfield

Preface

Traditionally, counselors have worked with personality and behavioral issues, whereas health-care personnel have focused on medical and health concerns. This book brings all these elements together, showing how counselors can help clients deal with lifestyle issues related to physical well-being and how health professionals can use counseling interventions in their work.

Often a book is written because an educator has been unable to find just the right resource to meet the needs of his or her students. This is the case with *Health Counseling*. As educators, we needed a book that could teach students how to use their counseling skills to address problems related to physical health. As clinicians, we wanted a book that would build a bridge between theory and practice, reviewing the literature on health issues but also focusing on clinical applications. We knew that counselors were being asked by their clients to help them with such common health concerns as weight control, smoking cessation, substance abuse, and sleep difficulties. We also knew that health-care professionals, trained to deal with physical problems, needed to add counseling to their repertoires of skills. We felt that a comprehensive text on health counseling, with a good balance of theory, research, and application, could help achieve these separate but complementary goals, and it was this belief that led us to plan and conceptualize *Health Counseling*.

This is the first book written specifically to prepare people for carrying out "health counseling." Health counseling is a process that takes place in many settings: schools, human service agencies, private practices, health-care organizations, businesses, and other environments. Its practitioners share an attitude toward helping that is holistic and integrative. They know that the focus of helping should be broad enough to encompass physical health as well as psychological and social well-being. They use a number of strategies to help their clients develop self-management skills and achieve optimal health. They recognize the importance of environmental as well as intrapersonal factors.

Part I of *Health Counseling* introduces our conceptual framework and discusses the practical strategies and skills that can be used to help clients initiate and maintain health-oriented behavior changes. In Part II, we apply the health-counseling model to a number of specific issues: weight control, smoking cessation, substance abuse, exercise, sleep, sexual health, chronic pain, and

coping with illness. Each chapter in this applications section surveys the theoretical and research literature related to the topic and also provides clinical input on assessment, treatment, maintenance, and prevention. Each applications chapter also includes case materials and pointers on available resources. Part III, the conclusion, speaks to the need for a wellness-oriented, comprehensive approach to prevention and intervention.

Acknowledgments

We had a great deal of help in preparing this manuscript. Special thanks go to Candace Ward Howell, Blythe Smith, Susan Lewandowski, and Dawn Stalbaum for their valuable assistance. We are indebted to the following reviewers for their helpful comments and suggestions: John D. Alcorn of Southern Mississippi University, Elizabeth Altmaier of the University of Iowa, Paul D. Blisard of the College of the Ozarks, David Van Doren of the University of Wisconsin at Whitewater, and John J. Zarski of the University of Akron. Len Sperry would also like to express his gratitude to Barry Blackwell, M.D., for mentoring during and since his Behavioral Medicine Fellowship and to his colleagues Dr. Sidney Shindell, Dr. William Greaves, and Dr. David Sheridan of the Department of Preventive Medicine at the Medical College of Wisconsin. We also appreciate the enthusiasm of Claire Verduin and the rest of the Brooks/Cole family; they are always open to creative projects that can take our profession in uncharted but valuable directions. We hope that this book will fit that category.

Judith A. Lewis
Len Sperry
Jon Carlson

Contents

Health Counseling

I

Introduction

1

Enhancing Physical Health: The Counselor's Contribution

He had much experience of physicians, and said "The only way to keep your health is to eat what you don't want, drink what you don't like, and do what you druther not."

Mark Twain

- Mary seemed agitated when she entered the counselor's office to complain about her company's new policy and its implications for her own behavior. Employees would no longer be allowed to smoke in the building where she had worked— and puffed—for more than ten years. Several times, Mary had tried to quit smoking on her own, but she had not been successful. Now she believed that she was at a turning point. She was unwilling to step outside during rain- and snowstorms when the urge to smoke overtook her, but she didn't believe that smokers' complaints would bring about a reversal in the new policy. What Mary needed from the counselor was help in making what she considered to be a very difficult adjustment: removing cigarettes from her life.
- John also needed a counselor's help. A recent physical examination indicated that both his blood pressure and his cholesterol level were becoming dangerously high. His physician suggested that changes in John's diet, along with a program of moderate exercise, would prevent health problems and might even help him avoid the need for medication. The physician, Dr. Jones, provided a hand-out with information about diet and exercise, but John believed that he was on his own in terms of setting his personal goals and developing new habits. Dr. Jones would not have time to work with John's specific health behaviors on an ongoing basis. Unfortunately, the hospital's cardiac rehabilitation unit was not available for preventive purposes. John knew that he wanted to modify his behaviors, but he realized that he did not really know how to proceed.
- The Barnes family also felt at a loss. Their adolescent daughter, Jane, had just been diagnosed with diabetes. The family had received a great deal of helpful information from the medical team, so they knew what part they needed to play in helping Jane improve her physical health. What they did not know was how to adjust emotionally to this family crisis and how to support Jane in her own efforts to maintain a positive self-concept during this crucial period in her development.
- Jim was another adolescent dealing with a crisis. Abrupt changes in his academic performance had prompted his school's Student Assistance Program to refer him for drug-abuse treatment. Jim received help in an inpatient setting, but he knew that this treatment represented only a beginning. Jim felt motivated to remain drug free, but the environments at school, at home, and in the community were all associated with substance use. He needed counseling to make the key transition back to his school setting and to prevent a return to his previous behaviors. The counseling process could help him develop new coping strategies for risky situations. Counseling could also help his family become a source of strength and support during this difficult period.

The concerns expressed by these clients are typical of the fresh challenges that counselors face in all settings. More and more, counselors find that their clients are asking for something new: assistance as they try to achieve healthier life-styles or adapt to changes in their physical well-being. *Health counseling* uses the skills of the counselor to help clients make the kinds of life-style changes that can enhance their physical health.

Addressing Physical Well-Being: A Natural Progression

Traditionally, counselors have focused on psychological and social issues, but they have not viewed themselves as competent to deal with their clients' physical well-being. In reality, however, it is a natural progression for counselors to move toward a more holistic approach. Mind and body are woven together so closely that counselors cannot realistically expect to focus on one at the expense of the other. As helpers, we can no more specialize in dealing with *either* the mind *or* the body than we can choose to work solely with emotions, solely with cognitions, or solely with overt behaviors. Each person's feelings, behaviors, and social milieu affect his or her physical health. At the same time, physical health can affect a person's ability to cope with a variety of stressors. Because these factors are locked together, we can be most effective as helpers if we approach counseling from a biopsychosocial perspective, (Engel, 1977; Schwartz, 1982), which recognizes the presence of biological, psychological, and social components in all aspects of individual well-being. Counselors—regardless of the settings in which they are employed—need to be able to help their clients make wellness-oriented behavior changes and cope with threats to their physical health. Health counseling is an action-oriented process through which a helper enables a client to make life-style changes that lead in the direction of optimal health. This process depends less on the helper's job title or employment setting than it does on his or her point of view. Health counseling takes place in schools, human services agencies, private practices, health-care organizations, and a variety of other settings. In short, it takes place wherever a helper with a biopsychosocial perspective can be found.

Linkages between Behavior and Health

The importance of health counseling becomes especially apparent when we consider the direct linkages between behavior and health. The most pressing health problems that our society faces today stem from health-compromising actions of individuals. A century ago, infectious diseases were the leading causes of death. Now, although diseases such as tuberculosis, measles, poliomyelitis, influenza, and pneumonia are still present, they can be treated through medical means that are at our disposal. In contrast, illnesses and disabilities related to life-styles show few signs of abatement. As Matarazzo (1982) has pointed out, the reduction in the incidence of infectious diseases "has occurred along with an increase during the same years in such conditions as lung cancer, major cardiovascular disease, drug and alcohol abuse, and motorcycle and alcohol-related automobile accidents" (p. 3). Even the most serious outbreaks of infectious diseases, such as the Acquired Immune Deficiency Syndrome (AIDS) epidemic, occur in the presence of high-risk behaviors. Undoubtedly, the afflictions that affect the largest number of people today are of the type that are more likely to be affected by behavioral interventions than by strict reliance on traditional medicine. And behavioral interventions are clearly in the counselor's bailiwick!

In the last half of the 1980s, nine chronic diseases—all largely preventable or controllable—accounted for more than half of the deaths in the United States ("Preventable diseases," 1990). These diseases—stroke, heart disease, diabetes, obstructive lung disease, lung cancer, breast cancer, cervical cancer, colorectal cancer, and cirrhosis of the liver—tend to be associated with such risk factors as cigarette smoking, poor diet, and insufficient exercise. Unintentional injury is another behaviorally affected cause of death that claims untold numbers of people, especially among the youngest members of the population. Among adolescents, the primary causes of mortality are accidents, homicide, and suicide. In members of this age group, disabilities related to vehicular accidents also take a high toll on individual well-being (Millstein, 1989). Adolescents are additionally at risk for death or long-term disability because of such life-style related problems as sexually tramsmitted diseases, early pregnancy, and substance abuse. In fact, problems related to adolescent health behaviors may be even more severe than we realize. The public tends to be aware of such immediate health risks as substance abuse and accidents but unaware of the degree to which other behaviors affect long-term health. As Millstein (1989) points out, "50% of the mortality among adults is a direct result of modifiable behavioral factors, many of which have their onset during adolescence" (p. 837).

In our society, people of all ages are at risk for the development of health-related problems associated with their behaviors and life-styles. According to Michael (1982), most Americans can improve their health and extend their life spans through "elimination of cigarette smoking, reduction of alcohol misuse, moderate dietary changes to reduce intake of excess calories and excess fats, moderate exercise, periodic screening for major disorders such as high blood pressure and certain cancers, adherence to traffic speed laws, and use of seat belts" (p. 937). Clearly, the association between behavior and health is well documented, direct, and—most important—amenable to intervention.

In addition to this overt mind-body connection, there is another set of interactions that is less likely to be readily understood but that, in the future, may turn out to be just as important. The relationships between diet and heart disease or between smoking and lung cancer are clear and understandable to most of us. Far less obvious is the notion that the immune system itself can be "compromised behaviorally" (Borysenko, 1984, p. 248). Very promising research conducted by Ader and his associates (Ader, 1981; Ader, 1989; Ader & Cohen, 1984) indicates that the immune system is not as autonomous as has generally been believed; rather, it is influenced by the central nervous system, which may act as a mediator between psychosocial factors and disease processes. Ader (1989) found that it was possible to condition immunosuppression in animals. Although comparable evidence is not available for humans, research that focuses on infectious diseases has indicated that "psychosocial factors appear to be capable of influencing both the likelihood of developing disease and the course of disease" (Ader & Cohen, 1984, p. 118). A number of studies—some going back over several decades—have identified linkages between social

or personality factors and such health problems as streptococcal disease (Meyer & Haggerty, 1962), respiratory illness (Boyce, Cassel, Collier, Jensen, Ramey, & Smith, 1977; Jackson, Dowling, Anderson, Riff, Saporta, & Turck, 1960; Jacobs, Spilken, Norman, & Anderson, 1970), and infectious mononucleosis (Greenfield, Roessler, & Crosley, 1959; Kasl, Evans, & Neiderman, 1979). Moreover, some evidence that is being accumulated indicates that people affected by stressful events, such as loss of a loved one, show measurable changes in immune responses (Bartrop, Luckhurst, Lazarus, Kiloh, & Penny, 1977; Schleifer, Keller, Camerino, Thornton, & Stein, 1983).

It is difficult to identify the specific mechanisms through which such linkages occur. It is increasingly apparent, however, that health is determined through interactions among genetic predisposition, environment, and behavioral factors (Borysenko, 1984). Of course, psychoneuroimmunology cannot, at this stage in its development, point counselors in the direction of preventive interventions, but the existence of the research does help to support the notion that psychosocial and biological factors are absolutely inseparable.

Linkages between Personal Characteristics and Health

The inseparability of mind and body is also brought to light when we consider the developing body of research linking personal characteristics and health. Again, the findings are not at this time so definite that they point toward very specific interventions. Yet, counselors need to be aware of the literature that identifies linkages between personality factors and health outcomes, if only because it provides still further evidence of the need for a holistic approach.

Researchers in health-related disciplines have been showing some success in identifying characteristics that may relate to positive or negative health events. Some individuals demonstrate characteristics that could make them vulnerable to the development of disease or dysfunction, whereas others exhibit attitudes or behaviors that appear to play a protective role. Among the personal factors that may affect general health are a "hardy personality style" (Kobasa, 1979; Kobasa, Maddi, & Courington, 1981), a "sense of coherence" (Antonovsky, 1987), a disposition toward optimism (Scheier & Carver, 1987), and a number of factors related to cognition and coping mechanisms. In addition, there appears to be a differentiation among the personality characteristics most closely associated with specific illnesses.

Hardiness
Kobasa (1979) used the concept of *hardiness* to explain the results of her study of business executives who had experienced a large number of stressful life events. Some of these individuals succeeded in maintaining their health despite high stress levels. What seemed to differentiate them from their less healthy peers was a collection of factors that she called the "hardy personality style." The components of this personality style include *commitment,* as opposed to aliena-

tion; *control,* as opposed to powerlessness; and *challenge,* as opposed to threat (Kobasa, Maddi, & Courington, 1981).

Hardy individuals show a high degree of commitment, involving themselves fully in life and work. They tend to believe in the importance and inherent interest of whatever they are doing. Far from feeling alienated, they maintain their curiosity about all aspects of life; they have a sense of purpose and believe that their lives are meaningful.

Their sense of commitment is closely related to their belief in the possibility of control. Hardy individuals perceive that they can influence events. They tend to take responsibility for their lives, showing an internal locus of control (Rotter, 1966; 1989) rather than attributing events to chance or to the actions of powerful others.

This attitude toward life tends to make the hardy individual welcome challenge and change. Such an individual assumes that change will always be a part of life and that the result will be positive growth and development. Far from seeing change as a threat, the hardy person sees it as a challenge and a source of stimulation.

The variables of commitment, control, and challenge are closely associated with one another. "Thus a hardy person's attempt to influence the course of some event (control) includes curiosity about how it happened and interest in what it is (commitment), plus an attempt to learn from it whatever will enhance personal growth (challenge)" (Kobasa, Maddi, & Courington, 1981, p. 369). This energetic approach to life may help hardy people to choose positive interpretations of life events that might prove stressful and health compromising to others. In contrast, people low in hardiness may be bored or threatened by the environment, feeling powerless to do anything about their lives and uncomfortable with change. "Because their personalities provide little or no buffer, the stressful events are allowed to have a debilitating effect on health" (Kobasa, Maddi, & Courington, 1981, p. 369). Constitutional predisposition and stressful life events contribute to the development of illness, but hardiness can play a role in mediating that relationship.

Kobasa (1987) has pointed out that, because the subjects of her original study included 900 male executives and only 20 females, "hardiness studies are essentially studies of personality and stress resistance in men" (p. 322). However, some subsequent studies have dealt with women and gender differences. Hardiness did appear to mediate the effects of stress on the well-educated, middle-class women who made up the sample in some studies. In a study of female secretaries, however, no such effect was found.

> Business executives may find themselves in jobs that allow them to exercise, and perhaps even to grow in, commitment, control, and challenge. Secretaries, on the other hand, may confront jobs which limit their expression of hardiness. It may indeed be the case, for example, that some bosses enjoy expressions of control at the expense of their secretaries' sense of control (Kobasa, 1987, pp. 324–325).

Thus, the construct of hardiness, like any factor, should be examined while keeping in mind questions about the effects of gender, culture, and economics.

Sense of Coherence

Antonovsky's (1979, 1984, 1987) concept of the sense of coherence also combines several variables to define a global, health-enhancing orientation. Antonovsky's work is based on an assumption that, given the stressfulness of life, health is more surprising and more mysterious than illness. "We all, by virtue of being human, are in a high-risk group" (1984, p. 117). Thinking "salutogenically," Antonovsky points out that, at any one time, all people can be placed somewhere on a continuum between total wellness and total illness. The question we need to address is not what causes illness (the pathogenic approach), but what facilitates an individual's position or movement along the health–illness continuum toward the wellness pole. His own research identified a general way of viewing the world that he termed the *sense of coherence*.

> The sense of coherence is a global orientation that expresses the extent to which one has a pervasive, enduring though dynamic feeling of confidence that (1) the stimuli deriving from one's internal and external environments in the course of living are structured, predictable, and explicable; (2) the resources are available to one to meet the demands posed by these stimuli; and (3) these demands are challenges, worthy of investment and engagement (Antonovsky, 1987, p. 19).

The components that make up the sense of coherence include comprehensibility, manageability, and meaningfulness. *Comprehensibility* involves the degree to which individuals feel able to understand (to comprehend) themselves and the world. A person with a high sense of comprehensibility believes that future events, if not predictable, are at least ordered and explainable. He or she finds that stimuli make cognitive sense, rather than being "chaotic, disordered, random, accidental, (and) inexplicable" (Antonovsky, 1987, p. 17). *Manageability* implies a belief that events are not only predictable but also controllable. The person with a high sense of manageability believes that resources for meeting life's demands can somehow be obtained. If he or she cannot control events, then legitimate others can. *Meaningfulness* is Antonovsky's emotional counterpart to comprehensibility. "People who are high on meaningfulness feel that life makes sense emotionally, that at least some of the problems and demands posed by living are worth investing energy in, are worthy of commitment and engagement and are challenges that are welcome rather than burdens" (Antonovsky, 1984, p. 119).

Antonovsky's conceptualization is that people who develop a strong sense of coherence are more likely to maintain or improve their health than are those with a weak sense of coherence. A number of explanations are possible. Perhaps the individual with the strong sense of coherence is more active in avoiding threat, more involved in health-promoting activities, more inclined to do the work needed to develop good coping mechanisms, and/or more likely to gather and exploit effective resources. In any event, such individuals are unlikely to give up in the face of health-endangering stimuli.

Dispositional Optimism

Scheier and Carver (1987) suggest that many of the characteristics that have been identified as differentiating between positive and negative health out-

comes may in fact be the result of a pervasive sense of optimism, or "generalized expectations that good things will happen" (p. 171). One plausible explanation for this phenomenon lies in the notion that people's behaviors are strongly affected by their beliefs in the outcomes that can be expected.

> In our view, people who see desired outcomes as attainable continue to exert efforts at attaining those outcomes, even when doing so is difficult. When outcomes seem sufficiently unattainable (whether through personal inadequacies or through externally imposed impediments), people reduce their efforts and eventually disengage themselves from pursuit of the goals. Thus, we see outcome expectancies as a major determinant of the disjunction between two classes of behavior: (a) continued striving versus (b) giving up and turning away (Scheier & Carver, 1987, p. 170).

Scheier and Carver reviewed several studies that seemed to bear out their conceptualization of the link between optimism and physical well-being. One of their own studies (Scheier & Carver, 1985) tracked college students during a particularly stressful time: the last four weeks of an academic semester. The subjects completed the Life Orientation Test, which provides a score for optimism, and were also asked to report on their physical symptoms both at the outset of the study and on the last day of classes. Optimism was negatively correlated with symptom reporting; people who scored high on optimism showed fewer symptoms over time.

The tentative conclusions of another of their studies (1987) also pinpoints the possible importance of dispositional optimism. After undergoing coronary artery bypass surgery, optimists showed better recovery rates than pessimists. Optimists were judged by members of the cardiac rehabilitation team as showing a faster rate of recovery, reaching recovery milestones more quickly, and showing healthier physiological responses. Six months after surgery, a strong correlation between optimism and self-reported quality of life remained.

A later study by Carver and Pozo (Adler, 1991) traced the progress of 60 women with breast cancer. Preliminary results indicated that optimists reported less distress than pessimists did throughout their medical ordeals. The researchers suspect that optimism made its contribution through its effects on coping techniques. Optimists used acceptance, humor, planning, reframing the situation in an active light, and active coping; pessimists tended to cope with distress through denial and behavioral disengagement.

Reker and Wong (1983) studied an elderly population. They, too, found a correlation between optimism and physical health. People who had been assessed as optimists two years earlier showed a higher degree of physical, psychological, and general well-being and reported fewer negative symptoms in comparison with pessimists.

The mechanism through which optimism acts on physical health is unclear, but the linkage of optimism with the use of effective, problem-focused coping strategies appears to be a promising line of research (Scheier, Weintraub, & Carver, 1986). "When confronting adversity optimists keep trying, whereas pessimists are more likely to get upset and give up" (Scheier & Carver, 1987, p. 191).

Cognitive Factors

Cognitive factors appear to play a central role in the individual's success in maintaining health and preventing or minimizing disease. As J. Seeman (1989) points out,

> If there is one dominant subsystem in its impact on health, it is the cognitive subsystem. Study after study (has) reported the commanding role of self-definition, self-perception, and sense of control in the maintenance and enhancement of health (p. 1108).

The individual's belief in his or her ability to exert control over events seems especially important. Both Kobasa's hardiness construct and Antonovsky's concept of the sense of coherence highlight the centrality of the healthy person's sense of control. Research findings that are focused specifically on the issue of control also provide support for the notion that a sense of control helps individuals stay healthy. For example, M. Seeman and T. Seeman (1983) conducted multiple interviews over a year-long period with more than 1000 individuals. On the basis of this study, Seeman and Seeman were able to measure correlations between sense of control and a number of health indices. They found that sense of control was associated with the following health-status measures:

> (1) practicing preventive health measures, e.g., diet, exercise, alcohol moderation; (2) making an effort to avoid the harm in smoking (by quitting, trying to quit, or simply not smoking); (3) being more sanguine about early medical treatment for cancer; (4) achieving higher self-ratings on general health status; (5) reporting fewer episodes of both chronic and acute illness; (6) evidencing a more vigorous management style with respect to illness; e.g., staying in bed less once a bed-confinement occasion has occurred; and (7) showing less dependence on the use of the physician (Seeman & Seeman, 1983, p. 155).

Research conducted by Rodin and Langer (Rodin & Langer, 1977; Rodin, 1986; Buie, 1988) indicates that experiences and perceptions of control affect the health status of older people. In one study, nursing home residents who were given choices and who were able to maintain control of day-to-day events showed greater health gains than did members of a control group whose needs were met through caring attention by staff members. Rodin and her associates also studied a group of older people who were not currently living in nursing home settings. For these people as well, control predicted immune function and a number of other health-related variables. A sense of personal control may be important not just in preventing illness, but also in improving the individual's ability to cope effectively with the presence of a disease or disability. Taylor, Lichtman, and Wood (1984), for instance, found that cancer patients who believed that they had personal control over the progression of the disease were able to make better adjustments and had better outcomes than those who expressed a sense of helplessness or denial.

In general, control seems to be an important factor for both men and women. Some studies, however, have shown gender differences sufficient to question whether generalizations about sense of control as a protection against

stress can be made with impunity. Possibly, there are differences in the kind and degree of control exerted by men and women.

> One can argue for a difference between control conceived of as (1) a sense of personal competence or mastery, and that defined as (2) generalized expectancies regarding control within oneself (rather than in others or fate) over a variety of personal, interpersonal, and broad sociopolitical domains. It may be that the former—that is, feeling effective in what it is that one has to do in life—is more important for women's stress resistance than it is for men's (Kobasa, 1987, pp. 317–318).

Bandura's (1982) concept of self-efficacy is closely related to questions of individual control. Efficacy involves a general ability to manage one's environment by mobilizing the cognitive and behavioral skills that are necessary for dealing with challenging situations. An individual's perceived self-efficacy involves his or her judgment about the adequacy of these skills. This judgment affects every aspect of the individual's performance. The person who lacks a sense of self-efficacy concerning a particular task is likely to give up quickly or even to avoid the challenge altogether. In contrast, the person with a strong sense of self-efficacy is likely to meet difficult challenges and to maintain positive behavior changes.

> In any given activity, skills and self-beliefs that ensure optimal use of capabilities are required for successful functioning. If self-efficacy is lacking, people tend to behave ineffectually even though they know what to do. . . . The higher the level of perceived self-efficacy, the greater the performance accomplishments. Strength of efficacy also predicts behavior change. The stronger the perceived efficacy, the more likely are people to persist in their efforts until they succeed (Bandura, 1982, pp. 127–128).

The perception of self-efficacy regarding health-enhancing behaviors may have a strong influence on well-being. Self-efficacy has been shown to affect people's ability to quit smoking and maintain the nonsmoking state (DiClemente, 1981; Curry, 1989), to avoid relapse in addictive behaviors (Marlatt & Gordon (1985), and to exert self-regulation regarding a range of preventive health measures (Schunk & Carbonari, 1984). "When knowledge of health risks is combined with a strong sense of efficacy for avoiding them, long-term maintenance of healthy lifestyles results" (Schunk & Carbonari, 1984, p. 244).

Although an individual's perceptions of control and self-efficacy are important, a number of other beliefs, especially about the nature of the situation being faced, can have a major impact on health-related behaviors and thereby on outcomes. The Health Belief Model, which was developed in the 1950s and had received major research attention by the early 1970s (Becker, 1974), has been the focus of a number of studies since that time. The Health Belief Model (HBM) was first developed by the United States Public Health Service in an attempt to determine why so few people participated in programs designed to prevent disease. The model is based on the notion that behavior is affected by the value that an individual places on a particular goal and by his or her estimate of the

likelihood that a specific action will help in the achievement of that goal. The model addresses the following cognitive dimensions (Janz & Becker, 1984):

1. *Perceived susceptibility:* the individual's feeling of vulnerability with regard to a particular illness or disability
2. *Perceived severity:* the person's evaluation of the seriousness of the medical or social consequences of the illness
3. *Perceived benefits:* the individual's belief that a specific action would be effective in preventing or overcoming the threat
4. *Perceived barriers:* the person's perceptions of negative effects that might balance the positive aspects of the specific behavior

The social psychologists who developed the model also took into account the importance of internal or external cues to action. They recognized the impact of demographic and psychosocial variables that might influence behavior indirectly through their effects on perception. Thus, the Health Belief Model posits that demographic and psychosocial variables affect the individual's perceptions concerning the seriousness of a disease and his or her susceptibility to it. If the individual perceives that he or she is at risk, the individual is more likely to adopt health-oriented behaviors. Whether this cue is internal (such as a symptom or physiological warning sign) or external (such as a public health media campaign), the likelihood that action will be taken depends on the person's perception of the action's benefits and liabilities. This perception may also be affected by a number of demographic and psychosocial variables.

Although the Health Belief Model was originally focused on preventive behavior, it has also been studied in relation to health-related behaviors that were initiated after the onset of an illness. Janz and Becker (1984) reviewed HBM studies that were published between 1974 and 1984 and were focused on sick-role behaviors as well as on preventive behaviors. With regard to preventive health behavior, the findings consistently supported the notion that individual perceptions of susceptibility, benefits, and barriers were significantly related to behavioral outcomes; perceived severity of the illness in question was less important. Studies of behaviors to aid recovery among people already diagnosed with illnesses showed that perception of severity was most important, second only to perceived barriers. Janz and Becker's summary of all HBM studies up to 1984 indicate that "each HBM dimension was found to be significantly associated with the health-related behaviors under study; the significance-ratio orderings (in descending order) are 'barriers' (89%), 'susceptibility' (81%), 'benefits' (78%), and 'severity' (65%)" (p. 41).

More recently, other conceptualizations have been developed in an attempt to learn how cognitive factors might affect people's health-related behaviors. For instance, Leventhal and his associates (Leventhal, Meyer, & Nerenz, 1980; Leventhal, Zimmerman, & Gutmann, 1984) conceptualized the relationship between people's representations of illnesses and the likelihood that they would adhere to medical regimens. According to this conceptualization, each individual is likely to have a cognitive representation of illness that includes both abstract and concrete components. Included in the individual's mental construction are perceptions about the symptoms associated with the disease,

beliefs about the causes and consequences of the disease, and expectations concerning its duration (acute, cyclic, or chronic). The researchers found that help-seeking behaviors and treatment compliance are affected by the patient's mental representation of the disease in question. For instance, people who believed that they could recognize their own hypertension by monitoring symptoms tended to take their medication only when they perceived symptoms of elevated blood pressure, despite the fact that hypertension is, in reality, asymptomatic. Similarly, patients who believed that hypertension was a chronic disease were more likely to remain in treatment than those who believed it to be an acute illness.

Meichenbaum and Turk (1987) have suggested that a large number of patient beliefs—either rational or irrational—may affect decisions concerning adherence to treatment. Among the possible reasons for noncompliance are such factors as uncertainty or even pessimism about the efficacy of the treatment being suggested; prior experiences with illness or with health care providers; belief that inconvenience or negative side effects of the treatment may outweigh the benefits; perceived stigma of being in treatment; desire to maintain a sense of control; competing demands that are seen as more important; and a "view of adherence as interfering with life-long belief systems, future plans, family relationship patterns, social roles, self-concept, emotional equilibrium, or daily life patterns" (p. 51).

Clearly, individual perceptions and beliefs have a major effect on health behaviors, even in situations in which treatment adherence would appear to be the only rational decision. Preventive health maintenance, which is characterized by vagueness in goals and a lower level of perceived need, presents an even greater challenge.

Coping Mechanisms

It is a generally accepted truism that stress plays an important role in health outcomes. This relationship is complex, however, because a number of factors mediate the effects of stressful events on the individual. One of the most important of these modifiers involves the ways in which people cope with stress (Cohen, 1984).

Lazarus and Folkman (1984) define *coping* as "the process of managing demands (external or internal) that are appraised as taxing or exceeding the resources of the person." (p. 283). This conceptualization makes clear that stress-related problems occur only when individuals interpret events or situations as demanding. Whether people find situations threatening depends on a number of factors: their view of their competence to handle the new demand, their previous success in dealing with similar situations, the degree to which they feel in control of events, their perceptions of being overloaded or of having conflicting needs, and the standards they set for their own performance. It is only when individuals perceive an event to be stressful that they react physiologically, activating the stress responses that can, over time, have negative effects on their health. "Broadly speaking, degree of stress depends mainly on the appraisal of how much appears to be at stake in the transaction . . . and the relative power of the environmental demand to do harm, compared with the power of the person to prevent or manage such harm" (Lazarus & Folkman, 1984, p. 290).

Stress-related problems result from a combination of three variables: external demands, individual perceptions, and physiological responses. Therefore, individuals can cope by making changes at any of these three points. First, they can alter their stress levels by exerting control over their environments, using problem-solving skills to confront potential stressors and to make their life situation less demanding. Second, they can alter their mental processes, learning to change their appraisals in a purposeful way. People who tend to see many stimuli as threatening can try to monitor their reactions and to substitute positive self-statements for their maladaptive cognitions. Finally, people can alter their physiological responses by learning relaxation techniques that can help them control the stress response and avoid the negative health consequences associated with long-term stress.

Any one of a number of coping strategies can be used at any of these points. In general, however, coping tends to be either "problem-focused" or "emotion-focused" (Folkman & Lazarus, 1980; Lazarus & Folkman, 1984). Problem-focused coping involves taking some kind of constructive action to mitigate conditions that are perceived as threatening, whereas emotion-focused coping attempts to regulate the individual's emotional response and thus to alleviate distress. The category of emotion-regulating responses includes denial of the existence or of the seriousness of the threat, as well as attempts to control nervous system activation. In fact, another way to categorize coping strategies is to make a distinction between active and avoidant strategies (Cohen, 1984).

Stress may affect people's health differentially, depending on the appropriateness and effectiveness of the coping strategies they choose. Because control, commitment, and optimism are associated with positive health, it is often assumed that active, problem-focused coping styles are most adaptive. In fact, it appears that there is no one coping mechanism that is always preferred. Suls and Fletcher (1985) found that avoidant strategies were associated with poor outcomes over the long term. In the short term, however, denial played a helpful role. Similarly, problem-focused coping strategies are adaptive when situations are amenable to change, whereas emotion-focused coping strategies are more effective when stressors are not subject to control. Thus, the coping mechanisms that succeed in mediating the effects of stress are the ones that work best in the situation at hand. The people who adapt most effectively may be the ones with several types of coping skills in their repertoires.

Characteristics Associated with Specific Illnesses

In their questions about the relationship between personal characteristics and health, researchers have been following two parallel lines. A number of studies have taken what Antonovsky would call a "salutogenic" approach, attempting to identify the positive characteristics that help to maintain health. This line of investigation has led to a growing awareness of the importance of such attributes as a sense of control, a tendency toward optimism, and an ability to cope effectively with stress. At the same time, researchers have continued to examine the relationships between specific personal attributes and disease-proneness, asking what characteristics might increase individual vulnerability to particular health problems.

The Type A behavior pattern, which is thought to have a relationship to

coronary heart disease among both men and women, is the most widely accepted and extensively researched example of such a behavioral risk factor (Spielberger, 1989). The Type A individual (Friedman & Rosenman, 1974) is characterized by hard-driving competitiveness, impatience, aggressiveness, hostility, overinvolvement in work, a strong need for control across all situations, and a sense of time urgency, The Type A personality is recognizable through such overt behaviors as excessive anger, irritability, and rapid speech and body movements; and it can be contrasted with the Type B pattern, which is characterized by a more relaxed approach to life. The usefulness of recognizing Type A behavior as a risk factor has become more apparent with the beginnings of some success in changing Type A individuals' behaviors and cognitions, and thereby preventing recurrences of myocardial infarction (Thoresen & Eagleston, 1985). Recent studies have led in the direction of increased precision in measuring and addressing the Type A pattern by showing that some of the characteristics associated with the syndrome overshadow others. In particular, it seems that the Type A individual's intense job involvement is not associated with heart disease (Spielberger, 1989), but that anger and hostility are more salient factors in placing him or her at risk for cardiac disease (Friedman & Booth-Kewley, 1987; Matthews, 1988; Spielberger, 1989).

Attempts have also been made to determine relationships between personality characteristics and cancer. The relationship between *risk behaviors* and the development of some cancers is known, but the role of *personality* as a predisposing factor is less clear. Temoshok and her colleagues (Temoshok et al., 1985) have posited a cancer-prone personality, which they have labeled Type C. The individual whom they view as vulnerable to cancer is emotionally repressed, apathetic, and even hopeless. Although other researchers have reported similar findings, their studies have largely focused not on the initial development of cancer, but on survival rates. For instance, Pettingale (1984) found that breast cancer patients who showed helplessness and passive acceptance of the disease are more likely to have recurrences than are those with more hopeful and expressive personalities. Jensen (1987) also followed up breast cancer patients and found that, over two years, cancer is more likely to spread if an individual demonstrates repression and an inability to express emotions.

Social and Cultural Factors

The health of individuals is drastically affected by their membership in specific populations. Consider, for example, the effects of gender on health and illness. Women live longer than men, but women are more likely to be subject to chronic illnesses and to have other health problems (Public Health Service, 1985; Strickland, 1988; Rodin & Ickovics, 1990). Women use health-care services more frequently, either because of the presence of more health problems or because of gender-driven differences in sick-role behaviors. Of course, there are also some problems that are unique to women, such as concerns related to pregnancy or breast disease; and some that affect women disproportionately, such as lupus, osteoporosis, and eating disorders (Rodin & Ickovics, 1990). Women are also subject to differences from men in how they are treated by medical personnel. Women are more likely to receive prescriptions for psy-

choactive medications and to undergo possibly unnecessary surgeries. At the same time, they are less likely than men to receive careful diagnostic workups when presenting the same symptoms. "Men get medical workups; women get tranquilizers" (Holt, 1990). Women have also been vastly underrepresented in health research, making the recent opening of the National Institutes of Health Office of Research on Women's Health a necessity.

Health problems are further exacerbated for minority women, who "suffer a disproportionate share of illness" and "experience higher infant and maternal mortality rates; greater prevalence of chronic diseases such as diabetes, hypertension, cardiovascular disease, and certain types of cancer; and a lower life expectancy than their White counterparts" (Manley, Lin-Fu, Miranda, Noonan, & Parker, 1984, pp. II–37). The differences between African-American males and white males are just as clear, with mortality rates for black males remaining 50 percent higher than those for white males (Rene, 1987). Cutting across ethnic and gender lines are the major barriers to health brought about by poverty.

> It is indisputable that health suffers when nutrition is poor, when living conditions are crowded and unsanitary, when the environment is polluted, when there is no respite from noise, when there is no meaningful work, when there is continuing stress related to unequal social treatment, and there are few ties to other human beings who are able to provide comfort, esteem, and mutual support. Until we can begin to change this total situation, poor health will be just another symptom of poverty, and resources will continue to be poured into secondary and tertiary level care for chronic health problems that are to a high degree preventable (Albino & Tedesco, 1984, p. 170).

At the microsystem level, access to social support of any kind is often considered to be as important as any other factor—including psychological state—that affects health. Studies that examine the relationships between social support and health have indicated that social support affects both the onset of health problems (S. Cohen, 1988; Gentry & Kobasa, 1984) and recovery from serious illnesses (DiMatteo & Hays, 1981).

Particular attention has been paid to the interactions among stress, social support, and health outcomes. Gentry and Kobasa emphasize the role of social support as a buffer, protecting people from the harmful effects of high and chronic levels of stress. Cohen, however, makes a distinction between (1) stress-buffering models, which posit social-support systems as protectors against the pathogenic influences of stressful events, and (2) main-effect models, which see support as an important predictor of health regardless of current stress levels. Cohen's conceptualization emphasizes that the individual's perception that social support is available is the most likely source of the stress-buffering effect, whereas social integration (the number and strength of social ties) is the primary cause of the more general main effects. In either situation, the links between social resources and health may be explained by the availability of useful information and advice; the role of social support in enhancing feelings of self-esteem, identity, and motivation; the presence of social controls and encouragement of health-enhancing behaviors; or the existence of tangible assistance in solving problems.

The preponderance of evidence indicates that social support, along with personality variables, cognitions, and coping mechanisms, can have a major impact on health outcomes. These personal factors may have direct, biological effects or may work more indirectly through their influence on health-related behaviors. Although these pathways may as yet be unclear, their results are certain. Psychosocial factors have a major impact on physical outcomes. Some psychosocial factors are amenable to change through interpersonal processes, making health-focused counseling a necessity.

The Health-Counseling Approach

The traditional medical model maintains an emphasis on physical symptomatology and a focus on illness rather than on wellness. This model no longer seems adequate to meet our society's health needs, now that we have come to recognize the interactions among psychosocial and physical factors and now that our most common ailments are amenable to prevention or control through behavior change. To augment the work of the medical establishment, we need a strategy that helps people maintain or improve their health through their own efforts. The health-counseling approach attempts to accomplish this task by helping people develop and practice health-enhancing behaviors.

The development of health-oriented behaviors seems to depend as much on specific skills as it does on factual information. Although people need to know something about the health issues that they are addressing, they also need to believe that they know *how* to change their behaviors. Because personal skills are so crucial, health counseling uses psychoeducational methods aimed toward skill building.

The literature concerning linkages between personal characteristics and health outcomes is equivocal or conflicted in some areas, but one clear message does emerge. A sense of personal control seems to be at the heart of many people's success in optimizing their health. Because this sense of control seems basic to health enhancement, we need to use interventions designed to increase clients' perceptions of control and self-efficacy.

It is also clear that health is at least partly a function of the interaction between an individual and his or her social environment. For this reason, health counseling tends to broaden the scope of the counseling process beyond the individual to include the social system. Interventions are designed to help the client build social support and, if possible, lessen environmental stressors.

The aim of health counseling is to build up the individual's ability to engage in self-management. Self-management, in turn, requires a repertoire of health-oriented skills, a belief in one's own ability to address life's challenges, and an environment that encourages positive development. Thus, three general emphases permeate the health-counseling process:

• a focus on educational skill building
• a focus on personal control
• a focus on the social environment

Skill building.   Thoresen (1984) points out that the health-enhancement literature tends to assume that people will be able to take better care of their own health if they have information and encouragement.

> Behaving in personally responsible ways—that is, exercising effective self-management—requires a number of skills that are not necessarily inherent in everyone's repertoire. . . . People need to be taught how to be more caring and more responsible for their own health and well-being, especially when the social environment commonly promotes irresponsible or nonhealthy behavior (p. 300).

Whether a client is working toward general health maintenance, toward risk reduction, or toward stabilization of an existing condition, he or she needs help with skill development—not just with cognitive input. Yet, as Thoresen has implied, health professionals frequently depend on the provision of information as their only psychoeducational vehicle.

Consider, for example, current practices regarding drug and alcohol abuse.

> "Educational" approaches in the form of lectures about the dangers of drugs and alcohol are used very widely, both as preventive tools and as treatment methods. In inpatient alcoholism treatment programs, for instance, a great deal of time is likely to be spent on lectures concerning the disease concept and the negative effects of alcohol. Although this approach may affect cognitive knowledge, it does not appear to have any measurable effect on behavior (Lewis, Dana, & Blevins, 1988, p. 182).

In view of the evidence that information alone neither prevents nor interrupts substance abuse, we should implement other educational options. People who have not yet developed problems related to substance use might benefit by developing life skills that have a preventive function. For instance, stress-management and relaxation skills might provide replacements for alcohol or drugs for dealing with anxiety; problem-solving and decision-making skills might forestall impulsiveness in drug use; interpersonal and life-planning skills might encourage participation in non–substance-related recreation; and assertiveness skills might help young people avoid the pressure to drink or use drugs in social settings. Clients being treated for existing drug or alcohol problems also need help in developing these skills, along with more intensive training that can help them single out situations that place them at risk for relapse, identify and practice methods for coping with these situations, and deal with personal cravings and with external pressures to use.

Self-efficacy and control.   The example of substance abuse also helps to illuminate the importance of strategies designed to enhance self-efficacy, or the individual's belief in his or her ability to meet a specific challenge effectively. "With regard to drinking, *self-efficacy* refers to a problem drinker's degree of confidence in his or her ability to control his or her drinking in situations that are generally associated with problem drinking" (Curry & Marlatt, 1987, p. 118). Whether the individual client's primary drug of choice is alcohol or another substance, he or she can be expected to deal with the problem most effectively if the sense of self-efficacy is high.

> When coping skills are underdeveloped and poorly used because of disbelief in one's efficacy, a relapse will occur. Faultless self-control is not easy to come by for pliant activities, let alone for addictive substances. Nevertheless, those who perceive themselves to be inefficacious are more prone to attribute a slip to pervasive self-regulatory inefficacy. Further coping efforts are then abandoned, resulting in a total breakdown in self-control (Bandura, 1982, pp. 129–130).

Unfortunately, many of the strategies in current use in treatment programs for alcohol- or drug-dependent clients emphasize powerlessness and loss of control, rather than power self-efficacy.

> It is ironic that the major strength of the disease model, absolving the addict of personal responsibility for the problem behavior, may also be one of its shortcomings. . . . If an alcoholic has accepted the belief that it is impossible to control his or her drinking (as embodied in the AA slogan that one is always "one drink away from a drunk"), then even a single slip may precipitate a total, uncontrolled relapse. Since drinking under these circumstances is equated with the occurrence of a symptom signifying the reemergence of the disease, one is likely to feel as powerless to control this behavior as one would with any other disease symptom (Marlatt & Gordon, 1985, pp. 7–8).

It is possible to work with substance-abusing clients in ways that emphasize the development of self-efficacy and that avoid notions of powerlessness. Such strategies begin at intake, with the counselor encouraging clients to take responsibility for their own treatment. Clients begin to build a sense of the possibility of control when they are allowed to decide on their own goals, beginning with the decision about whether to make any changes at all in their drinking or drug use. Once the commitment to change has been made, clients enhance their sense of the possibility of control as they identify situations that place them at risk for substance use and as they learn how to use coping methods that work for them. Each time these coping strategies are used successfully, self-efficacy is enhanced and long-term maintenance of the new behavior becomes a more likely outcome.

Clearly, an emphasis on skill building and a focus on control and self-efficacy are complementary. Effective implementation of skills enhances self-efficacy, and a sense of self-efficacy, in turn, encourages attempts to develop new competencies. If we think in terms of the example of substance abuse, we can see that the client who learns how to cope with situations that were previously associated with drinking or drug use becomes more aware of his or her efficacy and more optimistic about the possibilities of control with each success. At the same time, a client who is treated as a responsible person and as capable of making positive decisions is likely to be motivated to perform the hard work involved in embarking on new behaviors. His or her sense of self-efficacy may elicit an optimistic view of the possibility of control that is missing in treatments that emphasize powerlessness.

A self-management approach that focuses on skills and self-efficacy can be useful in a variety of health-related issues. One client may be learning to manage a chronic disease, such as diabetes; another may be attempting weight control or smoking cessation; still another may be addressing behavioral variables that put him or her at risk for heart disease. As does the substance-abusing client, these clients need to gain a belief in the possibility of control. Regardless of the specific health problem being addressed, the general principles underlying self-management hold true.

The self-management strategy also cuts across the methods used by the health counselor and the contexts in which service is provided. Self-management is an appropriate goal of an educational intervention focused on general life skills for people who have not shown signs of any particular health problem. It is just as applicable when the method being used is individual counseling for a client trying to cope with a serious illness, or for group counseling for people attempting to support one another in the eradication of health-jeopardizing behaviors. An examination of the general processes involved makes clear the generalizability of this approach.

> Training in self-management requires strong early support from the helper, with the client gradually relying more and more on his (or her) newly developed skills. These include skills in (1) self-monitoring; (2) establishment of specific rules of conduct by contracts with onself or others; (3) seeking support from the environment for fulfillment; (4) self-evaluation; and (5) generating strong reinforcing consequences for engaging in behaviors which achieve the goals of self-control (Kanfer, 1980, p. 344).

The focus, then, is on personal power and competence, not on dependence on professional assistance.

Systems Interventions

Although individual competence is important, "social environments can either facilitate or restrict people's competence development and adaptation" (Cowen, 1985, p. 38). Each person's health is affected by the environment, both directly through the presence or absence of health hazards, and indirectly through the effects of the setting on individual behaviors. If services that focus on clients' self-management skills are to have maximum impact, they should be joined by attempts to affect the wider social systems as well. Ideally, both macrosystem and microsystem interventions should be considered. *Macrosystems* "refer to the overarching institutions of the culture or subculture, such as the economic, social, educational, legal, and political systems. . . ." *Microsystems* involve "the complex of relations between the developing person and environment in an immediate setting containing that person (e.g., home, school, workplace)" (Bronfenbrenner, 1976, p. 3).

Interventions directed toward macrosystems occur largely at the policy-formation level, and they involve such strategies as imposing economic incentives or sanctions, creating barriers between individuals and risky products or situations, and placing controls on the advertisement or promotion of products related to unhealthy behaviors (Jeffrey, 1989). Smoking behavior, for instance, is affected on a populationwide basis through such strategies as taxation, limitations on settings in which smoking is allowed, and controls on cigarette advertising. Such strategies also have more direct effects on the health of nonsmokers because of the effect on the air around them.

In the context of health counseling, microsystem interventions focus on the healthy or unhealthy aspects of those environments that have the most immediate effects on individuals' lives. The workplace and the family are two examples of such powerful microsystems.

The importance of the workplace in enhancing individual health has become more and more apparent as corporate wellness programs have proliferated. Employers' recognition of their stake in maintaining employee health has fueled the growth of wellness and health-promotion programs, with the workplace being "recognized as an appropriate site for the encouragement of healthy lifestyles" (Lewis & Lewis, 1986, p. 139). Currently, most health-promotion programs offer at least some activities that focus on specific risk factors. Smoking-cessation clinics, weight-loss groups, drug and alcohol information, and exercise classes or facilities are elements of most such programs. Just as basic, however, is a general orientation toward wellness. Most programs try to encourage employees to take control of their own health by offering help with self-assessment and planning, along with encouragement aimed toward maintenance of health improvements. The element that should be added to workplace wellness programs is a recognition of the effects of environmental factors. "Identifying the effects of environmental factors on employees' health is just as important as strengthening individual coping mechanisms and self-responsibility" (Lewis & Lewis, 1986, p. 145) and, in fact, is complementary to self-management programs. For instance, if a wellness program includes training in stress-management techniques, it should also address questions related to stressful aspects of the workplace itself. Focus should be placed not just on increasing the adaptiveness of individual employees, but also on enhancing the organizational climate, on building social support mechanisms into the corporate environment, and on lessening such physical stressors as inadequate light, extreme temperatures, excessive noise, or noxious fumes. Similarly, if a company offers smoking-cessation programs as part of its wellness effort, it should also examine its policies concerning the locations where smoking is allowed.

The family is even more closely involved with individual health and well-being. Turk and Kerns (1985) say that the family is "the major context in which illness occurs and health is maintained" (p. 2). The power of the family to affect individual well-being becomes especially apparent when health problems occur, with family support serving as an important component in recovery (Roback, 1984; Turk & Kerns, 1985). In fact, "When patients are faced with disharmony in their families, family instability, or social isolation, they are less likely to cooperate with their medical regimens" (Friedman & DiMatteo, 1989, p. 77). Conversely, the illness or disability of a family member has a major impact on the family's functioning. Undoubtedly, health-counseling strategies should include work with the families of people who are facing chronic or acute health problems.

An Integrated Approach

Health counseling combines direct, skill-building strategies with environmental interventions. This integrated approach is helpful in dealing with a variety of health-related issues. Most of the chapters in this book are devoted to specific health-related problems or behaviors, but these chapters serve primarily as examples that illustrate the potential applications of health counseling. Any number of additional health-risk behaviors and problems exist and can be approached through similar combinations of strategies. Every applications chapter includes the same components, indicating the general applicability of the basic model. We begin with Chapter Two, which details the specific strategies and skills that underlie the health-counseling approach.

References

ADER, R. (Ed.). (1981). *Psychoneuroimmunology*. New York: Academic Press.

ADER, R. (1989, August). *Psychoneuroimmunology*. Paper presented at the 97th annual convention of the American Psychological Association, New Orleans.

ADER, R., & Cohen, N. (1984). Behavior and the immune system. In W. D. Gentry (Ed.), *Handbook of behavioral medicine* (pp. 117–173). New York: Guilford Press.

ADLER, T. (1991, February). Optimists' coping skills may help beat illnesses. *The APA Monitor, 22*(2), p. 12.

ALBINO, J. E., & Tedesco, L. A. (1984). Women's health issues. In A. U. Rickel, M. Gerrard, & I. Iscoe (Eds.), *Social and psychological problems of women: Prevention and crisis intervention* (pp. 157–172). Washington, DC: Hemisphere Publishing Corporation.

ANTONOVSKY, A. (1979). *Health, stress, and coping*. San Francisco: Jossey-Bass.

ANTONOVSKY, A. (1984). The sense of coherence as a determinant of health. In J. D. Matarazzo, S. M. Weiss, J. A. Herd, N. E. Miller, & S. M. Weiss (Eds.), *Behavioral health: A handbook of health enhancement and disease prevention* (pp. 114–128). New York: Wiley.

ANTONOVSKY, A. (1987). *Unraveling the mystery of health: How people manage stress and stay well*. San Francisco: Jossey-Bass.

BANDURA, A. (1982). Self-efficacy mechanism in human agency. *American Psychologist, 37*, 122–147.

BARTROP, R. W., Luckhurst, E., Lazarus, L., Kiloh, L. G., & Penny, R. (1977). Depressed lymphocyte function after bereavement. *Lancet, 1*, 834–836.

BECKER, M. H. (1974). The health belief model and personal health behavior. *Health Education Monographs, 2*, 324–508.

BLOOM, B. L. (1984). *Community mental health* (2nd ed.). Pacific Grove, CA: Brooks/Cole.

BORYSENKO, J. (1984). Stress, coping, and the immune system. In J. D. Matarazzo, S. M. Weiss, J. A. Herd, N. E. Miller, & S. M. Weiss (Eds.). *Behavioral health: A handbook of health enhancement and disease prevention* (pp. 248–260). New York: Wiley.

BOYCE, W. T., Cassel, J. C., Collier, A. M., Jensen, E. W., Ramey, C. T., & Smith, A. H. (1977). Influence of life events and family routines on childhood respiratory tract illness. *Pediatrics, 60*, 609–615.

BRONFENBRENNER, U. (1976). Reality and research in the ecology of human development. *Master lectures on developmental psychology*. Washington, DC: American Psychological Association.

BUIE, J. (1988, July). "Control" studies bode better health in aging. *APA Monitor*, p. 20.

COHEN, F. (1984). Coping. In J. D. Matarazzo, S. M. Weiss, J. A. Herd, N. E. Miller, & S. M. Weiss (Eds.), *Behavioral health: A handbook of health enhancement and disease prevention* (pp. 261–274). New York: Wiley.

COHEN, S. (1988). Psychosocial models of the role of social support in the etiology of physical disease. *Health Psychology, 7*, 269–297.

COWEN, E. L. (1985). Person-centered approaches to primary prevention in mental health: Situation-

focused and competence-enhancement. *American Journal of Community Psychology, 13,* 31–48.

CURRY, S. (1989, August). Motivation for behavior change: Testing models with smoking cessation. Paper presented at the 97th annual convention of the American Psychological Association, New Orleans.

CURRY, S. G., & Marlatt, G. A. (1987). Building self-confidence, self-efficacy and self-control. In W. M. Cox (Ed.), *Treatment and prevention of alcohol problems: A resource manual* (pp. 117–137). New York: Academic Press.

DiCLEMENTE, C. C. (1981). Self-efficacy and smoking cessation maintenance: A preliminary report. *Cognitive Therapy and Research, 5,* 175–187.

DiMATTEO, M. R., & Hays, R. (1981). Social support and serious illness. In B. H. Gottlieb (Ed.), *Social networks and social support.* Newbury Park, CA: Sage.

ENGEL, G. L. (1977). The need for a new medical model: A challenge for biomedicine. *Science, 196,* 129–136.

FOLKMAN, S., & Lazarus, R. S. (1980). An analysis of coping in a middle-aged community sample. *Journal of Health and Social Behavior, 21,* 219–239.

FRIEDMAN, H. S., & Booth-Kewley, S. (1987). The disease-prone personality: A meta-analytic view of the construct. *American Psychologist, 42,* 539–555.

FRIEDMAN, H. S., & DiMatteo, M. R. (1989). *Health psychology.* Englewood Cliffs, NJ: Prentice Hall.

FRIEDMAN, M., & Rosenman, R. H. (1974). *Type A behavior and your heart.* New York: Knopf.

GATCHELL, R. J., & Baum, A. (1983). *An introduction to health psychology.* Reading, MA: Addison-Wesley.

GENTRY, W. D., & Kobasa, S. C. O. (1984). Social and psychological resources mediating stress-illness relationships in humans. In W. D. Gentry (Ed.), *Handbook of behavioral medicine* (pp. 87–116). New York: Guilford Press.

GREENFIELD, N. S., Roessler, R., & Crosley, A. P. (1959). Ego strength and length of recovery from infectious mononucleosis. *Journal of Nervous and Mental Disease, 128,* 125–128.

HOLT, L. H. (1990, Oct.). How the medical care system has failed to meet women's needs. Paper presented at the Rush/North Shore Medical Center Women and Mental Health Conference. Evanston, IL.

JACKSON, G. G., Dowling, H. F., Anderson, T. O., Riff, L., Saporta, M. S., & Turck, M. (1960). Susceptibility and immunity to common upper respiratory viral infections—The common cold. *Annals of Internal Medicine, 53,* 719–738.

JACOBS, M. A., Spilken, A. Z., Norman, M. M., & Anderson, L. S. (1970). Life stress and respiratory illness. *Psychosomatic Medicine, 32,* 233–242.

JANZ, N. K., & Becker, M. H. (1984). The health belief model: A decade later. *Health Education Quarterly, 11*(1), 1–47.

JEFFERY, R. W. (1989). Risk behaviors and health: Contrasting individual and population perspectives. *American Psychologist, 44,* 1194–1202.

JENSEN, M. R. (1987). Psychobiological factors predicting the course of breast cancer. *Journal of Personality, 55,* 317–342.

JESSOR, R. (1984). Adolescent development and behavioral health. In J. D. Matarazzo, S. M. Weiss, J. A. Herd, N. E. Miller, and S. M. Weiss (Eds.), *Behavioral health: A handbook of health enhancement and disease prevention* (pp. 69–90). New York: Wiley.

KANFER, F. H. (1980). Self-management methods. In F. H. Kanfer & A. P. Goldstein (Eds.), *Helping people change* (pp. 334–389). New York: Pergamon Press.

KASL, S. V., Evans, A. S., & Neiderman, J. C. (1979). Psychosocial risk factors in the development of infectious mononucleosis. *Psychosomatic Medicine, 41,* 445–466.

KENDALL, P. C., & Turk, D. C. (1984). Cognitive-behavioral strategies and health enhancement. In J. D. Matarazzo, S. M. Weiss, J. A. Herd, N. E. Miller, & S. M. Weiss (Eds.), *Behavioral health: A handbook of health enhancement and disease prevention* (pp. 393–405). New York: Wiley.

KOBASA, S. C. (1979). Stressful life events, personality and health: An inquiry into hardiness. *Journal of Personality and Social Psychology, 37,* 1–11.

KOBASA, S. C. (1987). Stress responses and personality. In R. C. Barnett, L. Biener, & G. K. Baruch (Eds.), *Gender and stress* (pp. 308–329). New York: Free Press.

KOBASA, S. C., Maddi, S. R., & Courington, S. (1981). Personality and constitution as mediators in the stress-illness relationship. *Journal of Health and Social Behavior, 22,* 368–378.

LAZARUS, R. S., & Folkman, S. (1984). Coping and adaptation. In W. D. Gentry (Ed.), *Handbook of behavioral medicine* (pp. 282–325). New York: Guilford Press.

LEVENTHAL, H., Meyer, D., & Nerenz, D. (1980). The commonsense representation of illness danger. In S. Rachman (Ed.), *Contributions to medical psychology* (pp. 7–30). Oxford, England: Pergamon Press.

LEVENTHAL, H., Zimmerman, R., & Gutmann, M. (1984). Compliance: A self-regulation perspective. In W. D. Gentry (Ed.), *Handbook of behavioral medicine* (pp. 369–436). New York: Guilford Press.

LEWIS, J. A., Dana, R. Q., & Blevins, G. A. (1988). *Substance abuse counseling: An individualized approach.* Pacific Grove, CA: Brooks/Cole.

LEWIS, J. A., & Lewis, M. D. (1986). *Counseling programs for employees in the workplace.* Pacific Grove, CA: Brooks/Cole.

LEWIS, J. A., & Lewis, M. D. (1989). *Community counseling.* Pacific Grove, CA: Brooks/Cole.

MANLEY, A., Lin-Fu, J. S., Miranda, M., Noonan, A., & Parker, T. (1984). Special health concerns of ethnic minority women. Commissioned paper. *Report of the Public Health Service Task Force on Women's Health Issues, Vol. II* (pp. II-37–II-47). Washington, DC: U.S. Government Printing Office.

MARLATT, G. A., & Gordon, J. R. (1985). *Relapse prevention: Maintenance strategies in the treatment of addictive behaviors.* New York: Guilford Press.

MATARAZZO, J. D. (1982). Behavioral health's challenge to academic, scientific, and professional psychology. *American Psychologist, 37,* 1–14.

MATTHEWS, K. A. (1988). Coronary heart disease and Type A behaviors: Update on and alternative to the Booth-Kewley and Friedman (1987) quantitative review. *Psychological Bulletin, 104,* 373–380.

MEICHENBAUM, D., & Turk, D. C. (1987). *Facilitating treatment adherence: A practitioner's guidebook.* New York: Plenum.

MEYER, R. J., & Haggerty, R. (1962). Streptococcal infections in families: Factors altering individual susceptibility. *Pediatrics, 29,* 539–549.

MICHAEL, J. M. (1982). The second revolution in health: Health promotion and its environmental base. *American Psychologist, 37,* 936–941.

MILLSTEIN, S. G. (1989). Adolescent health: Challenges for behavioral scientists. *American Psychologist, 44,* 837–842.

PETTINGALE, K. W. (1984). Coping and cancer prognosis. *Journal of Psychosomatic Research, 28,* 363–364.

PREVENTABLE DISEASES TAKE HIGH TOLL. (1990, January 19). *Chicago Tribune,* p. 4.

PUBLIC HEALTH SERVICE (1985). *Women's health: Report of the Public Health Service task force on women's health issues.* Washington, DC: U.S. Government Printing Office.

REKER, G. T., & Wong, P. T. P. (1983, April). *The salutary effects of personal optimism and meaningfulness on the physical and psychological well-being of the elderly.* Paper presented at the 29th Annual Meeting of the Western Gerontological Society, Albuquerque.

RENE, A. A. (1987). Racial differences in mortality: Blacks and whites. In W. Jones & M. F. Rice (Eds.), *Health care issues in black America: Policies, problems, and prospects* (pp. 21–42). New York: Greenwood Press.

ROBACK, H. B. (Ed.). (1984). *Helping patients and their families cope with medical problems.* San Francisco: Jossey-Bass.

RODIN, J. (1986). Aging and health: Effects of the sense of control. *Science, 223,* 1271–1276.

RODIN, J., & Ickovics, J. R. (1990). Women's health: Review and research agenda as we approach the 21st century. *American Psychologist, 45,* 1018–1034.

RODIN, J., & Langer, E. (1977). Long-term effects of a control-relevant intervention with institutionalized aged. *Journal of Personality and Social Psychology, 35,* 897–902.

ROTTER, J. B. (1966). Generalized expectancies for internal versus external control of reinforcement. *Psychological Monographs, 80* (1, Whole No. 609).

ROTTER, J. B. (1989, August). *Internal versus external control of reinforcement: A case history of a variable.* Paper presented at the 97th annual convention of the American Psychological Association, New Orleans.

SCHEIER, M. F., & Carver, C. S. (1985). Optimism, coping, and health: Assessment and implications of generalized outcome expectancies. *Health Psychology, 4,* 219–247.

SCHEIER, M. F., & Carver, C. S. (1987). Dispositional optimism and physical well-being: The influence of generalized outcome expectancies in health. *Journal of Personality, 55*(2), 169–210.

SCHEIER, M. F., Weintraub, J. K., & Carver, C. S. (1986). Coping with stress: Divergent strategies of optimists and pessimists. *Journal of Personality and Social Psychology, 51,* 1257–1264.

SCHLEIFER, S. J., Keller, S. E., Camerino, M., Thornton, J. C., & Stein, M. (1983). Suppression of lymphocyte stimulation following bereavement. *Journal of the American Medical Association, 250,* 374–377.

SCHUNK, D. H., & Carbonari, J. P. (1984). Self-efficacy models. In J. D. Matarazzo, S. M. Weiss, J. A. Herd, N. E. Miller, and S. M. Weiss (Eds.), *Behavioral health: A handbook of health enhancement and disease prevention* (pp. 230–247). New York: Wiley.

SCHWARTZ, G. E. (1982). Testing the biopsychosocial model: The ultimate challenge facing behavioral medicine? *Journal of Consulting and Clinical Psychology, 50,* 1040–1053.

SEEMAN, J. (1989). Towards a model of positive health. *American Psychologist, 44,* 1099–1109.

SEEMAN, M., & Seeman, T. E. (1983). Health behavior and personal autonomy: A longitudinal study of the sense of control in illness. *Journal of Health and Social Behavior, 24,* 144–160.

SPIELBERGER, C. (1989, August). Stress, emotions, and health. Paper presented at the 97th annual convention of the American Psychological Association, New Orleans.

STRICKLAND, B. R. (1984). Levels of health enhancement: Individual attributes. In J. D. Matarazzo, S. M. Weiss, J. A. Herd, N. E. Miller, & S. M. Weiss (Eds.), *Behavioral health: A handbook of health enhancement and disease prevention* (pp. 101–113). New York: Wiley.

STRICKLAND, B. R. (1988). Sex-related differences in health and illness. *Psychology of Women Quarterly, 12,* 381–399.

SULS, J., & Fletcher, B. (1985). The relative efficacy of avoidant and nonavoidant coping strategies: A meta-analysis. *Health Psychology, 4,* 249–288.

TAYLOR, S. E., Lichtman, R. R., & Wood, J. V. (1984). Attributions, beliefs about control, and adjustment to breast cancer. *Journal of Personality and Social Psychology, 46,* 489–502.

TEMOSHOK, L., Heller, B. W., Sagebiel, R., Blois, M., Sweet, D. M., DiClemente, R. J., & Gold, M. L. (1985). The relationship of psychosocial factors to prognostic indicators in cutaneous malignant melanoma. *Journal of Psychosomatic Research, 29,* 139–154.

THORESEN, C. E. (1984). Overview. In J. D. Matarazzo, S. M. Weiss, J. A. Herd, N. E. Miller, & S. M. Weiss (Eds.). *Behavioral health: A handbook of health enhancement and disease prevention* (pp. 297–307). New York: Wiley.

THORESEN, C. E., & Eagleston, J. R. (1985). Counseling for health. *Counseling Psychologist, 13*(1), 15–87.

TURK, D. C., & Kerns, R. D. (Eds.). (1985). *Health, illness, and families: A life-span perspective.* New York: Wiley.

2

The Process of Health Counseling: Strategies, Skills, and Concepts

Health and intellect are the two blessings of life.

Menander

Were it simply a matter of providing patients with health-promotion information about life-style change, the task of health promotion would be relatively simple. Unfortunately, studies of the effectiveness of life-style-change programs indicate that there is no one-to-one relationship between a client's knowledge about the need and the means for change and a client's subsequent behavior change (Janis, 1983).It is for this reason that the knowledge base and the skills of health counselors have become so central to programs aimed at proper nutrition, exercise, management of stress, smoking cessation, and control of alcohol intake, to name a few (Jordan-Marsh et al., 1984).

In this book, health counseling is described more as an attitude toward counseling than as a new theory system or even as a counseling subspecialty. The "attitude" of health counseling reflects integrative, biopsychosocial, and proactive ways of viewing and working with clients. This holistic and biopsychosocial orientation means that the focus is on the whole client—physical health status, interpersonal and social competence, as well as psychological and emotional well-being—and not just on the psychological and emotional aspects that tend to be the focus of the majority of theories and systems of counseling. The biopsychosocial perspective has been articulated by Engel (1977) and is clearly based on systems thinking; it is called biopsychosocial therapy (Sperry, 1988) when related to treatment issues. In addition to having this holistic perspective, health counseling is proactive, meaning that not only it emphasizes restoration of previous levels of health and well-being or adjustment—which is primarily a reactive function—but it also emphasizes prevention and increasing an individual's level of development and functioning.

The need for professionals who are trained in health-counseling skills continues to increase. With additional training, professionals already skilled in individual psychotherapy can be prepared to practice effective health counseling. We hope that this book will be useful in this regard.

There are a number of similarities as well as differences between individual psychotherapy and health counseling. In this chapter, we begin with the exploration of these similarities and differences as they relate to strategy, skill, and concepts. Briefly stated, strategies for individual psychotherapy center on formal, ongoing, scheduled appointments—usually 50-minute sessions—in a private-practice or mental-health office or consulting room. On the other hand, strategies for health counseling are much more diverse, ranging from encounters that are scheduled and ongoing in a private-practice or physician's office to unscheduled, occasional sessions at the bedside or in a hospital clinic. Although specific counseling skills and interventions of psychotherapy and health counseling are quite similar, their focus tends to be different. And even though concepts such as adherence, psychoeducation, relapse prevention, and systems influence are common to both health counseling and psychotherapy, they are seldom discussed in the psychotherapy literature. Since these four concepts are so important to health counseling, they will be described in detail in this chapter and discussed further in subsequent chapters, in reference to topics such as nutrition, exercise, and smoking cessation.

In this chapter, we also describe the process of health counseling and highlight some of its important strategies, skills, and concepts. We begin by

comparing the practice of health counseling with medical care and with psychotherapy. We then describe two different strategies for relating to patients or clients. Subsequent sections focus on 13 counseling skills commonly utilized in both strategies, as well as on the concepts of treatment adherence, psychoeducation or patient education, relapse prevention, and systems influences. A detailed case example illustrates these points and provides the prospective health counselor with a "feel" for the process of health counseling.

A Comparison of Medical Care, Psychotherapy, and Health Counseling

Medical care, psychotherapy, and health counseling represent different ways of both viewing and working with clients. Although medical care, health counseling, and psychotherapy differ in their treatment goals, they have many similarities. We will briefly describe their differences and then indicate the similarities in the processes and in the interpersonal skills that are common to all three.

Medical care in a primary-care setting usually involves a relationship—with varying degrees of participation and involvement—between a patient who is experiencing acute or chronic symptoms and distress, and a skilled clinician who can provide relief of those symptoms or effect a cure. One or several visits might be necessary to achieve this goal. The methods used include diagnosing and labeling a treatable condition and then applying appropriate medical or surgical treatments to alleviate or cure the source of the symptoms and the distress.

In psychotherapy, a confidential and more intensive relationship develops between a client with emotional and behavioral symptoms and dysfunction and a skilled therapist. The therapist uses verbal and nonverbal methods to effect symptom relief and to improve the client's ability to cope with internal and external stressors and with relationships with others. Frank (1984) believes that the majority of psychotherapy patients are demoralized and that encouragement is the primary nonspecific therapeutic effect of treatment. Specific treatment methods are described as supportive, diagnostic, analytic, and reconstructive in nature. Although "talking therapy" is the mainstay of treatment, it may be supplemented with such adjuncts as dream analysis, biofeedback, hypnosis, or psychological testing. In addition, some medically trained psychotherapists may prescribe medications or other adjunctive somatic treatments. Traditional approaches to psychotherapy usually involve regularly scheduled sessions with the same therapist for months or even years. However, newer, brief therapy approaches involve shorter time frames—often 8 to 20 sessions.

Compared to psychotherapy, health counseling involves a more action-oriented and participative relationship between a client who needs to reduce health risks or change life-style patterns and a skilled counselor who can facilitate the patient's acquisition and maintenance of these health changes. The duration of treatment is usually a short term. This approach is more oriented toward prevention than is either medical care or psychotherapy. Treatment methods are basically action-oriented and not only involve information giving

and prescriptions for life-style change but also include a number of traditional psychotherapeutic interventions as well as interventions unique to health counseling.

A Strategy for Formal Health Counseling

Formal, planned health-counseling sessions often last about 30 minutes and may be scheduled weekly for six or more sessions, depending on the nature of the change program and the type of collaboration between the health counselor and the referring health provider. In some cases, the health-counseling sessions will be scheduled in tandem with the actual change program; in other cases, the session will be separate and distinct. In almost all cases, follow-up contacts or sessions will be arranged at 6, 12, and 18 months after the last session to evaluate progress, deal with compliance and relapse issues, and encourage permanency of the life-style change.

Three phases of the psychotherapy process have been adapted to the health-counseling process (Dinkmeyer, Dinkmeyer, & Sperry, 1987). The following section will describe a formal strategy for health counseling that involves developing the relationship and engaging the client, conducting the assessment, and reorienting and consolidating the life-style-change process.

Relationship

The relationship between the counselor and the client is developed in a fashion similar to that in individual psychotherapy. There are, however, some important differences involving timing and intentionality. In psychotherapy, the tasks of developing the relationship can be leisurely accomplished over the course of the first three or four sessions, but because of the very brief and focused nature of health counseling, the matter of achieving cooperation and a negotiated treatment agreement is the primary task of the first session. The first session is typically scheduled for 60 to 90 minutes and is the most important of all sessions. The purpose of this session is to engage the client in the change process by establishing a cooperative relationship between counselor and client and by negotiating a mutually acceptable change program. During this time, the health counselor must come to understand the client's reasons and degree of motivation for making the particular life-style change. If the change is sought primarily to appease a spouse, employer, or the family physician, this needs to be dealt with at the outset. If little or no intrinsic motivation can be elicited, the probabilities of noncompliance and limited success need to be openly discussed, and a consideration of continuing or stopping treatment is best made at this time. Next, three important questions are asked of the client.

The first question involves a functional assessment: "How does your (obesity, smoking, pain, and so on) interfere with your daily life?" This question is followed by asking about the life tasks of work, love, and friendship, including the individual's level of functioning and degree of satisfaction in each of these tasks. The extent of distress and impairment is often related to receptivity to change. The more distressed the individual, the more receptive he or she is to a

treatment program that will relieve that distress and impairment. The counselor must be alert to the payoff or gain that this dysfunction may provide the client and thus interfere with change efforts.

The second question involves the client's personal explanation for the symptom or condition: "What do you believe is the reason for your (obesity, stress, and so on)?" The answer to this and the follow-up questions will begin to suggest the individual's health beliefs, as well as the extent of the factual accuracy that the person has of his or her condition and prognosis. This will be an important indicator of the amount of information and education that the counselor will need to provide at a later time.

The third question helps to elicit the person's expectations for treatment in terms of his or her own as well as the counselor's involvement of time and effort, expected outcome, and satisfaction: "What specific changes are you expecting? By when? What kind of involvement are you willing to make to see that it occurs? What kind of involvement do you expect of me?" In addition, the counselor does well to evaluate the client's previous efforts to make life-style changes. Very specific information about the number of attempts, the length of time, the extent of success, the outside help, and the reasons for quitting or noncompliance are important factors in the client's current expectations for success or failure.

On the basis of the counselor's understanding of this background information—particularly the client's expectation for treatment and outcome—the counselor then proposes realistic expectations for a change program that states broad time lines, level of involvement, and expected outcomes; the counselor discusses these in relation to the client's expectations. The discussion that follows constitutes the negotiation process. The purpose of this negotiation is to achieve a mutually agreed-upon contract for change. Often, this agreement is put in writing and is couched in performance-based language.

Let's give an example of this phase. Eleanor S. is a 38-year-old mother of three who was referred by her doctor to a health counseling specialist at the behavioral medicine clinic of Excel Health Plan, a local Health Maintenance Organization (HMO). Her physician, who had assumed care for Eleanor when she and her husband switched into the HMO some two months before, had determined that Eleanor was 55 pounds over her ideal weight and had placed her on a 1200 calorie Blackburn diet (Berland, 1983). He had provided her with detailed instructions for this high-protein diet and had indicated that if she followed the program closely, she could expect to lose 2 to 3 pounds per week. She was expected to see her phsyician biweekly to monitor her weight, vital signs, and certain blood levels. After four weeks and a slight weight increase, the referral for health counseling was made. In the first session, the counselor learned that Eleanor had gained 45 pounds over the past eight years of marriage, and most of that gain had occurred in the last 18 months while working part-time for a local realtor. She related that her husband had encouraged her to develop a career once the children were in school, but now she felt that he was subtly discouraging her.

Eleanor's answers to the three screening questions suggest that she has good insight and motivation for change. Her obesity does not seem to affect her

daily life unduly. She attributes her recent weight gain to the stressfulness of keeping up with all her home duties while trying to keep on top of new realty listings. She also notes that although on weekdays she was successful at following most of the diets she tried—including the Blackburn diet—she would "fall off" on weekends. Usually, her husband would "reward" her by taking her to exotic restaurants on Saturday night, and on Sundays, there was a standing invitation for a seven-course meal at one of their relatives' home. She notes that her parents cannot understand why she would want to lose weight. She believes that she could probably be successful on her doctor's diet if she could "control my cravings better" and find time for the exercise part of the prescribed diet program.

A specific change program was then negotiated between the counselor and Eleanor, in which she would meet for 20 weekly sessions and then for follow-up sessions at 6-month intervals for the following 2 years. A goal of 45 pounds of weight loss over the 20 sessions, which is approximately 2 to 3 pounds per week, was negotiated. She also committed herself to a graduated exercise program along with a behavioral and cognitive restructuring plan. At least three conjoint sessions with Eleanor's husband were also planned. She would continue to be monitored medically by her Excel Health Plan physician, who would confer regularly with the counselor.

Assessment

The assessment phase in health counseling tends to be more focused and, in many cases, is briefer than is the assessment phase in personal psychotherapy. In this phase, the counselor attempts to understand the person's present health behaviors in terms of personal and contextual factors. As such, the standard procedure of obtaining a complete social and developmental history and assessment of personality and cognitive factors may not be possible or even necessary.

At a minimum, it is useful to do at least a brief assessment of personality style, health beliefs, and past and current gain or payoffs for the current health condition or symptoms. In addition, it is useful to evaluate the extent and accuracy of the individual's knowledge about his or her condition. The client's earliest recollection of health or experience of illness is useful for assessing his or her health beliefs and attitudes toward health and illness (Sperry, 1986). This is done by asking the person to recall singular experiences when he or she was ill or that involved other family members or relatives who were ill. Often, responses will provide valuable insights into the person's body image and personality regarding cognitions or beliefs about self and others, and particularly about themes of entitlement, superiority/martyrdom, and authority figures.

In terms of contextual factors, it would be helpful to do a brief assessment of the client's family of origin, with a focus on family values related to health and illness behaviors, and to learn about the health and illness behaviors of other family members or relatives who could have served as social models for the client. It is essential that the counselor assess the client's cultural health status, which, according to Allen (1981), involves the "silent" attitudes and norms of one's family, social and ethnic groups, and community that influence and

reinforce certain health behaviors and not others. Allen indicates that we all are influenced by cultural norm indicators for exercise, smoking, stress, weight control, nutrition, alcohol and alcohol abuse, safety, and mental health, and he has developed several paper-and-pencil inventories to elucidate these cultural norms.

Let's return to our case example. On the basis of Eleanor's early recollections, health beliefs, family health values, spousal behavior, and cultural norms, the health counselor developed this formulation: Eleanor views her inner self as small and incapable yet encapsulated in a large, outer body shell that makes her appear strong and competent in some situations but vulnerable to external influences in other situations. She views the world as demanding and sometimes cruel, especially to the sick and obese, and believes that women are to be subservient to authority figures, particularly men. Therefore, her goal is to strive to be strong and competent and yet to avoid conflict and displeasing others at all costs. Thus, overeating serves as a safety valve for the conflict between her expectations and those of authority figures. Her payoffs for being obese as a child involved special parental attention and rewards of desserts for her unquestioned obedience. Modeling for overweight was universal in Eleanor's family of origin.

Turning to contextual factors, it becomes clear that Eleanor's spouse is a negative support system for her weight-management program, as he subtly and not so subtly sabotages her weight-loss efforts by taking her out for high-calorie meals. A conjoint session revealed his jealousies and fears that he might lose her to another man if she lost too much weight; Mr. S. himself was moderately overweight. He was not particularly happy that she was successful in the realty business, but the thought that she might leave him was unbearable. On the other hand, Eleanor has a college friend, with whom she now works, who was successful at a weight-loss and management program and who was willing to provide the social support necessary for Eleanor's program. Eleanor had eastern European roots and a tradition of believing that "You're not worthwhile unless you're strong enough to work; and you're not strong and healthy unless you're stout and proud of it." She checked the following items from the inventory of cultural norms (Allen, 1981):

"It's expected that if you lose weight through dieting you'll gain it back sooner or later."

"Sweets are a special reward for good behavior."

"Everybody loves a fat person."

"Sweets are just as nutritious as other food types."

These norms undoubtedly reinforced her self-view and worldview.

Reorientation

There are two main levels of intervention: the individual level and the systems, or family, level. At the individual level, encouragement is the basic, nonspecific intervention. Specific interventions involve information and instruction giving, cognitive restructuring, and behavior modification, which includes the setting of behavior goals, monitoring and pattern identification, stimulus control, reinforcement, and relapse prevention training.

Intervention at the systems level has the express purpose of increasing client compliance and minimizing relapse. Dropout rates from life-style-change programs are as high as 80% when there is no health counseling provided. Enlisting the aid of social-support systems like the family, co-workers, or friends is a critical task for both client and counselor. Not surprisingly, the more uninvolved and dysfunctional the family or the marital partner, the more the health counselor can anticipate problems in implementing any change program. To the extent that family members can be incorporated in the change program, the more likely the program is to be successful. For example, Brownell (1984) reports that when the obese client's spouse attended weight-loss sessions in which the spouse was also encouraged to modify his or her own eating habits, weight loss and maintenance was greater than for the control group studies. Brownell also found that an unwilling spouse can, and often does, sabotage the client's treatment program. Similarly, it has been shown that in exercise pro-grams, the spouse's attitudes toward the change program are probably more important than the client's (Dishman, Ickles, & Morgan, 1980).

If family members can be directly involved in individual or group sessions, they should be encouraged or even required to participate. If this is not possible, the family's indirect support should be enlisted. Doherty and Baird (1983) describe "family compliance counseling" as one way of enlisting this support, and describe the following steps. After the change program has been negotiated, the client is asked to come to the next session with his or her family. The counselor begins the session by providing information about the client's health condition to all family members and answering whatever content questions they may have. This is done to develop a common mindset and to set the stage for the family's commitment to the change program. The counselor then asks for the family's reaction to the client's health problem and then about the proposed change program. Next, the counselor helps the family make a contract for compliance to the change program. The counselor does this by asking the client whether he or she would like help from the family. If the response is affirmative, the counselor asks the client questions about what kind of help he or she would like and continues until a family contract emerges. The counselor may provide specific health promotional literature to family members that could clarify and increase their involvement in the program. Finally, a follow-up session is scheduled for the purpose of evaluating the client's progress and the family's support contract.

Let's return to our case example. Eleanor and the counselor have already negotiated the contract for change and the assessment has specified the change strategies. At the behavioral level, Eleanor was quick to learn, and she applied a number of behavioral methods for changing her eating behaviors and for learning and practicing some relapse prevention skills. Because lack of assertive-ness, especially in the marriage, was defined as a major issue, skill training was begun in the third session. Stimulus prevention or environmental engineering was stressed from the beginning. Eleanor had to avoid situations in which she would be "forced" by social convention to overeat, such as Sunday meals with her overeating relatives. She partially solved this by scheduling social activities

with her children during that time and inviting her relatives to her house for a light dinner that she prepared. She and her friend joined a beginner's aerobics class at a local YWCA.

At the cognitive level, Eleanor worked with the counselor to challenge and restructure some of her personality-style cognitions and health beliefs in a more socially useful direction. The counselor reframed her occasional relapses as slips rather than as failures. At the social-support level, three conjoint marital sessions were helpful in reducing Mr. S's fears about Eleanor leaving him should she slim down. And, after some communication and skill training, he became more sensitive to her needs to assert her independence. He further supported her when both sets of parents were upset with the change in their Sunday schedules. By the fifth session, Mr. S. was willing to go on the same diet plan as his wife, which aided her compliance with the program. Eleanor's friend was invaluable in helping her stick to her weight-loss and maintenance program on the job, as well as in helping her with menu planning. At the physiological level, she continued to be monitored biweekly by her physician, who conferred periodically with the counselor. By the twentieth session, Eleanor had shed 55 pounds, and 12 months later she was within 8 pounds of her ideal weight. Her husband also approximated his ideal weight, and they both reported improved personal and marital functioning.

A Strategy for Less Formal Health Counseling

Health and mental-health personnel can also utilize a strategy for health counseling that is particularly suited for less formal and less structured counseling encounters. When the client encounter is limited to only a few meetings, telephone calls, or even a single occasion, the ERIC strategy has been particularly useful (Sperry, 1987).

Briefly, ERIC is a "mental map" that guides the counselor's relationship with the client so that each planned or unplanned encounter, such as return telephone calls, can be primarily therapeutic and not simply conversational. ERIC is the acronym for four progressive levels or steps of therapeutic communication. The rules for using this map are simple: (1) begin each client encounter at the first level of ERIC and move to subsequent levels only when the situation requires, and (2) in subsequent encounters with the same client, begin again at the first level, but expect to focus more time and effort at subsequent levels. ERIC can be described as follows.

E – Refers to *engaging* the client in a relationship of respect and confidence and *exploring* the client's world. This is shown by the counselor's utilization of nonverbal and verbal cues, such as active or empathic listening. During this process of engagement, the client's problem or concern is explored. This exploration involves the antecedents and consequences of the problem along with the client's beliefs about and *expectations* for resolving it.

R – Refers to *reformulating* the client's concern into a diagnostic category or solvable entity. This usually involves *reassurance* and *reframing*. It can require *renegotiation* when previous treatment plans did not account for the client's understanding and expectations, which may have set the stage for noncompliance or for a negative set for treatment outcomes. The purpose here is to come up with a mutually developed treatment plan or contract.

I – Refers to the *initial intervention* that follows from a mutually developed treatment plan. It usually involves information and permission giving, and it may involve *instructing* the patient in learning *"interference" strategies* to reverse, for example, anxious or dysphoric feelings or ruminative thoughts that significantly interfere with daily functioning. Such basic interference strategies as controlled breathing, affirmations, and thought stopping can be taught to a client in a few minutes.

C – Refers to *continued intervention*. This level is needed only when initial interventions have not been sufficient or when compliance with the treatment plan is an issue. Outside *consultation* or referral may then be indicated. Otherwise, other *counseling interventions* can be implemented.

As few as one or as many as four levels of progression may be utilized in a single encounter, depending on client need or circumstance. For instance, the client's concern may be adequately addressed at the first level with simple engagement skills or processes, such as when the counselor's active listening allows the client to "get something off his chest" so that he feels understood and encouraged to go on with his life without further professional help. At other times, it may be that progression to the second level is needed. For example, the counselor may need to reformulate the client's perception of certain physical symptoms into a diagnosable and easily treatable illness or to reframe the client's perceived "failure" in a behavior modification program as a correctable "lapse." Let's now look at the way the levels of therapeutic communication apply to health counseling.

In health-promotion counseling, the counselor engages the client by empathically listening and nonverbally attending to her or him. Usually, a preventive prescription for diet change, exercise, or stress management has already been made, and counseling has been recommended because of the client's noncompliance—that is, inability to implement the prescribed change. The counselor explores the client's need for and reservations about life-style change, her or his explanation of the current health predicament and previous compliance issues, and the specific expectations for the current treatment. Reformulating and negotiating a viable treatment contract are critical. Instances of noncompliance are inevitable when trying to change long-standing habits. Since clients will frame these as failures, the counselor must reframe these as correctable lapses. Such reframing encourages and supports the client's efforts to change. Relapse prevention (Marlatt & Gordon, 1985; Sperry, 1986) is one of the most important initial interventions in this type of counseling. Contracting for change, attention to compliance issues, and specific skill training in self-monitoring and assertiveness, among others, are important continuing interventions.

Interviewing Skills in Health Counseling

There are five general categories of interviewing skills: empathic, exploring, engaging, reframing, and instructional responses. In the following sections, we give descriptions and examples for 13 specific skills in these 5 categories.

Empathic Responses

Empathy has been described as the ability to understand another individual's feelings and ideas and to communicate that understanding to the individual by nonverbal as well as verbal means (Riccardi & Kurtz, 1983). In a health-care setting, communicating empathy is an important means of establishing rapport, showing support, clarifying clients' problems, and collecting information. We will first describe the nonverbal means of conveying empathy and then the verbal means.

The counselor asks a client: "Have you been following your diet prescription regularly?" This rather straightforward and simple question could be expressed in several different ways, each producing different meanings for the listener. The counselor could be frowning or looking expectantly at the client, standing over the client or seated at eye level, speaking in a businesslike tone of voice or one that is soothing and encouraging. Irrespective of the verbal message, communication at another level is occurring. It is estimated that only 7% of a communication is transmitted through verbal speech; 22% is communicated through nonverbal speech, such as tone of voice and inflection; whereas 55% is communicated through what is popularly called "body language." DiMatteo and his associates (DiMatteo, Taranta, Friedman, & Prince, 1980) report that physicians who were judged to be more expressive of and sensitive to nonverbal communication skills received higher satisfaction ratings from their patients. This and other studies suggest that the counselor's nonverbal behavior can either facilitate the counselor/client relationship—and thus the treatment outcome—or detract from it.

Nonverbal communications can be either negative or positive. A counselor can communicate negative nonverbal messages through expressionless, blank faces, infrequent eye contact or staring, turning the body 45 degrees or more away from the client, and sitting away from the client in a slouched position with legs crossed and arms folded across the chest. Sitting or standing too close to the client (within 2 feet) or too far away (9 feet) also conveys a negative message. Incongruence between verbal messages and nonverbal behaviors, such as saying "I'd really like to know more about your job" while sitting with arms across the chest and body turned away from the client, negates the message.

Positive nonverbal messages are communicated when counselors face their clients directly and at the same eye level, position themselves a comfortable distance from patients—about 3 to 4 feet away—maintain eye contact without staring, lean forward, and assume a relaxed body posture. Interest in clients is also communicated when counselors gently nod and respond with animated facial expressions. Finally, responding in complete sentences without verbalized pauses ("uhs"), rambling, hesitation in delivery, and asking only one question at a time also communicate respect for clients.

The main verbal behaviors that convey empathy are called *active listening,* because the counselor actively attends to a client's words and feelings rather than passively waiting for the client to stop speaking. The four main skills of active listening are: clarifying, paraphrasing, reflecting, and summarizing responses.

Clarifying is a way in which the counselor makes a client's previous message explicit, confirms the accuracy of what the counselor heard, or clears up any ambiguity of the message. Clarifying usually rephrases all or part of the client's previous message in a question that begins "Are you saying that . . .?" or "Do you mean . . .?" The following example illustrates how clarification helps clients clarify their own thinking.

Client: "I wish I didn't have to fill out these diet forms! This doesn't make much sense to me."

Counselor: "Are you saying that you don't see any purpose to filling out these forms?"

Client: "No. I just don't think they can possibly help me with my problem at this point."

Paraphrasing is a way of rephrasing or reflecting the content of the client's message in the counselor's own words. By responding to the content of the message, counselors help clients focus on important information that could easily become clouded with emotions. For example:

Client: "I can follow this diet when I'm at home, but with the kind of job I have that puts me on the road five or six days a month, I have to eat in restaurants, and then I really blow my diet."

Counselor: "You're saying that you have success on the diet when you can eat at home, but you're not very successful when you eat away from home."

Paraphrasing highlights the content of the statement, namely that diet compliance is situation specific; it is not a response to the client's feelings about his or her job. These feelings may be very important but, in this exchange, they only distract from the important topic of compliance.

Reflecting rephrases the affective or feeling component of the statement. When counselors respond to feelings, they encourage the client to express additional feelings or to experience the emotion more intensely.

Client: "I don't know. Staying on this diet seems so useless. I don't think I'll ever slim down."

Counselor: "You feel very discouraged about your prospects for slimming down."

Client: "Yeah. It really is discouraging. I've been thinking about dropping the diet. What's the use in kidding myself?"

The reflecting response unearthed the client's ambivalence about continuing with the diet. This provided the counselor with an opportunity to deal with these feelings of discouragement and ambivalence before the lack of progress caused both the client and counselor to become disheartened.

Summarizing is a more complex skill than the previous ones, yet it builds on them. Here the counselor recognizes the pattern or themes in several of the client's messages and then links these themes into a single statement that reflects both feeling and content. Summarizing puts together two or more paraphrases or clarifications to condense several patient messages or even the entire session. Following is an example.

Client: "I really want to stay on this diet. But, there are so many things that pull me back to food and my old ways of eating. I mean, my friends, the places I hang out, my family . . . you name it. But even so, I know it's best for me to lose weight, and I want to stick with this program."

Counselor: "You are really feeling torn. On the one hand, you want to lose weight and you know its best for you, but on the other hand, you're reluctant to part ways with people and circumstances that pull you toward food and overeating."

Exploring Responses

Exploring responses are the principal communication skills in the exploratory phase. They are counselor-oriented rather than client-oriented. They move beyond the client's frame of reference and help the client see the need for action and behavior change through a more objective frame of reference (Egan, 1986). Two kinds of exploring responses are probing and confronting.

Probing responses are critical for securing specific information, such as the effect that clients' problems have on their daily lives, clients' explanation for why they have these problems, their past attempts to change their health behavior, and their expectations for the current program. Three kinds of probing responses are useful in health-care settings: open-ended, closed, and focused questioning.

Open-ended questions encourage patients to begin to talk and elaborate on their symptoms or their "story." These questions usually begin with "What," "When," "Who," or "How" and are phrased in such a way that they cannot easily be answered by a yes or no. This kind of question is most effective at the beginning and during the early stages of the exploration. Some examples follow:

Counselor: "What problems (or concerns) bring you here today?"

"How does being obese interfere with daily living?"

"How did your diet charting go this week?"

"What do you think keeps you from losing weight?"

Whereas general or open-ended questions broaden the focus of inquiry, *closed questions* narrow the focus to gather specific information. Sometimes specific or closed questioning is needed to probe for more explicit meaning or to clarify data. These kinds of questions are prefaced with words like "Do," "Is," "Did," "Can," or "Could" and are phrased to encourage one-word or short-phrase answers. This form of questioning is very effective in the review of systems in a medical history or in screening examinations, where the purpose is to assess risk factors, precipitants (events that trigger a symptom or a condition), and social-support systems. This form of questioning has its place, but when

counselors use it exclusively, it inhibits discussion, fosters a dependent client role, and allows clients to avoid sensitive topics. Some examples are:

Counselor: "Is your husband aware that taking you to restaurants frustrates your diet program?"

"Do you see any solution to this particular frustration?"

Focused questions narrow or define a topic by asking for a specific response. These are used when patients have difficulty responding to an open-ended question, or when the goal is to characterize a symptom or to elicit descriptive data concerning a clinical sign or issue. Focused questions usually begin with "Have you . . .," "Do you . . .," or "Can you . . ."

Counselor: "Can you tell me more about the health status of your parents?"

"Can you describe that sensation of bloating?"

Closed questions such as "Are your parents obese?" or "Do you feel bloated?" do not elicit the quality of response that the focused questions are likely to prompt.

There are some general guidelines for wording all types of probing questions. According to Cormier, Cormier, and Weisser (1984), questions should be phrased:

- simply, avoiding medical jargon
- concisely
- singly—ask one question at a time, rather than stringing two or three questions together
- in a nonaccusatory way, beginning with "What" or "How" rather than "Why"
- not as leading questions that suggest symptoms, illness, or a diagnosis

A *confronting response* points out a distortion or discrepancy in the client's communication. In popular usage, the word *confrontation* often has hostile or punitive overtones, but it does not carry such a meaning or intent in health counseling. Counselors judge neither feelings nor behavior, and they do not imply that a client is wrong. Rather, they calmly and noncritically point out discrepancies in what the client is communicating. These discrepancies can be between a client's messages and actions or between a client's verbal statement and nonverbal message.

Since confronting responses can have a powerful effect on the client and on the course of the interview, they must be carefully used. Generally, confrontation is most helpful in the latter parts of the interview, after empathy and trust have been established. The confronting response should be descriptive and concrete rather than judgmental and vague. It should be directed toward situations and behaviors that the client can change rather than toward those beyond the client's control or means; for example, certain dietary changes or supplements may be unrealistic for clients with limited incomes. A confronting response should be a request rather than a demand for change, made only when there is sufficient time to hear and understand the client's reaction to the situation. Clients may react to confrontation with denial, anger, confusion, feigned acceptance, or genuine acceptance. This example of a confronting response points out the discrepancy between verbal statement and behavior.

Client: (a 35-year-old woman who has just admitted she has not completed the daily diet and exercise diary) "I need to lose this weight because it's clear I was passed over for this promotion because of my obesity. Can't you do something to change this quickly?"

Counselor: "On the one hand, you're indicating you want to get your weight under control as soon as possible. But on the other hand, you've said you have had a hard time remembering to do the things that will help you achieve your goal."

Engaging Responses

It is usually necessary to orient clients to the treatment process and to the counselor's frame of reference. This involves what is called *engagement,* and one way of fostering this is with role-structuring responses.

Because much of the process and outcome of health counseling is affected by the client's attitudes at the start of treatment, it is important to describe the treatment program, its potential outcomes, and the roles and expectations of both client and counselor in the treatment process. Frank (1984) has called this process the "role induction interview." Patients who receive such an orientation are less likely to drop out of treatment and are more likely to benefit from it (Goldstein, 1973).

Counselor: "It will be helpful if I mention what I believe the weight management program should involve. We will spend time together to discuss your concerns about your weight and what you would like to do about them. Then we will work as a team to try to meet these goals. The treatment plan we come up with, and that you carry out—with my assistance—both in and outside these sessions can help you change your eating and other health behaviors that will result in weight loss and maintenance. This is not a 'quick fix' approach, but it has been very successful. I'd like to know your reaction and your own expectations."

Reframing Responses

Reframing responses offer an alternative to the client's view of a situation, including the nature of the problem, the client's progress, and the client's expectation for success in the program. A standard medical diagnosis is an example of reframing; the physician reframes the symptoms and signs into a diagnosis. Reframing is a powerful tool because it redefines what appears to be an incomprehensible, unbearable, or untreatable concern as a comprehensible, bearable, and treatable problem. Reframing has a significant place in health-promotion counseling, particularly when clients feel that they have failed to adhere to a treatment regimen. The reframing of perceived failures as correctable lapses can reduce patient embarrassment and discouragement. Here we will describe only one form of reframing, the ability-potential response.

The ability-potential response points to the client's current potential for achieving something (Cormier & Cormier, 1979). This sort of encouragement is particularly valuable in health-promotion and life-style-change programs when

clients become discouraged about the prospects for change. Ability-potential responses encourage clients who lack initiative or self-confidence to follow through with a desired change. They can also expand a client's awareness of personal strengths. This response should be reserved for times when a client has indicated a readiness for change but is hesitant to begin without some encouragement. It is best used when there is a basis for affirming the client's ability to pursue a desired goal, rather than as a pep talk to counteract discouragement from previous failure. In most cases, it is best to clarify and reflect these feelings of discouragement before affirming the person's ability to change. In this example, with a 45-year-old male who has tried several weight loss plans, the counselor has used reflecting and paraphrasing before using the ability-potential response:

Client: "Right now, I'm not sure I can drop this weight and keep it off. I've tried! But its really getting to me, and it's affecting my family. I just don't feel I can do it, or for that matter, do anything else right."

Counselor: "You're really discouraged right now. And because of that, you're not sure you can be successful at anything. But the fact is that you've been tobacco-free for over ten years, and you were able to lose and keep off 40 pounds for nearly ten months. With a track record like this, you've got a lot going for you, and a lot to build on."

Instruction

A basic counseling skill that is directed at behavior change is called *instruction*. There are two kinds of instruction, information giving and instruction giving (Cormier & Cormier, 1979). We will describe the first type in some detail and develop the second type more fully in the following chapter.

Communicating data or facts to a client at an appropriate time and in an effective manner serves to inform a client of possible options, to help the client evaluate these options, and to correct inaccurate information. Informing and instructing are the cornerstones of patient education. They involve much more than transmitting information; timing and delivery are critical. For each client, the counselor must identify what information to give and when and how to provide it. Effective instruction giving is a skill that can be learned, and the following guidelines should be helpful. First, identify the kind of information that will be useful to the client, and assess the accuracy and the extent of present knowledge. Second, wait for the client's cues of readiness, and don't force the information prematurely. Third, limit the amount of information given at one time, and deliver the information in a sensitive and friendly manner. Finally, ask for and discuss the client's feelings and biases about the information. Here is an example.

Counselor: (after reviewing the client's clinical picture and lab results) "Well, Mr. Burns, these results confirm both of our suspicions that you have diabetes. What's your reaction?" (after counselor and client discuss this) "Can you tell me what you know about diabetes?"

Client: "Sure. One of my friends has it so I know the symptoms and the causes. And, I know there is more than one way to treat it."

Counselor: "That's correct; there are generally three ways to treat diabetes: diet, exercise, and medication. Usually, we try diet and exercise first. Because there's so much information about all three, I'd just like to discuss diet for now, to see if it would be a reasonable approach to start. How does that sound to you?"

Client: "Well, I don't want to go to medication except as a last resort. What would diet be like?"

Counselor: (The counselor explains carbohydrate intake, insulin requirements, blood sugar levels, and their relationship to weight loss. The counselor then asks for the client's reaction to this information).

Instructing means verbally directing a patient on how to perform a specific task or follow a treatment regimen. As we pointed out earlier, instructing must be integrated with other interpersonal skills if the clients are to understand, cooperate with, profit from, and be satisfied with the treatment regimen and their relationship with the counselor. This skill is a major theme of the following chapter, so it will not be elaborated here. However, we can briefly state that to be effective, instructions must be specific, concise, and delivered as suggestions rather than as commands. Counselors should confirm that clients have understood the directions and, when possible, should give clear, written instructions for clients to take home. When appropriate, oral instructions should be supplemented with demonstrations. Adherence to instructions is more likely if they are limited to positive or rewarding consequences, such as sustained weight maintenance, social compliments, or an increased sense of self-control.

Compliance and Adherence

Compliance refers to how faithfully a client follows the advice and direction of a treatment provider (Sperry, 1986). Recently, this term has acquired a pejorative connotation, implying a passive and subservient client in relation to an active, authoritarian health-care provider. As a result, adherence, cooperation, and mutual participation have become preferred designations. In any event, treatment compliance is a problem encountered by all health-care professionals. It encompasses a wide variety of client behaviors, such as failure to begin treatment, premature termination, or minimally completing the treatment regimen, particularly regarding medication or life-style-change prescriptions. Compliance also encompasses a number of behaviors on the part of the treatment provider, such as emotional and time involvement with the client, clarity and specificity of language, and awareness of patient needs and expectations for treatment. Statistics from the life-style-change literature suggest that treatment adherence is one of the most critical health-care issues of the day. What is the practical significance of this issue for the counselor?

As more counselors become involved with life-style-change and other health-care programs, the issue of nonadherence takes on new dimensions. Nonadherence presents numerous and perplexing concerns and challenges for health counselors. Since financial compensation is often based on actual ser-

vices provided clients, nonadherence can dramatically affect clinical practice. Increasing adherence increases not only the client's satisfaction with the treatment rendered but also the counselor's job satisfaction. It is not surprising, then, that the research on adherence in life-style-change programs has increased significantly in the past few years. Unfortunately, this work is not easily available to practicing counselors. Thus, we offer a brief review.

Medical programs.   Composite averages of over 200 studies reviewed by Sackett and Haynes (1976) suggest that 50 percent of patients do not take prescribed medications in accordance with instructions. Furthermore, about 20 to 40 percent of recommended immunizations are not obtained, and about 20 to 50 percent of medical appointments are missed. Even being hospitalized does not guarantee treatment adherence. Under- and overdosage of medications and failure to follow prescribed diets are commonly reported in hospital studies (Kirscht & Rosenstock, 1979).

Life-style-change programs.   Life-style-change programs span the spectrum from smoking and weight-management treatment to exercise programs for health and for post–heart attack adults. The statistics are as dismal as are those for medical compliance. Sachs (1982) finds that the average dropout rate for all types of exercise programs is 30 to 70 percent. In spite of reported improvements in figure, mood, and a general sense of well-being, 50 percent of individuals who start an exercise program drop out within six weeks to six months (Ward & Morgan, 1984). Cox (1984) notes that corporate wellness programs typically recruit no more than 15 to 20 percent of employees, and of these, 50 percent or more drop out within the first six months—at considerable cost to the corporation. Smoking-cessation programs by comparison, are considered unusually effective if more than one-third of entrants have reduced their smoking at the end of six months (Kirscht & Rosenstock, 1979).

Statistics such as these often shock health-care providers, who assume that good adherence is the norm. They reason that if treatment is worthwhile, its benefits cannot be gained in the absence of adherence. Various attempts have been made to explain nonadherence. Blackwell (1982b) notes that there is little consensus on features that consistently influence adherence, despite research on more than 200 variables. However, most would agree that the main determinant involves the client, the health conditions, the treatment regimen, the treatment setting, and the provider/client relationship.

The majority of adherence studies have focused on the characteristics of clients. Many researchers anticipated that a noncompliant personality type would be identified. Unfortunately, as in the search for the cancer-prone personality, no such profile for nonadherence was found (Blackwell, 1973). Rather, studies suggest that, under certain circumstances, every client is a potential defaulter. Clients' health beliefs, presence of aggressive or passive-aggressive behavior patterns, dependence, and denial are associated with nonadherence (Backeland & Lundwall, 1975). No single client attribute—with the possible exception of scores on the self-motivation inventory (Dishman, Ickles, & Morgan, 1980), which have adequately predicted compliance with exercise—

combined with biological factors or with personality factors is as predictive as are situational variables and provider/client factors. One possible explanation for this abundance of studies that link adherence to client characteristics is the underlying belief that the client is basically to blame for nonadherence to treatment!

Blackwell's reviews (1973, 1982a, 1982b) suggest that only recently has there been a recognition that adherence is multiply determined. Reviewing a number of situational variables, Blackwell indicates that the duration of the health conditions—as well as the repetition of relapse and the presence of specific kinds of symptoms—influences adherence, as does the complexity of the treatment regimen and its side effects. The more complicated and inconvenient the regimen and the more the perceived discomfort, the less the adherence. Adherence is also strongly influenced by perceived or actual shortcomings in the treatment setting, as well as by the extent of supervision, social support, and follow-up supplied by the health-care provider or team. Finally, Blackwell and others suggest that the provider's attitudes and behaviors as evident in the provider/client relationship may be critical among the multiple variables that predict adherence.

There is a modest but growing literature on the aspect of mutuality, collaboration, or cooperation in the provider/client relationship as it relates to treatment adherence. For the most part, these studies are descriptive or correlational rather than experimental in design. This, of course, poses considerable limits on statements of causality. One group of these studies describes the informational techniques and the extent of explicitness regarding client behaviors that are necessary to ensure adequate levels of adherence. A second group of these studies views compatibility of client and provider expectations for treatment as a critical variable for adherence. These studies focus on the provider behaviors that are necessary for this mutuality of expectations of goals to occur. A third group of these studies links the client's assumptions of responsibility for treatment to maximal adherence. A final group of studies deals with the affective tone of the provider/client relationship before and during the treatment regimen. Adherence is seen as dependent on the social support supplied by the provider, as well as that provided by other clients and members of the treatment team (Garrity, 1982).

Psychoeducation

Psychoeducation, also known as patient education, encompasses any health-education experience planned by both health-care provider and client to meet the client's specific learning needs, interests, and capabilities (Squyres, 1980). Thus, psychoeducation is a process of education and activity based on an intentional exchange and sharing of information such that the patient's behavior is positively affected. It is best explained as a communication activity occurring within the context of a counselor/client encounter that influences client behavior toward improved health. Psychoeducation includes a variety of strategies designed not only to facilitate behavioral change, but also to help individuals to

identify their social support and to maintain their achieved behavior over a long period of time. It is much more complex than the printed handouts or audiovisual aids so often associated with it. In short, personal interaction is the key dimension.

The purpose of psychoeducation is to provide individuals with enough information and motivation to help themselves understand the factors that promote and/or threaten health, so that they may have a better opportunity to make informed choices in their lives (Levant, 1986). In addition, it provides the support as well as the technical assistance necessary to help individuals carry out their choices.

Assessing Client's Needs

The most challenging task in the psychoeducation process is to identify what the client actually needs to do or to know. A structured approach can help health counselors analyze the presenting problem or risk in terms of behavioral causes and to determine the educational or psychoeducational technique most appropriate for the treatment goals and desired outcomes. This type of assessment leads to the articulation of educational objectives. *Educational objectives* are based on the individual's behaviors, or absence of behaviors, that influence or cause a particular health problem. If the individual's health-related behavior is appropriate, reinforcement may be the only client-education intervention required. However, if some deficiency is obvious, it will be necessary to identify that behavior and the appropriate actions that may help to resolve it.

Establishing the cause of the performance deficit is most important. Is it a knowledge gap, a skills deficiency, an emotional factor, a social or environmental variable, or some combination of these? Assessment of an individual's knowledge and skills regarding a particular positive health behavior or life-style prescription is essential. Knowledge about the individual's family or significant other can also be relevant in psychoeducation. The individual's attitudes, beliefs, or emotions may also be a predisposing factor that interferes with appropriate health behavior. An individual may be so influenced by religious or cultural doctrine or so preoccupied with peripheral concerns, such as attaining a perfect physique, that noncompliance is inevitable. In addition, health counselors should assess social and environmental constraints that influence health behavior. Counselors cannot create ideal environments for clients or dictate what clients should do, but they can help clients to recognize mitigating factors, to weigh the pros and cons for change, to identify alternative options, and to learn to gain more self-control over their personal environment and their life.

Psychoeducation Techniques

Learning facts and skills is a prerequisite to the client's successful involvement in the maintenance of good health. Some basic educational principles for transferring information and teaching new skills are listed below.

Some Basic Principles of Psychoeducation

1. Psychoeducation cannot accomplish more than behavioral change.
2. Combination of strategies is required for all learning.

3. The client cannot be taught in isolation from family, friends, peers, or employers.
4. Audiovisual and printed ads cannot substitute for personal instruction.
5. Psychoeducation begins were the client is now, relates new information to previous knowledge, and adapts available aids to individual needs.
6. Psychoeducation encompasses the KISS principle: keep it simple and short. Patient education should be specific, brief, and direct, and should avoid overkill.
7. Clients should be encouraged to write down critical or complex information and then repeat it.
8. Clients should be encouraged to practice skills in simulated settings and implement them in real-life situations.
9. Effective psychoeducation recognizes that follow-up is essential.

Counseling and psychological support of clients is essential in the psychoeducational process. Social support, family sessions, self-care instruction, and ongoing reassurance are common interventions utilized by the counselor in the course of psychoeducation.

Sources of Material and Information

An abundance of printed materials useful in psychoeducation is available from a number of sources. These include governmental agencies and departments, voluntary community agencies, pharmaceutical firms, and insurance companies. For instance, the American Lung Association offers a considerable amount of audiovisual and printed materials on smoking cessation. In addition, there are a number of companies that specialize in health-education materials. For instance, Trainex and Professional Counseling Aids, Inc., market a variety of elaborately packaged learning systems for sale or rent. They, and other such firms, make available a resource catalog of these materials. One of the most comprehensive listings of psychoeducational materials is *The Guide to Health Information Resources in Print.* It is available from Health Information Library, PAS Publishing Company, Daly City, CA 94015.

Types of Psychoeducational Materials

The most common type of psychoeducation material is the patient handout. It is usually a simple one- to two-page information sheet that is either commercially available, or developed by the health counselor himself/herself, or adapted from any number of sources. The annual publication *Innovations in Clinical Practice* has a section on client handouts that can be copied and made available to clients. For example, a recent selection was on "Tips for Dealing with Insomnia."

Newsletters and magazines that focus specifically on health and patient education are becoming more available. Health newsletters published by several university health departments are offered to the general public on a subscription basis. The *Harvard Medical School of Health Letter* and the *Harvard School of Mental Health Newsletter* are two examples. Tufts University and the University of California at Berkeley offer similar letters on the topic of nutrition. The magazine *Medical Self-Care,* published quarterly, is an excellent background resource for both health counselors and clients.

Self-help organizations are another form of psychoeducation. Individuals with a particular condition or problem can be referred to any number of groups that share information and provide mutual support. The most common self-help groups are based on the 12 Step Model: AA, ACOA, Overeaters Anonymous, Procrastinators Anonymous, and Smokers Anonymous, to name a few. In addition, there are a number of self-help groups related to health behaviors that are not based on the 12 Step Model. Examples are TOPS (Take Off Pounds Sensibly), cardiac support groups, and cancer support groups. The community bulletin-board section of most metropolitan-area newspapers will list the various support groups available in the community. A similar and extended list is usually available in the community resource directory for particular communities and are available to most health-care providers.

Relapse, Education, and Prevention

Earlier, we defined relapse prevention as an intervention consisting of specific skills and cognitive strategies that prepares the client in advance to cope with the inevitable "slips" or relapses in compliance to change programs (Marlatt & Gordon, 1985; Sperry, 1986). Health counseling that does not recognize and emphasize the importance of relapse education and prevention is ineffective counseling. The subsequent chapters of this book will each include a specific section on relapse, education, and prevention strategies specific to the content of that chapter—be it weight management, smoking cessation, or exercise. In this section, we briefly review four different models of relapse education and prevention training (Daley, 1989). These different relapse-prevention models grew out of both inpatient and outpatient programs, often from those involving substance dependence. However, we believe the concepts embodied in these models have relevance to many other life-style-change and health-promotion programs.

Addict Aftercare: Recovery Training and Self-Help Model

This relapse-prevention model assumes that addiction, besides being a disease, is a way of life within a distinct subculture. It is further assumed that recovery requires that the addict not only stop substance use but also develop a new way of life. Developing a new way of life includes the development of new skills, and the recovery program responds to several critical recovery challenges. To avoid relapse, the client must learn: to handle substance cravings; to socialize differently in order to build a new social network; to adjust to substance-free activities and satisfaction; to cope with physical pain or stress without returning to substance use; to initiate and sustain interpersonal relationships to meet intimacy needs; to refuse substance-use offers and to respond to occasional slips without suffering a full-blown relapse.

The aftercare program for meeting these challenges consists of four components: (1) recovery-training sessions; (2) fellowship meetings; (3) substance-free social and community and activities; (4) a network of senior ex-addicts.

Recovery-training sessions focus on particular aftercare recovery issues. It is an educational tool, rather than a substitute for therapy or for 12 Step

Programs. These sessions help addicts to examine their experiences and to think and learn facts and ideas about recovery and healthy life-styles. These groups consist of between 6 and 30 members who meet for a minimum of an hour and a half. Written handouts and group exercises are used to actively involve all members. The primary purpose of these sessions is for members to learn facts and ideas about recovery and healthy life-styles, to prepare for predictable difficulties, and to respond to the inevitable relapses.

As do other relapse prevention models, addict aftercare addresses the reality of relapse by discussing this possibility before troubles arise. The developmental model encourages honest reporting of actual substance-use episodes. These relapses are carefully assessed and discussed so that members learn to develop strategies to stop substance use. Systematic research on addict aftercare discloses that 32 percent of participants were abstinent during the year-long follow-up, in contrast to the 18 percent abstinence of those not in the program.

The primary source of information on addict aftercare is F. Zackon, W. McAuliffe, and J. Ch'ien, *Addict Aftercare: Recovery Training and Self-Help,* DHHS Pub. No. (Adm) 85-1341 (Rockville, MD: National Institute on Drug Abuse, 1985.)

Cognitive-Behavioral Model

The relapse-prevention model developed by Dr. Helen Annis and her colleagues at the Addiction Research Foundation of the University of Toronto incorporates tenets of Bandura's self-efficacy theory. The two important elements of this cognitive-behavioral model are efficacy expectation and outcome expectation. *Efficacy expectation* refers to the belief that one has the ability to execute a certain behavior pattern. Clients who believe that they can cope with substance-related situations are more likely to do so than those who lack this belief. An outcome expectation refers to a judgment about the likely consequences of such a behavior. For instance, the judgment of an alcoholic may control his desire to drink because he believes that this will result in acceptance by his spouse.

According to self-efficacy theory, procedures for helping clients to begin changing may not be the most effective ones for generalizing behavior change or for maintaining long-range treatment effects. Self-efficacy theory presumes that treatment interventions are effective only if the client's expectations of personal efficacy are increased. Treatment effects that generalize into the future would be the result of strong efficacy expectations—for example, the client's confidence that he or she can successfully cope with alcohol-related situations. Conversely, low efficacy expectations indicate poor coping behaviors in difficult situations.

The behavioral model treatment has two phases. The first phase concentrates on initiating behavior change, and the second phase concentrates on maintaining and expanding these positive changes. During the second phase, the client takes a more active role in designing performance paths that lead to self-directed mastery experiences. As treatment progresses, the client assumes greater personal responsibility for change.

This relapse-prevention program involves six hours of assessment, followed by eight outpatient sessions over a three-month period. Outpatient treatment consists of a 1½-hour group session involving four to seven clients. This group is followed by 10 to 15 minutes of individual counseling for each client, during which time previously assigned homework assignments for performance tasks are reviewed and new performance tasks are planned.

Early research findings from two randomized control trials show that the cognitive-behavior model for relapse prevention was effective in helping most clients make dramatic changes in reducing alcohol consumption. Also, these studies exposed that clients who received this specialized relapse prevention improved in several areas of personal and social functioning.

The primary source of information of the cognitive-behavioral model is Helen Annis, "Relapse Model for Treatment of Alocholics," in *Treating Addictive Behaviors,* edited by W. Miller and N. Heather (New York: Plenum, 1986), 407–433.

Marlatt's Relapse-Prevention Model

Marlatt and his colleagues (Marlatt & Gordon, 1985) from the Addictive Behaviors Research Center at the University of Washington have developed one of the most comprehensive theoretical and clinical models of relapse prevention. This model has been applied to impulse control problems, such as sexual compulsions, and to impulsive aggressive acts, such as child abuse and rape, as well as to chemical dependency and weight control.

Marlatt believes that addictive behaviors are acquired habit patterns that can be changed by learning new procedures. Essentially, he views relapse prevention as a self-management program that helps the individual maintain changes in substance as well as behavioral addictions. A relapse-prevention approach effectively engages the client in the recovery process, giving him or her the primary responsibility for making changes. In short, recovery from addictive behaviors is a learned task that involves acquiring new skills.

This model of relapse prevention is predicated on three key assumptions about human behavior change. The first assumption is that the cause of the addictive habit and the process of behavior change are governed by different principles. The second assumption is that changing an addictive habit involves three distinct stages: (Stage 1) making a commitment and becoming motivated to change, (Stage 2) implementing change, and (Stage 3) achieving long-term maintenance of change. The third key assumption is that maintenance accounts for the greatest proportion of variance in long-term treatment outcomes. In other words, clients have a much easier time getting sober than staying sober for a long time. Relapses most often occur during the maintenance stage.

Marlatt and his colleagues have identified several determinants of relapse. These fall into one of two general categories: intrapersonal and interpersonal factors. Examples of intrapersonal factors are negative emotional states, urges, and temptations; examples of interpersonal factors include conflicts in relationships and social pressure to use substances. These researchers have found that the majority of relapses in adults occur in response to stressful situations,

while the individual is in a negative emotional state, and following some interpersonal conflict or social pressure.

The first step in relapse prevention is to help the client anticipate high-risk situations and predict how she or he will cope. An individual's high-risk situation can be identified by examining past situations, by discussing the problem behavior (that is, the substance or behavioral addiction), or by fantasizing relapse situations.

Recovery strategies should address each client's unique high-risk factors. The counselor first helps the client identify situations that pose future relapse risks. Self-monitoring records, self-efficacy ratings, autobiographical data, and a review of past relapses are some of the materials that can be used to assess these risks. It is also helpful for the counselor to assess the client's coping skills by observing the client in an actual problem situation. Simulation and role playing have been effectively used as assessment tools.

Cognitive factors in relapse.   Three cognitive factors interact in the relapse process. They are self-efficacy, outcome expectancy, and attribution of causality. *Self-efficacy* and *outcome expectancy* are similar to Annis's model of relapse prevention. *Attribution of causality* refers to a cognitive process that becomes important only when a person engages in a taboo behavior, such as a substance or behavioral addiction. It is the person's perception of the cause of the initial lapse to the addictive behavior. The addiction or relapse may be attributed to internal or external factors. Attributions of causality are important because they influence subsequent behaviors. For example, an individual who believes that an initial lapse will lead to a total loss of control and that this was caused by personal weakness (called the *abstinence violation effect*) is more likely to continue using substances. If this individual believes that the relapse began because he or she made the mistake of not applying relapse skills, he or she is more likely to stop the lapse before it gets out of control.

Marlatt and his colleagues indicate that both skill-training strategies and cognitive-reframing strategies are important in relapse prevention. Skill-training strategies help clients learn to cope with high-risk situations through behavioral and cognitive responses. Dry runs, covert modeling, and relapse rehearsals are examples of skill-training methods useful to clients. Cognitive-retraining strategies teach clients techniques such as alternative cognitions, coping imagery, and reframing reactions to initial episodes of addictive response. Cognitive skills might include learning to think of the long-term "seeing through the urges." If a relapse occurs, it can be framed optimistically, and with constant restructuring, the relapse can be viewed as a simple mistake rather than a fatal error or moral shortcoming. Marlatt notes that relapsers who view the relapse as a failure and who blame themselves are more likely to have complete relapses. Those who learn from the experience and act as "Monday morning quarterbacks" have a greater chance of recovering from the relapse. Finally, Marlatt notes that life-style-intervention techniques, such as exercise, meditation, or relaxation, are designed to strengthen total coping ability as well as to diffuse urges and cravings.

The basic source on this cognitive behavioral model is G. Marlatt and J. Gordon, Eds., *Relapse Prevention: A Self-Control Strategy for the Maintenance of Behavior Change* (New York: Guilford, 1985).

Psychoeducational Model

Daley (1989) has developed an educational model of relapse prevention based on his clinical experience with individuals, families, and groups in a residential chemical-dependency treatment program. This program involves group sessions that are task-oriented and consist of a combination of lectures, large-group discussions, and small-group tasks that are structured and precisely focused. Written handouts are used to provide information and to engage clients in self-assessment and relapse-prevention planning activities.

The goal of these relapse-prevention groups is to provide clients with information on relapse prevention and intervention and to instill in clients the attitude that sobriety in relapse prevention is a continuing process that requires long-term commitment to recovery. As do the other models of relapse prevention, the psychoeducation model also introduces clients to several cognitive and behavioral coping strategies.

Group sessions may be held daily and last between one and two hours. Topics covered in the course of these groups include: understanding the relapse process; handling of cravings to use substances; identification and handling of high-risk situations; use of leisure time and sobriety; relapse intervention; social pressure to use substances; and anger management and sobriety.

The primary resource on the psychoeducational model is D. Daley, "Relapse Prevention with Substance Abusers: Clinical Issues and Myths," *Social Work, 45,* 2 (1987):38–42.

Systems Factors in Health Counseling

We have previously argued that a knowledge of health-promotion principles does not translate to health-behavior changes. And we advocated that health changes require specific health-counseling interventions and strategies. We must add one more factor to the equation: systems influences. As you will see in the remaining chapters of this book, the influence of peers, family, spouse, and subculture cannot be ignored when assessing and intervening in any of the areas of life-style or health-behavior change. For instance, in weight-control programs, the health counselor quickly becomes aware of how the obese patient's spouse can sabotage the best-conceived treatment interventions, if that spouse's influence and collaboration with treatment have not been considered (Brownell & Foreyt, 1985). Similarly, Allen (1981) argues that the counselor's failure to account for the impact of subcultural norms can, for all practical purposes, sabotage the treatment plan. In short, systems factors play a significant role not only in assessment and intervention but also, as we will repeatedly demonstrate, in the reduction of relapse and the enhancement of treatment adherence.

GARRITY, T. (1982). Medical compliance and the clinician-patient relationship: A review. *Social Science and Medicine, 15,* 215–222.

GOLDSTEIN, A. P. (1973). *Structured learning therapy.* New York: Academic Press.

GOTTMAN, J., & Leiblum, S. (1974). *How to do psychotherapy and how to evaluate it.* New York: Holt, Rinehart & Winston.

HAYNES, B. (1984). Compliance with health advice: An overview with special reference to exercise programs. *Journal of Cardiac Rehabilitation, 4,* 120–123.

JANIS, I. (1982). *Counseling on personal decisions: Theory and research on short-term helping relationships.* New Haven: Yale University Press.

JANIS, I. (1983). *Short-term counseling: Guidelines based on recent research.* New Haven: Yale University Press.

JORDAN-MARSH, M., Gilbert, J., Ford, J., & Kleeman, C. (1984). Life-style intervention: A conceptual framework. *Patient Education and Counseling, 6,* 29–38.

KIRSCHT, J., & Rosenstock, I. (1979). Patient problems in following recommendations of health experts. In G. Stone, F. Cohen, & N. Adler (Eds.), *Health psychology: A handbook.* San Francisco: Jossey-Bass.

KRISTELLER, J., & Rodin, J. (1984). A three stage model of treatment continuity: Compliance, adherence and maintenance. In A. Baum, S. Taylor, & J. Singer (Eds.), *Handbook of psychology and health: Social aspects of health.* Hillsdale, NJ: Erlbaum.

LEVANT, R. (1986). *Psychoeducational approaches to family therapy and family counseling.* New York: Springer.

MARLATT, G., & Gordon, J. (1985). *Relapse prevention: A Self-Control Strategy for the Maintenance of Behavior Change.* New York: Guilford Press.

OLDRIDGE, N. (1984). Efficacy and effectiveness: Critical issues in exercise and compliance. *Journal of Cardiac Rehabilitation, 4,* 119.

RICCARDI, V., & Kurtz, S. (1983). *Communication and counseling and health care.* Springfield, IL: Charles C Thomas.

SACHS, M. (1982). Compliance and addiction to exercise. In R. Cantu (Ed.), *The exercising adult.* Lexington, MA: Collamore Press.

SACKETT, D., & Haynes, R. (Eds.). (1976). *Compliance with therapeutic regimens.* Baltimore: Johns Hopkins University Press.

SHULMAN, B. (1964). Psychological disturbances which interfere with the patient's cooperation. *Psychosomatics, 5,* 213–220.

SILVERMAN, W. (1982). Investigating the drop-out phenomenon in community health centers. *Quality Review Bulletin, 8,* 3–6.

SIMONDS, S. (1982). Individual health counseling and education: Emerging directions from current theory, research and practice. *Patient Counseling and Health Education, 4,* 129–136.

SPERRY, L. (1985). Treatment noncompliance and cooperation: Implications for psychotherapeutic, medical and lifestyle change approaches. *Individual Psychology, 41,* 228–236.

SPERRY, L. (1986). The ingredients of effective health counseling: Health beliefs, compliance and relapse prevention. *Individual Psychology, 42,* 279–287.

SPERRY, L. (1987). ERIC: A cognitive map for guiding brief therapy and health care counseling. *Individual Psychology, 43*(2), 237–241.

SPERRY, L. (1988). Biopsychosocial therapy: An integrative approach for tailoring treatment. *Individual Psychology, 44*(2), 225–235.

SQUYRES, W. (1980). *Patient education: An inquiry into the state of the art.* St. Louis: C. V. Mosby.

SZASZ, T. S., & Hollender, M. H. (1956). A contribution to the philosophy of medicine: The basic models of the doctor-patient relationship. *Archives of Internal Medicine, 97,* 585–592.

WARD, A., & Morgan, W. (1984). Adherence patterns and health: Men and women enrolled in an adult exercise program. *Journal of Cardiac Rehabilitation, 4,* 43–159.

References

ALLEN, R. (1981). *Lifegain.* New York: Appleton-Century-Crofts.

ANSBACHER, H., & Ansbacher, R. (Eds.). (1956). *The Individual Psychology of Alfred Adler.* New York: Basic Books.

BACKELAND, F., & Lundwall, L. (1975). Dropping out of treatment: A critical review. *Psychological Bulletin, 82,* 738–783.

BERLAND, T. (1983). *Rating the diets: Consumers Guide,* 1983 edition. New York: Signet Books.

BEUTLER, L. (1983). *Eclectic psychotherapy: A systematic approach.* New York: Pergamon Press.

BLACKWELL, B. (1973). Drug therapy: Patient compliance. *New England Journal of Medicine, 289,* 249–252.

BLACKWELL, B. (1982a). Treatment adherence. *British Journal of Psychiatry, 129,* 513–531.

BLACKWELL, B. (1982b). Treatment compliance. In J. Greist, J. Jefferson, & R. Spitzer (Eds.), *Treatment of mental disorders.* New York: Oxford University Press.

BROWNELL, K. (1984). The psychology and physiology of obesity: Implications for screening and treatment. *Journal of American Dietetics Association, 84,* 406–414.

BROWNELL, K. D., & Foreyt, J. P. (1985). Obesity. In D. Barlow (Ed.), *Clinical handbook of psychological disorders.* New York: Guilford Press.

CORMIER, W., & Cormier, L. S. (1979). *Interviewing strategies for helpers: A guide to assessment, treatment and evaluation.* Pacific Grove, CA: Brooks/Cole.

CORMIER, W., Cormier L. S., & Weisser, R. (1984). *Interviewing and helping skills for health professionals.* Boston: Jones & Bartlett.

COX, M. H. (1984). Fitness and life style programs for business and industry: Problems in recruitment and retention. *Journal of Cardiac Rehabilitation, 4,* 136–142.

DALEY, D. C. (1989). Relapse prevention: *Treatment alternatives and counseling aids.* Blaze Ridge Summit, PA: TAB Books.

DiMATTEO, M., & DiNicola, D. (1982). *Achieving patient compliance: The psychology of the medical practitioner's role.* New York: Pergamon Press.

DiMATTEO, M., & Friedman, H. (1982). *Social psychology and medicine.* Cambridge, MA: Oelgeschlager, Gunn, and Hain.

DiMATTEO, M. R., Taranta, A., Friedman, H., Prince, L. M. (1980). Predicting satisfaction from physicians' nonverbal communication skills. *Medical Care, 18,* 376.

DINKMEYER, D., Dinkmeyer, D., & Sperry, L. (Eds.). (1987). *Adlerian counseling and psychotherapy.* Columbus, OH: Merrill.

DISHMAN, R., Ickles, W., & Morgan, W. (1980). Self-motivation and adherence to habitual physical activity. *Journal of Applied Social Psychology, 10,* 155–132.

DOHERTY, W., & Baird, M. (1983). *Family therapy and family medicine.* New York: Guilford Press.

DREIKURS, R. (1956). Adlerian psychotherapy. In F. Fromm-Reichman & J. Moreno (Eds.), *Progress in psychotherapy.* New York: Grune & Stratton.

DREIKURS, R. (1967). Minor psychotherapy: A practical psychology for physicians. In R. Dreikurs (Ed.), *Psychodynamics, psychotherapy and counseling.* Collected papers. Chicago: Alfred Adler Institute.

EGAN G. (1986). *The skilled helper: A model for systematic helping and interpersonal relating.* Pacific Grove, CA: Brooks/Cole.

ENGEL, G. (1977). The need for a new medical model: A challenge to biomedical science. *Science, 196,* 129–136.

EPPERSON, D., Bushway, D., & Warman, R. (1983). Client self-termination after one counseling session: Effects on problem recognition, counselor gender, and counselor experience. *Journal of Counseling Psychology, 30,* 307–315.

FRANK, J. D. (1984). Therapeutic components of all psychotherapies. In J. M. Myers, (Ed.), *Cures by psychotherapy: What affects change?* New York: Praeger.

FRIEDMAN, H., & DiMatteo, M. (Eds.). (1982). *Interpersonal issues in health care.* New York: Academic Press.

FROELICH, R. E., Bishop, F. M. (1979). *Clinical interviewing skills.* St. Louis: C. V. Mosby.

References

ALLEN, R. (1981). *Lifegain.* New York: Appleton-Century-Crofts.

ANSBACHER, H., & Ansbacher, R. (Eds.). (1956). *The Individual Psychology of Alfred Adler.* New York: Basic Books.

BACKELAND, F., & Lundwall, L. (1975). Dropping out of treatment: A critical review. *Psychological Bulletin, 82,* 738–783.

BERLAND, T. (1983). *Rating the diets: Consumers Guide,* 1983 edition. New York: Signet Books.

BEUTLER, L. (1983). *Eclectic psychotherapy: A systematic approach.* New York: Pergamon Press.

BLACKWELL, B. (1973). Drug therapy: Patient compliance. *New England Journal of Medicine, 289,* 249–252.

BLACKWELL, B. (1982a). Treatment adherence. *British Journal of Psychiatry, 129,* 513–531.

BLACKWELL, B. (1982b). Treatment compliance. In J. Greist, J. Jefferson, & R. Spitzer (Eds.), *Treatment of mental disorders.* New York: Oxford University Press.

BROWNELL, K. (1984). The psychology and physiology of obesity: Implications for screening and treatment. *Journal of American Dietetics Association, 84,* 406–414.

BROWNELL, K. D., & Foreyt, J. P. (1985). Obesity. In D. Barlow (Ed.), *Clinical handbook of psychological disorders.* New York: Guilford Press.

CORMIER, W., & Cormier, L. S. (1979). *Interviewing strategies for helpers: A guide to assessment, treatment and evaluation.* Pacific Grove, CA: Brooks/Cole.

CORMIER, W., Cormier L. S., & Weisser, R. (1984). *Interviewing and helping skills for health professionals.* Boston: Jones & Bartlett.

COX, M. H. (1984). Fitness and life style programs for business and industry: Problems in recruitment and retention. *Journal of Cardiac Rehabilitation, 4,* 136–142.

DALEY, D. C. (1989). Relapse prevention: *Treatment alternatives and counseling aids.* Blaze Ridge Summit, PA: TAB Books.

DiMATTEO, M., & DiNicola, D. (1982). *Achieving patient compliance: The psychology of the medical practitioner's role.* New York: Pergamon Press.

DiMATTEO, M., & Friedman, H. (1982). *Social psychology and medicine.* Cambridge, MA: Oelgeschlager, Gunn, and Hain.

DiMATTEO, M. R., Taranta, A., Friedman, H., Prince, L. M. (1980). Predicting satisfaction from physicians' nonverbal communication skills. *Medical Care, 18,* 376.

DINKMEYER, D., Dinkmeyer, D., & Sperry, L. (Eds.). (1987). *Adlerian counseling and psychotherapy.* Columbus, OH: Merrill.

DIHMAN, R., Ickles, W., & Morgan, W. (1980). Self-motivation and adherence to habitual physical activity. *Journal of Applied Social Psychology, 10,* 155–132.

DOHRTY, W., & Baird, M. (1983). *Family therapy and family medicine.* New York: Guilford Press.

DREIKRS, R. (1956). Adlerian psychotherapy. In F. Fromm-Reichman & J. Moreno (Eds.), *Progress* psychotherapy. New York: Grune & Stratton.

DIKU R. (1967). Minor psychotherapy: A practical psychology for physicians. In R. Dreikurs (E *Psychodynamics, psychotherapy and counseling.* Collected papers. Chicago: Alfred Ad Institute.

EGA (1 5). *The skilled helper: A model for systematic helping and interpersonal relating.* Pacific ov CA: Brooks/Cole.

ENG (17). The need for a new medical model: A challenge to biomedical science. *Science,* 12–136.

EPPE , Bushway, D., & Warman, R. (1983). Client self-termination after one counseling Effects on problem recognition, counselor gender, and counselor experience. of Counseling Psychology, 30,* 307–315.

FRAN 4). Therapeutic components of all psychotherapies. In J. M. Myers, (Ed.), *Cures by* FRIEL py: *What affects change?* New York: Praeger.

DiMatteo, M. (Eds.). (1982). *Interpersonal issues in health care.* New York: FROE ss.

hop, F. M. (1979). *Clinical interviewing skills.* St. Louis: C. V. Mosby.

GARRITY, T. (1982). Medical compliance and the clinician-patient relationship: A review. *Social Science and Medicine, 15,* 215–222.

GOLDSTEIN, A. P. (1973). *Structured learning therapy.* New York: Academic Press.

GOTTMAN, J., & Leiblum, S. (1974). *How to do psychotherapy and how to evaluate it.* New York: Holt, Rinehart & Winston.

HAYNES, B. (1984). Compliance with health advice: An overview with special reference to exercise programs. *Journal of Cardiac Rehabilitation, 4,* 120–123.

JANIS, I. (1982). *Counseling on personal decisions: Theory and research on short-term helping relationships.* New Haven: Yale University Press.

JANIS, I. (1983). *Short-term counseling: Guidelines based on recent research.* New Haven: Yale University Press.

JORDAN-MARSH, M., Gilbert, J., Ford, J., & Kleeman, C. (1984). Life-style intervention: A conceptual framework. *Patient Education and Counseling, 6,* 29–38.

KIRSCHT, J., & Rosenstock, I. (1979). Patient problems in following recommendations of health experts. In G. Stone, F. Cohen, & N. Adler (Eds.), *Health psychology: A handbook.* San Francisco: Jossey-Bass.

KRISTELLER, J., & Rodin, J. (1984). A three stage model of treatment continuity: Compliance, adherence and maintenance. In A. Baum, S. Taylor, & J. Singer (Eds.), *Handbook of psychology and health: Social aspects of health.* Hillsdale, NJ: Erlbaum.

LEVANT, R. (1986). *Psychoeducational approaches to family therapy and family counseling.* New York: Springer.

MARLATT, G., & Gordon, J. (1985). *Relapse prevention: A Self-Control Strategy for the Maintenance of Behavior Change.* New York: Guilford Press.

OLDRIDGE, N. (1984). Efficacy and effectiveness: Critical issues in exercise and compliance. *Journal of Cardiac Rehabilitation, 4,* 119.

RICCARDI, V., & Kurtz, S. (1983). *Communication and counseling and health care.* Springfield, IL: Charles C Thomas.

SACHS, M. (1982). Compliance and addiction to exercise. In R. Cantu (Ed.), *The exercising adult.* Lexington, MA: Collamore Press.

SACKETT, D., & Haynes, R. (Eds.). (1976). *Compliance with therapeutic regimens.* Baltimore: Johns Hopkins University Press.

SHULMAN, B. (1964). Psychological disturbances which interfere with the patient's cooperation. *Psychosomatics, 5,* 213–220.

SILVERMAN, W. (1982). Investigating the drop-out phenomenon in community health centers. *Quality Review Bulletin, 8,* 3–6.

SIMONDS, S. (1982). Individual health counseling and education: Emerging directions from current theory, research and practice. *Patient Counseling and Health Education, 4,* 1–136

SPERRY, L. (1985). Treatment noncompliance and cooperation: Implications for psychotherapeutic, medical and lifestyle change approaches. *Individual Psychology, 41,* 228–2

SPERRY, L. (1986). The ingredients of effective health counseling: Health beliefs, compliance and relapse prevention. *Individual Psychology, 42,* 279–287.

SPERRY, L. (1987). ERIC: A cognitive map for guiding brief therapy and health counseling. *Individual Psychology, 43*(2), 237–241. treatment.

SPERRY, L. (1988). Biopsychosocial therapy: An integrative approach for t dividual Psychology, 44*(2), 225–235. is: C. V. Mosby.

SQUYRES, W. (1980). *Patient education: An inquiry into the state of the a*icine: The basic

SZASZ, T. S., & Hollender, M. H. (1956). A contribution to the philosophy, 585–592. models of the doctor-patient relationship. *Archives of Internal* en enrolled in an

WARD, A., & Morgan, W. (1984). Adherence patterns and health: Me adult exercise program. *Journal of Cardiac Rehabilitation,*

II

Applications

3

Weight Control

Clogged with yesterday's excess, the body drags the mind down
with it, and fastens to the ground this fragment of divine spirit.

Horace

Obesity is one of our nation's most common and persistent problems. Epidemiological studies show that over one-half of American adults are more than 20 percent over their ideal weight (Miller & Stephens, 1987). Americans spend more than $10 billion a year on commercial weight-loss treatments, and the increasing level of media attention to crash diets, weight-loss clinics, and exercise suggests that this figure can only increase. Interestingly, this massive investment in weight-reducing treatment has failed to produce any decrease in the frequency of obesity, which has actually risen over the past 30 years.

Obesity has not always been regarded as a problem. In the past, and in most second- and third-world countries, obesity was and is a sign of health and wealth. It appears that when food becomes scarce, personal fat stores are an advantage. In Western society, obesity came to be seen as a medical problem in the late eighteenth century (Schwartz, 1986). Over the next century, aesthetic preferences changed, and slim, svelte figures came to be valued. This trend has continued, as shown by the steady decrease in the body size of fashion models (Garner et al., 1980), which has helped to create an image of an ideal body shape that few women have a chance of achieving.

Today, the problem of obesity tends to be viewed in both medical and psychological terms. Actuarial studies by life insurance companies have demonstrated that higher body weights are associated with lower life expectancy, and numerous independent studies have confirmed this observation (Van Itallie, 1979; Lew & Garfinkel, 1979). Obesity is associated with higher morbidity as well as with increased mortality, including the greater incidence of diabetes, hypertension, gall bladder disease, orthopedic problems, and complications during surgery (Rimm et al., 1975; Kannel & Gordon, 1979). Not surprisngly, there is little doubt that obesity contributes substantially to the cost of health care. A review of the literature confirms the perception of the negative stereotype of obesity, which ranges from criticism and public ridicule accorded obese children to the active prejudice, particularly against obese females, in occupational settings. Obese individuals can be expected to be teased and taunted, treated as less intelligent than they are, and rejected from training or jobs in favor of less qualified but slimmer individuals. At a personal level, excess weight is associated with low self-esteem and low body satisfaction. Embarrassment about body shape can make overweight individuals reluctant to engage in sexual relationships or to take part in activities in which their body shape is exposed, taking a further toll on physical and emotional well-being (Wardle, 1989).

Of all the areas of life-style change, losing and maintaining weight loss is undoubtedly the most difficult and perplexing area. Weight loss is a life-style change because it requires more than simply losing weight or changing eating behaviors. Often, the changes require altering a person's life well beyond diet modification. For example, just one relatively simple dietary change, such as reducing the daily consumption of soft drinks, might involve a series of un-expected changes: changes in shopping habits to modify the routine purchase of soft drinks; the development of assertiveness skills to handle well-meaning friends who continue to prefer soft drinks; acquisition of time-management skills, as other beverages may not be so readily available as the conveniently

located soda machine; knowledge acquisition concerning the nutritional content of soft drinks vis-à-vis other beverages; and some experimentation and emotional considerations in finding a suitable replacement for the soft drink (Laquatera & Danish, 1988). It is no exaggeration, then, to suggest that weight loss is a complex, difficult life-style change.

This chapter provides an overview of both the theoretical and the clinical information on weight control. We begin by examining obesity in terms of etiology, theories of obesity, and classification of obesity. As in other chapters, biopsychosocial factors are emphasized, particularly as they relate to weight gain and weight loss. Various approaches to the assessment and treatment of obesity are then reviewed which, as in previous chapters, emphasize a comprehensive, biopsychosocial view of the process of change. We include two different treatment protocols that health counselors have found useful in working with weight-control issues. Further, because relapse prevention is such a critical issue in weight-control management, we present an extended discussion of this issue, including primary prevention measures. Finally, we offer two detailed cases and an extended resource section at the chapter's end.

To begin, we need to define and clarify two terms that we use in this chapter. Obesity and overweight are not synonymous terms. *Obesity* specifically refers to excess body fat stores, whereas *overweight* refers to excess body weight (Stunkard, 1984).

Biopsychosocial Factors in Weight Control

Causes of Obesity

Obesity develops when one's daily caloric intake exceeds one's metabolic requirements. Also, obese individuals may be less efficient in utilizing the calories that they ingest. Ultimately, the regulation of the valves between intake and metabolic requirement is uncontrolled by higher brain processes. The pathophysiology underlying this controlling mechanism is still not fully understood. However, a very promising line of research suggests that obesity is related to both the number and the size of fat cells (Bjorntorp, 1986).

Hypertrophic Obesity. *Hypertrophic obesity* refers to an increase in body weight that is associated with an increase in fat-cell size but not in fat-cell number. Adults with normal body weight have approximately 30 to 35 billion fat cells, and each cell weighs about 0.4 to 0.6 micrograms. When an individual gains weight and becomes mildly obese, weight gain is associated with an increase in fat-cell size up to 1.2 micrograms. With calorie restrictions and increased physical activity, fat-cell size and body weight can return to normal.

Hyperplastic obesity. Severe obesity is characterized not only by an increase in fat-cell size, but often by an increase in fat-cell number, called *hyperplastic obesity.* An obese person of 300 pounds or more may have as many as 100 to 150 billion fat cells. Moderately obese individuals will have an increase in cell number, but usually not to the same extent as does the severely obese individual.

Whereas hypertrophic obesity appears to be completely reversible, hyperplastic obesity is not. Once the body has produced new fat cells, it appears to retain them for life. Therefore, individuals with severe hyperplastic obesity tend to remain overweight despite rigorous dieting and exercise. For such individuals to return to their ideal weight, they would have to reduce the size of their individual fat cells so far below normal limits (that is, to 0.1 to 0.2 micrograms) that they would literally be in a state of semistarvation. Chronic dieters report that they experience general apathy, depression, and total preoccupation with food while on semistarvation diets. Given these circumstances, severe hyperplastic obesity often requires radical treatment, such as gastric bypass surgery, or stomach stapling. In short, obesity that begins in childhood usually involves both hypertrophic and hyperplastic fat cells; all obesity that begins after the age of 20 is usually characterized by hypertrophic obesity. Once formed, fat cells are permanent and are not decreased in number by weight reduction, which probably explains why childhood obesity often persists into adulthood and why this weight loss is so difficult.

Genetic and psychosocial determinants also play a role in the development of obesity. There is a high correlation between obesity in parents and the subsequent obesity in their children. Overeating may be an inappropriate response to a variety of different stimuli, such as the sight of appetizing foods, the time of day (as in bedtime snacking), or particular social settings (for example, TV watching). For some individuals, overeating is used as a method of coping with stress or boredom. Finally, less than 2 percent of obesity is attributed to endocrine or gland problems; of these types, hypothyroidism and hyperadreneocorticism are the most common (Bjorntorp, 1986).

A Classification Schema of Obesity

Classification schemata arose from the observation that obese clients differ in their response to treatment. Stunkard (1984) has proposed a schema for three types of obesity that have practical clinical significance. The three types are:

1. *Mild obesity.* In this type, a client is 20 to 40 percent over his or her ideal weight. For instance, 90.5 percent of all obese women meet this criterion. This type represents hypertrophic obesity; a diet program with a behavioral or cognitive-behavioral approach to weight control appears to be the treatment of choice.

2. *Moderate obesity.* In this type, a client is 41 to 100 percent over his or her ideal weight. About 9 percent of obese women meet this criterion. This type can represent elements of both hypertrophic and hyperplastic obesity. Diet therapy, particularly with a very-low-calorie diet (VLCD), needs to be combined with a behavioral or cognitive-behavioral approach for weight loss and maintenance to be successful.

3. *Severe Obesity.* In this type, a client is more than 100 percent or 100 pounds above his or her ideal weight. Only 0.5 percent of obese women meet this criterion. This type represents both hypertrophic and hyperplastic obesity in which many are hyperplastically obese. Treatment with behavioral or cognitive-behavioral techniques alone has not been shown to be effective. Treatment of

these individuals is most difficult. As a rule, these individuals have tried and failed at several programs. Typically these clients have lost many pounds, sometimes as much as 50 to 100 pounds, and then regained that weight. Clients and professionals can become discouraged because even significant weight loss makes little or no difference in appearance or in self-concept. Gastric bypass surgery, or stomach stapling, is the treatment of choice for many severely obese clients, but only after less invasive forms of treatment have failed. Sometimes a combination of a VLCD diet and a behavioral approach has been found effective with some, but not all, clients. When this combination program has failed, the choice is between surgery and helping the individual to adapt socially and psychological to his or her obesity.

Theories of Obesity

Various physiological and psychological theories have been proposed to explain the phenomenon of obesity. No one theory is presently able to account for all or even most of the factors involved in the interaction between physiological and sociopsychological processes. While we await a comprehensive, biopsychosocial explanation of obesity, it is worthwhile to review some of the more noteworthy theories.

Set-Point Theory

Keesey (1986) proposed that individuals have a "set point" at which their weight is held within a particular range. The amount of fat one carries is automatically regulated, and some individuals genetically have more fat than others. The set-point mechanism, which may receive information from fat cells, hormones, and enzymes, strives to maintain a given amount of weight, fat, lean body mass, and related factors. Obesity is thought to result from a homeostatic process that acts to maintain body weight and fat at a high level. An attempt to lose weight is then opposed by strong biological processes. An obese individual starting a diet to overcome the set point, or a thin person overeating to gain weight, fights a difficult battle. Various studies (Keesey & Corbett, 1984) attest to the remarkable tenacity of the body to maintain a fairly constant weight range and a preordained amount of fat.

The theory of set points has yet to be proved. Since there are many factors that can change one's set point, the utility of this theory has been questioned. However, the notion that the body may regulate weight is helpful when approaching clients who consistently remain in a specific weight range.

Fat-Cell Theory

In a previous section, we described hypertrophic and hyperplastic obesity. We noted that in weight loss, fat cells can reduce in size but cannot be eliminated (Bjorntorp, 1986). It has been speculated that, when people strive to achieve a specific fat-cell size, their efforts to decrease fat-cell size below the average will result in lipid depletion. The cell can then initiate a physiological mechanism to replenish the energy stores. Thus, fat-cell theory maintains that weight loss

beyond the point in which cells reach their normal size will be met with great resistance. Accordingly, advocates of this theory attempt to modify the individual's diet to decrease high-fat and sweet foods, while increasing the individual's physical activity.

Weight-Cycling Theory

The "yo-yo" phenomenon, in which weight is lost and regained many times, is the basis of the weight-cycling theory. Research indicates the body can increase its efficiency in food utilization, which can create dieting-induced obesity. The weight-cycling theory postulates that food-utilization efficiency increases as weight is lost, regained, and then lost again. As increased efficiency is maintained in each successive loss and gain, the results are slower losses, more rapid regain of each loss, and decreased resting metabolic rate. In short, as the individual diets, the body compensates by losing weight more slowly with each diet, and less time is required to regain the weight once dieting ceases. Therefore, with decreased metabolic rate, the same body weight is maintained on fewer calories than before dieting began. Presently, it is unknown whether prolonged weight maintenance and exercise produce an upward adjustment of the resting metabolic rate and a decrease in efficiency in formerly obese patients (Brownell, Greenwood, Stellar, et al., 1986). Clinically speaking, if the weight-cycling theory is correct, it is of the utmost importance to ensure that the client's motivation is high before embarking on any weight-control treatment. Otherwise, exposing the patient to repeated dieting may only make weight loss more difficult in the future.

Biological Factors in Obesity

Buckmaster and Brownell (1989) indicate that there are five factors involved in weight control. They are: (1) exercising; (2) nutrition training, (3) changing the act of eating, (4) cognitive retraining, and (5) developing support systems. From a biopsychosocial perspective, all five are integral in understanding the change process. Nutrition training and exercise are clearly biological factors and will be discussed in detail in this section.

Exercise

Clients who exercise while engaging in a behavioral treatment program maintain their weight loss better than patients who do not exercise (Pi-Sunyer, 1989). It appears that even moderate amounts of exercise are useful. For example, it has been shown that obese children who increase their energy expenditure by 200 to 400 calories by walking more or by using stairs rather than elevators are more likely to maintain their weight loss than are those who participate in programmed aerobic activity (Epstein, Wing, Roseke, et al., 1982). When modifying a client's activity level, treatment must begin with a level of exercise that is reasonable given the individual's physical condition and attitude about exercise. As with eating, self-monitoring and reinforcement are important components of changing exercise behavior. In addition to physiological benefits,

there are considerable psychological benefits to regular exercise. These and other matters related to exercise are described in further detail in another chapter of this book.

Nutrition

Because improper nutrition can lead to loss of lean body tissue, as well as to other physical problems, nutrition is important for optimal weight reduction and maintenance. Generally speaking, most weight-management groups do not forbid particular foods, since mandated abstinence only seems to enhance the desire and craving for certain foods. Also, most programs tailor diets to incorporate clients' food preferences. Not to do so only encourages the client to return to old eating patterns and thus regain any weight lost on the prescribed diet.

Simply prescribing a more nutritious diet is usually not enough to guarantee weight maintenance. Individuals need to increase their nutritional literacy as well. For this reason, many weight-control programs educate participants in the fundamentals of nutritional science in the form of lectures, individual consultation, or reading materials. In this section, we briefly overview some basic information about nutrition.

Helpful diets are those that provide sufficient amounts of all essential nutrients for the body's metabolic needs. In addition to water, food contains five types of chemical components that provide specific nutrients for bodily functioning. The five types of components are:

1. *Carbohydrates.* These include simple and more complex sugars that constitute major sources of energy for the body. Simple sugars include glucose, which is found in products made of animal products, and fructose, which is found in fruits and honey. Complex sugars include sucrose, such as in table sugar; lactose, which is in milk products; and starch, which is in many plants.
2. *Lipids.* Lipids, or fats, also provide energy for the body. Lipids include saturated and polyunsaturated fats, as well as cholesterol.
3. *Proteins.* These are important mainstays in the body's synthesis of cell structures. Proteins are composed of organic molecules called amino acids. About 10 of the 20 or so known amino acids are essential for body growth and functioning and must be provided by the diet.
4. *Vitamins.* These are organic chemicals that regulate metabolism and functions of the body. They are used in converting nutrients to energy and producing hormones, as well as for breaking down waste products and toxins. Some vitamins are fat soluble. These are vitamins A, B, E, and K. They dissolve in fats and are stored in the body's fatty tissue. The remaining vitamins are water soluble, which means that the body stores very little of them and excretes excess quantities as waste.
5. *Minerals.* Minerals are found in organic substances such as calcium, phosphorus, sodium, iron, potassium, and zinc. Each mineral is important in body development and functioning. For example, phosphorous and calcium are basic components of teeth and bone tissue, whereas potassium and sodium are involved in neuron transmission.

Food also contains fiber, which, although not considered a nutrient, is still needed in the process of digestion. Individuals can get all the nutrients and fiber they need through diets that contain a variety of foods from the four basic food groups (Nelson, 1984; Suitor & Hunter, 1980). Most nutritional approaches emphasize four basic food groups. The four groups are: the meat or protein group, the milk group, the fruit and vegetable group, and the grain group.

Psychological Factors in Obesity

According to the Buckmaster and Brownell schema (1989), modification of eating behavior and cognitive training would be considered psychological factors in weight control. To these, we would add life-style convictions and other psychodynamic aspects of weight control.

Modification of Eating Behavior

The first application of behavior modification to weight control was reported by Ferster and his associates (Ferster et al., 1962), nearly 30 years ago. Traditional behavioral techniques were utilized in early behavioral weight-control programs to minimize excessive eating. Such techniques were self-monitoring, stimulus control, preplanning, slowing eating, and so on. For example, in self-monitoring, the client was asked to keep a daily record of calories consumed. These records were then checked by the health counselor to assess their accuracy and to detect problem areas. Stimulus-control techniques often included always sitting in the same place when eating, not engaging in other activities (such as reading or watching television) while eating, eating from a smaller plate, or storing food out of site. Preplanning was another commonly used technique. With this technique, clients were helped to anticipate the what, when, and where of meals. For instance, if the client decided in advance to eat at home at 5:30 P.M. and had the proper ingredients available, the likelihood of eating other foods would be decreased. Preplanning also reduced the chance of impulsive eating. Slowing the act of eating allowed the client to experience satiety, or a sense of fullness, before overeating. The purpose of these techniques was to help the clients develop an awareness of their eating habits, as well as learn how the structure of their environment can minimize eating cues that might lead to excessive eating. Unfortunately, these early applications of behavioral techniques were not particularly effective and have been mockingly oversimplified as "put your fork down and chew each mouthful 20 times."

Today the behavioral or, more correctly, cognitive-behavioral, approach deals with all behaviors that affect weight loss, weight gain, and weight maintenance. The same principles that could be applied to eating—such as shaping, goal setting, self-monitoring for feedback, reinforcement, stimulus control—can be used for changing exercise patterns, food selection, and self-defeating thoughts and for engendering social support from others in the client's environment.

Cognitive Training

The cognitive component of weight control includes setting goals, restructuring dysfunctional beliefs about eating, improving self-image, coping with mistakes, and developing motivation. Emphasis is placed on the client's attitudes toward treatment, especially in the later stages when relapse prevention is of particular concern. The cognitive component in weight-control programs seeks to emphasize primarily positive attitudes and enhance adherence to the exercise, lifestyle, and nutritional parts of the program (Brownell & Foreyt, 1985).

Psychodynamic Aspects

Although there has been only limited interest in obesity by psychoanalytic and psychodynamic therapists, there are a few contributions from this orientation that a health counselor may well heed. An early concept that emerged from psychoanalytic theory was the *oral character* structure. Conflicts over the satisfaction of libidinal and aggressive needs, met through sucking or biting, were believed to be related to obesity. Hilde Bruch's (1973) ongoing experience with obese individuals offers an important perspective on motivation for weight loss. Bruch divided her obese patients into three groups: those without significant psychological problems; those whose obesity was "interwoven with their whole personality development," which she called *developmental obesity;* and those who became obese as a reaction to some traumatic event, called *reactive obesity.*

Bruch described the reactive form of obesity as characteristic of relatively psychologically mature individuals who eat more when they are worried, tense, or anxious. Reactive obesity usually develops after the death of a family member, separation from home, loss of a love object, or other situation involving the fear of abandonment. These individuals have difficulty coping with their aggressive feelings and tend to become depressed. They overeat in response to their feelings of aggression and other undesirable emotions.

Bruch found that individuals who were developmentally obese suffered from disturbances in psychological functions. Developmental obesity is often evident by late childhood or early adolescence. Rather than develop a positive concept of their body image, obese adolescents tend to have serious adjustment problems, whereby inactivity and overeating become integral parts of their personal development. They are not fully aware of themselves as separate from the important figures in their environment, and they feel a lack of control over their sensations and actions. In addition, they fail to achieve a sense of ownership of their body or a sense of themselves as active participants in the outcomes of their lives. Thus, their initiative and automomy appear poorly developed. For the developmentally obese individual, commitment to a sustained, systematic, but gradual weight-loss program is very difficult for them because of their unrealistic expectations for quick, painless cures.

In short, Bruch believes that, in contrast to reactively obese patients, developmentally obese patients seldom have the motivation to commit themselves to a serious weight-management program.

Closely related to the psychodynamic approach, as well as to the cognitive approach, to obesity is the view of Adlerian psychology. In the Adlerian view,

individuals with obesity or other eating disorders develop mistaken convictions or cognitions about themselves, other people, and life. Obesity is understood as the purposeful maintenance of body weight through overeating. It is viewed as a life-style that protects, excuses, and silently communicates dependency and fear of dependency, or independence and fear of independence. Nearly always, obesity serves a family function: the unconscious goal of the obese person is to focus attention away from a parental or family problem and onto themselves. The obese individual focuses on food rather than issues, weight rather than judgment, and unreality rather than decision. The eating disorder then comes to symbolize the control issues, denial, avoidance, excesses, and emptiness of the family (Casper & Zachery, 1984).

Social Factors in Obesity

Social factors play an important role in both the etiology and treatment of obesity. Among the most influential social factors are social-support systems and cultural values. Research shows that social support can decrease attrition or early termination from treatment programs, improve weight loss, and improve weight-loss maintenance (Morton, 1988). Family and spouse interactions and spousal involvement in obesity programs have generated much interest in research in this field.

Marital factors can determine whether an individual will succeed in treatment. Clients' social networks may greatly help or hinder their progress. For instance, a spouse may act as the "gatekeeper" of food that enters the house, may overtly or covertly encourage or discourage the client to lose weight, and invariably changes the homeostasis in the marital relationship and in their sexual intimacy.

In short, spousal interactions may be a causal factor in obesity. On the basis of extensive survey research, Stuart and Jacobson (1987) offer some intriguing reasons why married women overeat. These researchers note three characteristic uses of food in marriage. First, Stuart and Jacobson found that some of their respondents felt that, once married, they could relax, stop worrying about keeping their weight down, and enjoy the trust and security of their marriage. When things were going smoothly and weight didn't interfere with their self-esteem, they had little motivation to lose the weight they inevitably gained. For the majority of wives who had not been overweight before marriage, the responsibilities and stresses of being a wife and a mother translated into weight gain. And, it was noted that women who didn't consistently hold outside jobs had a more difficult time losing weight than did those who worked outside the home. Finally, when marital and sexual problems were present, weight problems were compounded. Specifically, women in unhappy marriages gained 2.5 times more weight than did women who reported being in happy marriages—42.6 pounds gained over 13 years of unhappy marriage compared to 18.4 pounds in happy marriages.

These researchers also found that being overweight could serve four

purposes in a marriage. First, overweight served to allay a woman's fears of becoming too sexually attractive or even promiscuous. Second, weight gain served to diminish a husband's sexual interest and to inhibit the woman's own sexual desire; the end result was that consciously or not, weight gain served as a means of avoiding intimacy. Third, weight gain served to control anger and to neutralize the husband's efforts to overcontrol his wife. These women internalized anger by "swallowing" it. Some gained weight to rebel at their husband's insistence that they become thin. Thus, the women's bodies became the battleground in a power struggle that neither they nor their husbands could win. Finally, weight gain was used to hide a woman's fear that she would be a failure— or a success—in life. As such, weight became a convenient scapegoat for insecurity and other problems in the woman's life.

In short, many women want to be thin, but they need to overeat to nourish their empty lives, to soften the threat of failure or success, and to shield themselves against the demands for sex or against the control of their husbands. Unfortunately, these purposes serve to confirm the role of the wife as a victim.

Particularly surprising were Stuart and Jacobson's findings about the husband's view of his overweight wife. Insecure husbands often blocked and sabotaged their wives' efforts to lose weight. Utilizing both survey data and their clinical observations, these researchers noted a number of reasons why a husband preferred that his wife remain overweight. These husbands were unwilling to change their comfortable routines to tackle their own weight problems or to deal with their own addictive behavior, such as drinking or gambling. Some used their wife's weight to divert attention from marital or sexual problems in their relationship. Furthermore, some men feared that their wives would become unfaithful or leave them if they lost too much weight.

Finally, Stuart and Jacobson found that approximately half of the women wanted their husband's positive collaboration and support in losing weight, and the other half did not. The researchers' experience as marital therapists confirmed that when a woman wants and expects her husband to collaborate in her weight-loss program, she will more likely than not lose weight and maintain the weight loss.

Family Influences

Mahoney and Mahoney (1976) have described four negative patterns that can characterize the eating atmosphere in a family in which one member is attempting to lose weight. In Pattern I, family members tease the individual about being overweight and criticize attempts at weight loss. In Pattern II, family members openly discourage weight-loss efforts and openly sabotage these efforts. Strategies in the next two patterns are more indirect and insidious. In Pattern III, family members ignore the individual's change efforts and somehow communicate their pessimisim. Finally, in Pattern IV, family members verbally encourage the individual's efforts but nonverbally discourage and even sabotage them. Knowledge of patterns like these can be very helpful to health counselors and their patients.

Sociocultural Influences

Another important social factor involves family cultural norms. Allen (1981) describes family cultural norms as unspoken social and cultural influences that unconsciously influence a person's attitudes toward his or her body in relationship with others and, most importantly, health beliefs and behaviors. Allen has generated a list of sociocultural norm indicators that relate to weight control. Some examples are:

- People tend to view children who are slightly overweight as healthier and better cared for than children who aren't.
- Parents encourage children not to leave food on their plate, even if it is more than they want or need.
- People think or say, that "everybody loves a fat person."

These indicators are discussed further in the section "Social-Support Systems Assessment."

Assessment

Biological Assessment

Assessment in the area of weight control is usually carried out in stages. Often, an initial screening is done to collect basic background information, frequently collected on paper-and-pencil forms and inventories. The first interview then focuses on the assessment of the client's general psychological state and motivation for treatment. Finally, a self-monitoring phase is generally needed to record details of eating and activity patterns. (The patient typically completes these forms between sessions.) The biological assessment includes at least three dimensions: the client's weight history, assessment of fatness, and assessment of fitness.

Weight history. Weight history can provide important information, including clues as to the degree of fat-cell hyperplasia and hyperthrophia. The counselor usually begins by asking when the client first became significantly overweight. Childhood onset of obesity is generally associated with greater body weight as an adult and with excess fat-cell numbers. On the other hand, weight gain in an adult who was previously at a normal weight is generally not associated with an increase in fat-cell numbers. Therefore, the prognosis for returning to ideal body weight is more favorable in people with adulthood-onset than in those with childhood-onset obesity. This is not to say that individuals who have been severely overweight since childhood may not lose significant amounts of weight; however, they are likely to fall far short of reaching ideal weight and to have greater difficulty maintaining the weight loss.

The counselor next asks whether there is a family history of obesity. Studies of twins and adoptees suggest that obesity is highly related to heredity. If neither parent is obese, the likelihood of one of the children becoming obese is only 8 percent; if one parent is obese, the likelihood rises to 40 percent; and if both parents are overweight, the probability jumps to 80 percent. Severely

overweight clients with positive family histories of obesity, as well as onset in childhood, almost invariably have hyperplastic obesity.

The counselor then inquires about the client's dieting history. Clients who are moderately or severely overweight and have repeatedly lost and regained weight are likely to have excess fat-cell numbers. In addition, behavioral and emotional factors may also contribute to this rebound in body weight.

Assessment of fatness.   There are a number of ways of assessing fatness, and the method chosen is usually determined by available resources. First, an accurate recording of the patient's weight is made, preferably using a balance with a beam rather than a spring scale. The client's weight can then be compared with a standard weight chart to determine ideal weight. The counselor can also compute the percentage of overweight or calculate the client's body mass index.

Circumference measurements can also be useful to identify subsequent changes in shape. Hip, waist, and thigh measurements are usually sufficient. Algorithms for converting girth measures to estimates of total body fat are available (see McArdle et al. 1981). Subcutaneous fat, which usually represents half of the total body fat, can also be measured using skin-fold calipers applied at specific locations. Algorithms can then be used to calculate total body fat from skin-fold thickness (see Durin & Wormensley, 1974). Although there is some controversy over the accuracy of skin-fold measurements, this method has been particularly useful for clients with anorexia nervosa but not with extremely obese subjects.

Finally, where resources are available, determination of fat-cell number can be assessed. This begins by determining the amount of body fat using hydrostatic weighing or other subtle techniques. Next, a biopsy is performed on fat tissue taken from the client's body, usually from the buttock. From this, a determination of the weight of the average size fat cell and the weight of total body fat can be estimated.

Assessment of fitness.   It is useful to make some estimate of fitness in order both to plan an appropriate exercise program and to provide a baseline against which to assess change. Fitness can easily be determined using the step test, in which the patient is asked to step up and down a 13-inch-high step at a rate of about 80 steps per minute. Pulse rate is recorded both immediately after finishing the exercise and then again after a recovery period. These results are then used to classify the initial fitness level and can be repeated after implementing the treatment program (Katch & McArdle, 1983).

Medical evaluation.   Moderately and severely overweight individuals should be referred for a thorough medical evaluation before undertaking a weight-reduction program. Furthermore, the health counselor should fully apprise the physician of the details of the weight-reduction program that is planned for the client. Such clients often take medication or have a history of illness that may contraindicate the use of some approaches, such as a VLCD or surgery. In addition, patients need to be medically monitored during their diet

to assess changes or complications in such indicators as cholesterol level, blood glucose level, blood-pressure level, and electrolytes. It is also advisable for even mildly obese individuals to consult with their physician before dieting, even though there are fewer risks of complications. As with the more severely overweight individuals, it is useful to track changes in blood pressure, cholesterol, and other measures of health.

Psychological Assessment

Whereas the biological assessment focuses on the effects of food on the body, psychological assessment focuses more on what, how, and why a person eats particular types and amounts of foods. This section describes a number of methods for assessing these concerns.

Eating diary.   The mainstay of most treatment programs for obesity is a food record or the eating diary. This diary can vary from a simple list of foods eaten to a complex record involving ratings of hunger and recordings of the environment in which the eating took place. Most records or diaries require the client to indicate caloric intake. This may mean that foods must be weighed or portions estimated. Some clients are prepared to weigh all their foods at least for a few days, although the benefits of such accuracy may be outweighed by the drawbacks of reactivity. In other words, patients may eat differently during this period. For most patients, it is sufficient for the counselor to provide a standard calorie guide so that the patient's caloric intake can be estimated.

The more comprehensive eating diaries require that—in addition to the listing of foods eaten, calories consumed, place of eating, and rating of hunger—the client record the mood states that preceded each eating and the cognitive self-talk involved before, during, or after the meal.

Eating in response to emotional disturbances (called emotional eating) or eating more when food cues occur (external eating) are common features of eating styles in individuals of all weight levels and are not specific to obesity. However, emotional eating and external eating need to be assessed and modified as part of the treatment program. This is especially necessary after prolonged dietary restrictions, when emotional or external cues can result in relapse. If the food binging is excessive, the impact of days of dietary restriction can be lost in only a few hours. An eating diary can provide some evidence for this kind of nonregulatory eating, but it is best supplemented with a standardized assessment instrument, such as the *Dutch Eating Behavior Questionnaire* (Van Strien et al., 1986), which includes scales for external and emotional eating. As with other aspects of the assessment, the aim is to identify areas of potential behavior change as well as for potential problems.

There are various formats for an eating diary; one is shown in Figure 3-1. Such a diary provides useful behavioral and cognitive information about a client's eating patterns. The client is asked to complete a daily food-intake diary for at least one week. The diary in Figure 3-1 is a composite of those used in most weight-treatment programs. The first week of the diary provides the health counselor with sufficient information to determine general patterns of eating.

Common eating patterns exhibited by patients include abstinence from

Date: _____

Food/Quality	Time	Degree of Hunger (0–5)	Place	Activity	Mood	Self-Talk	Calories

Figure 3-1. Eating diary form

eating until late in the day, followed by periodic snacking until late evening. Another pattern involves eating three full meals but also several large snacks between meals. A less common pattern consists of eating three meals a day without snacking, but the food choices for these meals are very high in caloric content. When this increase in caloric intake is not matched by an increase in exercise, the result is an increase in fat stores and, subsequently, an increase in body weight.

Whereas the diet-book writer and the registered dietician may focus on food type, quantity, and calories, the health counselor is even more interested in the other five dimensions of the eating diary. Each of the factors of time of eating, place of eating, level of activity, degree of hunger, prevailing mood, and self-talk while eating all are important eating behaviors that can become a target for habit change.

Initial interview.   During the course of the initial interview and usually following the weight history, the health counselor turns to how the client's weight affects and is affected by intimate relationships, social functioning, and occupational and leisure pursuits. Although psychological inventories generally do not predict weight loss, the MMPI, MCMI, or similar instrument may be routinely administered at the onset of treatment. Results of such testing can alert the health counselor to personality or emotional factors that may emerge during the course of treatment. In addition to assessing the client's current psychosocial functioning, the counselor should address several issues specifically related to weight and weight loss.

The counselor may begin by eliciting the client's feelings about his or her size and the way it affects his or her social life, work, and other people's reactions. Further information may be assessed with the use of the *Stanford Eating Disorders Questionnaire* (Agras, 1987).

The counselor then inquires as to why the client has decided to lose weight at this particular time. Although this question may be answered rather perfunctorily, the counselor should remember that the client has probably been overweight for several months or years and something has recently occurred to motivate him or her to enter treatment. Clients frequently seek therapy because of medical problems, the insistence of an upset spouse, or hopes that their social life and job opportunities will improve with weight loss. In many instances, the obese client has experienced disappointment, anger, sadness, and so on, and these issues should be examined before initiating a weight-loss regimen.

The counselor then asks for whom the client is losing weight. In many instances, clients indicate that they are losing weight for themselves to feel better physically and psychologically. The counselor follows up by determining whether the client has a realistic understanding of his or her condition, its health implications, and the role that these can play in treatment. On the other hand, clients who are losing weight solely because of a doctor's orders or at a spouse's insistence have a more guarded prognosis. Treatment is seldom successful if clients do not see the need for it and are merely appeasing a physician or a spouse. When the client's motivation is based on the spouse's insistence, the health counselor would do well to meet conjointly with the client and the

spouse to determine what marital issues are underlying the insistence on weight loss. These can include avoiding intimacy, testing love, or rebelling against a domineering spouse.

Next, the counselor elicits the client's expectations for treatment. Clients are often interested in weight loss as a means to an end. If the end can be clearly articulated at the outset of treatment, such as improving one's social life or finding a new job, the counselor can take steps to increase the likelihood that these expectations will be met. Some obese clients are shy and unassertive, as are some persons of normal weight. Therefore, no matter how good they look after a substantial weight loss, their social lives are unlikely to improve, particularly if their expectations are unrealistic. Some clients may expect to return to their ideal weight in a matter of weeks or months. The counselor needs to spend as much time as necessary educating the client about the health risks of rapid weight loss; the need for slow, gradual weight loss with subsequent change in eating patterns and self-body image; and the ways in which magical thinking and unrealistic expectations foster relapse.

Finally, the counselor inquires about the client's previous experience with dieting, weight loss, and weight-loss maintenance. Typically, clients who seek help with weight control have experimented with six or more diets or with formal weight-loss programs before their current consultation. It is important to review these efforts to determine what worked, what went wrong, and what needs to happen differently to improve the client's chances for success in this treatment endeavor. Clients often bring with them negative expectancies that they anticipate the counselor will confirm. All expectancies, negative and positive, need to be examined at the outset so that the counselor can realistically determine whether he or she has something to offer this client that is different from what other professionals or programs have offered in the past.

In addition to answering the global assessment questions about what the client needs and under what circumstances, and what the client's goals and expectations for treatment are, the counselor does well to ask why the person eats to excess and why he or she maintains the image of an obese person. An assessment of the client's health beliefs and health behaviors as well as past and current gains or payoffs for obesity can provide important information. We have found that an assessment of the client's early memories or recollections are useful in elucidating the client's health beliefs. This is done by asking the individual to recall singular experiences in childhood or early adolescence that involved food and body weight. These responses often provide valuable insight into the client's body image and maladaptive beliefs or convictions about entitlement, inferiority, inadequacy, and control.

Social-Support Systems Assessment

Because social factors appear to play a significant role in the etiology and treatment of obesity, it is important to assess their impact (Brownell & Foreyt, 1985). Earlier, we suggested that family, social, and cultural factors affect not only the process of weight gain and loss but, more importantly, weight maintenance. Therefore, it is essential that the counselor assess the spouse's expectations and feelings about the client's desire to lose weight. In addition, the

counselor should inquire as to the spouse's degree of encouragement and cooperation, as well as any overt or covert indications of sabotage of the client's weight-control program.

The counselor will also find it useful to characterize the eating atmosphere that surrounds the family of the client who wishes to begin a therapeutic weight-control program. Mahoney and Mahoney's (1976) criteria for family Patterns I through IV (see p. 67) is quite useful in this regard. Combining this information with previously elicited family-weight history and spousal support can be used to anticipate problems in the course of treatment, particularly regarding relapse.

Next, the counselor should assess the client's cultural health status, which, according to Allen (1981), consists of the "silent" attitudes of one's family, social and ethnic group, and community that influences and reinforces certain health behaviors and not others. Allen indicates that we all are influenced by cultural-norm indicators for nutrition and weight control. As mentioned earlier, Allen has developed an inventory to elucidate these norms, and the following are some additional representative norm-group items that a patient might endorse:

- People who are a few pounds overweight are healthy and happy.
- Sweets are a special treat and are therefore more "rewarding" than nutritious foods.
- Overindulgence in food is associated with relaxation, pleasure, and good social relationships.
- Hosts and hostesses should encourage guests to eat more food than would be desirable for them.
- It is natural for individuals to be slightly overweight, particularly for the elderly.
- It is okay to eat when you are lonely or feeling hurt.
- Feeding children more than they need for growth and health shows that you really love them.
- It's normal to lose weight through dieting but to gain it back again.

Treatment Issues and Strategies

General Treatment Considerations

Perhaps the first and most important consideration is who should be treated. In most clinical settings, it is assumed that if a client requests a weight-loss program, he or she should be offered the treatment. However, this may not be advisable in all cases. Some clients, particularly young women with bulimia or anorexia who harbor an obsessive concern about their weight, should not be accepted automatically for weight-control treatment. Weight reduction may still be indicated, but only after the weight obsession has been dealt with in therapy. Often, these individuals are only mildly overweight, if at all, have a history of continuous dieting, have negative body images, and report thinking about their weight in an obsessive fashion. This information can be collected in the initial assessment.

There may also be individuals who are quite overweight who should be encouraged to accept their condition rather than to suffer through the rigors of a weight-control program. Acceptance rather than weight reduction can be a wise course to follow for some clients, particularly those who have repeatedly tried and failed to follow the best available treatment. These may be people whose obesity is primarily of the hyperplastic type. A more humane and ethical course of treatment may focus on helping them accept their body size. Focusing on acceptance may be better than continuing to fail at diets, using financial resources that could be better spent, and incurring the negative reactions of disappointed family members, friends, and fellow employees (Brownell & Foreyt, 1985).

A final concern regarding who should be treated involves the "new" weight client. By "new" we refer to the individual who has never sought professional help for weight loss. Since many obese people lose weight on their own and maintain that weight loss for years, some counselors believe that these individuals should first try to lose weight on their own. Accordingly, these clients can be counseled to choose a good, well-balanced diet and to gradually increase their activity level; they may be successful by themselves. If they are not able to lose much weight or to maintain the weight loss, then they may be candidates for formal, professional treatment.

At least four general treatment issues need to be considered by the counselor before initiating specific interventions. These include: individual versus group treatment, self-help versus commercial groups, therapist and client variables, and the crises stages in the process of weight loss.

Group versus individual treatment.   The issue of group versus individual treatment for obese individuals has received relatively little attention in the scientific literature, despite its obvious importance. Each approach has different social effects on most individuals, such that the same treatment may benefit a person in one setting and be ineffective in another (Brownell & Foreyt, 1985).

A study by Kingsley and Wilson (1977) compared group versus individual treatment of trained counselors and found that, although the two approaches did not differ at the end of the formal treatment, the group approach was superior during the follow-up period. Generally speaking, group treatment is cost-effective as well as effective in providing peer support and encouragement, which is different in nature from that provided by the counselor/client relationship. Clients often feel more at ease discussing their problems among others with similar concerns. Clients may accept advice better from a fellow group member than from the professional. Finally, clients in a group can often generate creative solutions to specific problems that may not arise in individual treatment.

There are some circumstances in which individual sessions may be more appropriate for a particular client. This is particularly true when a client has emotional difficulties that are not appropriate for a group or that may require more attention that the group can provide. Some clients may not be able to

profit much from group process because of their shyness and reluctance to talk openly. Others may be too suspicious and guarded and may be unwilling to disclose personal information, particularly their weight status. Finally, there are those clients who easily create negative group contagion, which is destructive to the group process. For the benefit of other group members, these clients should be seen individually. Clients with borderline and/or antisocial features may be appropriate for severe-personality-disorder groups (Linehan, 1987), but they tend to do poorly in task-oriented groups such as weight-control groups.

Group treatment and individual treatment are not mutually exclusive. Some clients do well in groups if they receive periodic individual sessions. Others may do well in groups but require individual treatment during a crisis period. And then there are those clients who need individual treatment to start the process of behavior change but who then can make the transition into group treatment. Counselors experienced in both individual and group treatment can usually make this determination at the onset. Finally, some health counselors have experimented with a combination of individual treatment and an adjunctive self-help group treatment, such as Overeaters Anonymous (OA). In any event, a careful and comprehensive assessment of the client's needs and status should govern the decision of group versus individual treatment.

Self-help versus commercial groups.   Health counselors trained in an obesity clinic that operates within a university department of psychology or a medical school know that their clinics often provide treatment that is free or for a nominal fee. Subsequently, many counselors are wary of commercial weight-control programs because of the high fees they charge, or they may be wary of self-help groups, but for different reasons. Often this distrust results from lack of knowledge of these groups, the absence of published research on treatment outcomes, and a disdain for profit enterprises for commercial groups or the etiological bias of certain self-help groups. Inasmuch as the vast majority of dieters seek out treatment from self-help and commercial groups, these groups are an important part of treating obesity from a public health perspective. Subsequently, self-help commercial groups can be a valuable resource for the counselor.

A detailed overview of these groups is beyond the scope of this book. However, reviews of the outcome literature by Colletti and Brownell, (1982) and by Stuart and Mitchell (1980) show that the major shortcomings of these groups is attrition. Approximately 50 to 80 percent of participants drop out of these groups within six weeks. For example, the average individual who joins Weight Watchers has joined three times before. For those who remain in the program, weight losses are usually only moderate. The high attrition from these groups can be viewed as an indictment of the self-help commercial approaches. Yet, since some of these groups are offered at no cost or at low cost, some patients who are minimally motivated may join and then drop out.

The therapeutic issue is to decide which patient profits from which approach. This requires that the counselor become acquainted with details of the various programs by calling or visiting them and by obtaining information from patients who have participated in these groups.

Several factors distinguish these groups both in their procedures and in the way in which they view obesity. For instance, Overeaters Anonymous (OA) is modeled after Alcoholics Anonymous (AA). The participants are referred to as compulsive overeaters, and they are encouraged to call upon a higher power for strength and to rely on a sponsor to help them cope in times of crisis. On the other hand, Take Off Pounds Sensibly (TOPS) has no spiritual overtones and stresses a buddy system, gentle competition, and group support. Not surprisingly, middle-class gregarious women find TOPS both attractive and helpful. Weight Watchers utilizes specific diets, markets, and food products and relies on regular weigh-ins for motivation.

Assuming that the health counselor and the client jointly determine that a self-help commercial group would be appropriate, the challenge is to match the client to the best possible group. This can be done by discussing the details of the different approaches with the client and encouraging him or her to speak to others who have been in the program. Finally, it should be noted that clients also can benefit from joining a self-help group after a course of individual or clinic treatment (Brownell & Foreyt, 1985).

Therapists and client variables.   Therapists can exert an important influence over the success or failure of a client's weight loss program. Relatively little research has been reported on what qualities make therapists effective in weight-loss treatments. Jeffrey, Wing, and Stunkard (1978) found that clients of experienced therapists achieve greater weight loss than do clients of novice therapists, and Levitz and Stunkard (1974) found that professional therapists produced better results than did lay therapists. Brownell and Foreyt (1985) found that the most effective therapists are able to show empathy, positive regard, respect, warmth, and genuineness and that they possess a detailed knowledge of nutrition, physiology, and the psychology of weight loss.

There has been very little research to identify client variables that predict treatment outcomes in weight-control programs Brownell and Foreyt (1985) note that men seem to lose more weight in treatment programs than do women and that individuals with a relatively short history of obesity are more successful at weight loss than are individuals who have a longer history of obesity. They also note that behavioral treatment programs do not appear to be very helpful for morbidly obese individuals—that is, those who weigh over 300 pounds or who are 100 percent above their ideal weight.

The stages of crises in the weight-loss process.   Fawzy (Fawzy et al., 1984) describes some phases of weight loss in morbidly obese clients that the counselor may find to be clinically useful information. Fawzy distinguishes three crises—disorientation, mid-fast motivational burnout, and normalization—that, he reports, occur over the course of five months when clients are placed on a protein-sparing, modified fast (PSMF) diet. In the first crisis, the individual is preoccupied with dreams and fantasies of food, unpleasant physical sensations, and magical thinking that he or she will become problem-free after reaching the ideal weight. Fawzy notes that there are some family stressors on the client that

are associated with the early demands of fasting, but he does not specify them. In the next crisis, boredom, noncompliance, and cheating are prominent. In the third crisis, magical thinking fades, and progressive encounters with an expanded range of food choices can trigger old eating patterns. Fawzy mentions that, as family members recognize physical changes in the client, they put new demands on the individual for change in personal and social behavior. Even though Fawzy's characterization is far from complete, it may not generalize either to those who are not moderate or morbidly obese or to other weight-loss protocols. Yet, this scheme does suggest some therapeutic markers that health counselors can utilize for assessing the client's progress and anticipating problems and crises.

Biological Interventions

Three types of biological interventions are commonly utilized in a weight-control program. They are exercise, nutritional prescription, and bypass surgery.

Exercise.   When discussing weight-control programs, we can talk about life-style exercise and a formal exercise prescription (Brownell, 1985). Life-style exercise is simply an increase in physical exertion during the course of one's day-to-day activities. It may include parking the car some distance from one's destination to increase walking or using the stairs rather than an elevator or escalator. Climbing stairs is one of the few "necessary" daily activities that require a significant expenditure of energy. Increases in activity can significantly decrease the risk of heart disease and at the same time increase the likelihood of long-term adherence to and a positive attitude toward exercise. After the third or fourth week clients are asked to increase the activity level in their life-style. More specifically, they are asked to choose a behavior they will monitor for a week and to report on their progress at the next session.

On the other hand, a formal exercise program consists of regularly engaging in significant physical exertion, such as running, aerobics, swimming, and cycling, or taking part in regular sporting events. An integral part of a weight-control program is the exercise prescription. The health counselor, in collaboration with the client, should decide on the kind of exercise that is most compatible with the client's physical ability, health, and interests. Whether the exercise prescription involves walking, swimming, soft aerobics, or stationary bicycling, exercise should begin at the outset of treatment. The distance walked or swam and the time involved in aerobics or bicycling should depend on the client's physical condition. A very overweight person is not likely to be able to run more than a few yards at first, but, with practice, the distance should steadily increase. Thus, some may start running half a mile every other day, whereas others may begin with half a block. Progress should be charted so that improvement can be ascertained readily by both counselor and client.

Monitoring exercise levels is important. For a walker or jogger, a pedometer can enhance compliance by giving the person immediate feedback. Increased activity should also be rewarded in some way, at least by making a

preferred sedentary activity contingent on some less-preferred and more-vigorous exercise activity. Self-control procedures, such as self-monitoring, goal setting, and reinforcing new behaviors, are useful to the exercise component of the weight-loss program. Finally, social support can encourage adherence to exercise. Family support is particularly important, as some family members may discourage or sabotage the client's efforts to engage in vigorous activity because they are embarrassed about his or her appearance (Wardle, 1989).

Nutritional prescription.   Since obese clients typically derive more than 40 percent of their calories from fat, most nutritionists recommend a diet that derives no more than 30 percent of calories from fat, 12 percent from protein, and 58 percent from carbohydrates (Buckmaster & Brownell, 1989).

Health counselors and weight-control programs are divided on the issue of prescribing specific diets. Some routinely refer their patients to a registered dietician for a diet prescription. Others believe that prescribing a diet sets the stage for abandoning the program when the inevitable dietary transgression or relapse occurs. Instead, these counselors ask female clients to limit their calories to 1200 per day and male clients to limit themselves to 1500 calories per day. Caloric intake is adjusted to reflect the individual's energy expenditure, but the specifics of the diet—within the boundaries of good nutrition—are left to the client. These nutritional changes are subsequently woven into the client's entire life-style.

A weight-control program that incorporates a 1200- to 1500-calorie diet with a behavioral-modification component should produce an average weight loss of 11 pounds in 10 to 12 weeks; a 25-pound weight loss should be realized after 25 weeks of treatment (Wilson & Brownell, 1980). For the mildly obese patient, these results are more than sufficient.

However, for the moderately obese person who needs to lose 60 to 100 pounds, or for the morbidly obese individual who needs to lose 100 or more pounds, such a treatment program is not appropriate. These people are likely to require more aggressive treatment based on a very-low-calorie diet (VLCD). Such diets provide 300 to 600 calories a day and produce an average weight loss of 2 to 3 pounds per week. VLCDs are designed to produce the same large weight losses as fasting but reduce the loss of lean body mass common in starvation diets. VLCDs reduce lean body mass loss by providing dietary protein. Current VLCDs take two forms. One is the protein-sparing, modified fast (PSMF) diet developed by Dr. Blackburn (1978) and his colleagues, which provides the client with the equivalent of 70 to 100 grams of protein per day. This protein is obtained from lean meat, fish, and fowl. Carbohydrates are prohibited and fat is restricted to only that present in a protein source. The other type of VLCD relies on a milk- or egg-based protein formula to serve as a liquid diet. These commercially prepared diets provide a daily ration of approximately 35 to 70 grams of protein, 30 to 45 grams of carbohydrates, and about 2 grams of fat. Optifast and Medi-fast are two medically supervised liquid-protein diets; Ultra Slim Fast is a similar over-the-counter preparation. The PSMF is supplemented by vitamins and minerals, particularly potassium, calcium, and sodium. Both

approaches produce similar weight losses, but some studies have shown that patients prefer the PSMF diet over the liquid-protein diet (Wadden, Stunkard, Brownell, & Day, 1984).

Gastric surgery. There is a great degree of enthusiasm for gastric bypass surgery among morbidly obese clients. In this operation, the stomach is reduced to a small pouch by a series of sutures or staples. This pouch has a volume of about 50 ml, which is about one-seventh the size of a soft-drink can. The pouch dramatically limits the client's food intake, thus leading to weight loss. If the client ingests more than the pouch will hold, vomiting will result, which is the main complication of the surgical procedure.

The results of this surgery can be very dramatic. Clients not only eat less but are also likely to experience a change in food preference. They eat smaller amounts of high-density fats, high-density carbohydrates, high-calorie beverages, and high-fat meats. In addition, the postoperative course for clients who have had gastric surgery is more benign psychologically than is dieting. Morbidly obese clients who have a grossly negative body image report more positive evaluations of their body several months after their surgery, even though they are still somewhat obese. Clients have exhibited increased mobility, stamina, assertiveness, and self-confidence and tend to be less self-conscious and withdrawn in social situations. They also begin to explore social and occupational activities formally inaccessible to them.

On the down side, morbidly obese clients who have had dysfunctional marriages before the surgery tend to be more likely to divorce. This probably results from clients improved self-confidence and their unwillingness to continue playing the victim role in the relationship. In addition to the complication of vomiting mentioned above, rupture of a suture line and stretching of the gastric pouch may require follow-up surgery. Finally, the mortality rates of gastric surgery are 0.5 to 3 percent. What this means is that up to 3 percent of clients who undergo the procedure may die as a result of it (Halmi, 1980).

The best candidates for the gastric surgery procedure are individuals who are at least 100 percent or 100 pounds above their ideal weight, have a history of repeated failures with other weight-control methods, and are free from alcoholism, substance abuse, or psychiatric disorders that would prevent them from cooperating with post-surgical treatment. Clients should also have realistic expectations for the operation, accept the needs for extreme caloric restrictions after the surgery, and realize their responsibility for long-term weight reduction.

Psychological Interventions

The best weight-control programs are multimodal and tailored to the needs of the individual patient or group. A behavioral or cognitive-behavioral component is an essential part of all multimodal programs. The main behavioral components are self-monitoring, stimulus control, response prevention, and cognitive restructuring.

Self-monitoring. Self-monitoring is an integral part of the weight-control program, and it provides the basis for frequent discussions in treatment

sessions. Once treatment has begun, self-monitoring becomes a long-term necessity, requiring that the health counselor set the expectations as well as monitor the client's compliance with the self-monitoring assignment. For example, the eating diary sheets should be collected regularly and the data recorded on a weight chart and compliance record so that the client can see a tangible record of change. The importance of accuracy and truthfulness on the diary sheets should also be stressed from time to time, since the patient might prefer to omit certain details. These problems can be minimized if the treatment program is presented as a collaborative endeavor.

Eating behavior is affected by numerous environmental cues. These obviously vary, but they include being offered food, being in an environment in which eating takes place, buying food, engaging in activities that are commonly associated with eating, and being presented with a variety of foods. A good eating diary should reveal these environmental cues. Behavioral approaches offer two choices for dealing with them. Either the environment is modified so that exposure to the situation that cues eating is limited—stimulus control—or systematic, unreinforced exposure is offered so that the association is broken— response prevention (Wadden et al., 1984).

Stimulus control.   Stimulus control is appropriate for situations in which environmental modification is practical and possible. Possible changes include persuading family members not to buy food for or offer food to the client, confining eating to only one room in the house, and increasing the length of meals by putting down eating utensils after each mouthful or following the slower eating pace of a family member. Once the environmental cues are isolated and stimulus control methods are begun, the new behaviors must be monitored and systematically reinforced so that they are maintained (Stuart, 1980).

Many aspects of the meal structure itself might also be modified to contribute to a lower food intake. Palatability of food is one important determinant of food intake. Since people eat more of the food they like, clients should be counseled to avoid highly preferred food at times when their self-control may be low. Variety is another critical feature. People tend to eat more when provided with a wider variety of food. Accordingly, limiting the number of different tastes and textures in a meal can help to limit intake.

Response prevention.   The essence of response prevention is that a behavior should be possible but not performed; in other words, food should be available but not eaten. Clients are often disturbed by occasions when they eat even though they are not hungry, particularly when there is a compulsive quality to their eating. Clients need to be told that eating in the absence of hunger, also called nonregulatory eating, is common and is not necessarily a sign of poor willpower or lack of control. On the other hand, a reduction of food intake does require an increase in self-control, and self-control can be increased through exposure and response prevention training. During counseling sessions, the clients can be exposed to the cue conditions either with an in vivo or by an imaginal exposure regimen. This regimen might include looking at advertisements of foods or evoking emotion-arousing images. Between sessions, home-

work may be assigned in which the patient practices response prevention by going into food stores or bakeries and not buying anything (Wardle, 1989).

Cognitive restructuring. Because cognition plays an important role in mediating behavior change, particularly in response to transgressions such as food binging, cognitive-restructuring techniques have an important place in weight-control treatment. Negative thoughts about the difficulty of dieting, the unfairness of some people being naturally thin, and so on have the potential to both induce a negative mood and increase noncompliance in treatment. After a minor transgression, negative thoughts such as "Now that I have ruined my diet for the day, I might as well abandon the whole thing" often trigger binge eating.

The usual techniques of cognitive therapy (Beck, 1976) can be used to develop alternative and more adaptive thoughts to substitute for the negative ones. Cognitive restructuring begins by helping clients discover their predictable negative self-talk and develop arguments against them. Health counselors will readily learn that obese clients are easily discouraged by self-talk such as "It takes too long to lose weight" and "I find myself obsessed by thoughts of food." The counselor must coach clients to interrupt such thoughts and to replace them with more optimistic ones, such as: "A pound a week adds up over time"; and "If I can just cut down on snacks, I will be ahead of the game"; and "I can replace thoughts of food with images of places I like to be and people I really like being with." If the eating diary sheets require that clients to list the negative self-talk they engage in while eating, the counselor can then help them dispute the negative thoughts, restructure them, and replace them with more positive thoughts and self-affirmations (Brownell, 1985).

Social Interventions

Richard Stuart (1984) coined the term *indirection* as an alternative to the directive approach taken in most health-counseling programs. Because he believes that most life-style problems are integrally related to the context in which they occur, he initiates treatment efforts within the marital relationship. The first stage of treatment, then, is to modify the marital relationship. Only then can the second stage of intervention, which focuses on the issue of weight control, be realized.

Brownell and Foreyt (1985) believe that it is important to involve the spouse in weight-control treatment, even though it is not always possible to elicit his or her cooperation. They suggest approaching the spouse as an ally in aiding the client's progress and treatment. A phone call from the counselor can convey to the spouse that he or she is important to the client and that the counselor would benefit from the perspective of the person who knows the client best. This approach must be explained to the client so that the spouse is receiving consistent messages. Once the spouse is involved, both client and spouse can be trained in specific ways to deal more effectively with each other.

Weight Control Treatment Protocol

The behavioral or cognitive-behavioral component of most weight-control programs uses essentially the same techniques but with slightly different protocols. Programs usually differ in the sequence in which topics and techniques are covered and in the relative emphasis on specific components. The treatment

protocol developed by Brownell (1979; 1985) is probably the model program on which most others have been based. Brownell provides an extensive treatment manual that gives a step-by-step description of a 16-week training program (1979). Brownell's program can be utilized in either a small-group or an individual format. His LEARN program (acronym for *L*ifestyle, *E*xercise, *A*ttitudes, *R*elationships, *N*utrition) is a refined version of the original program that contains a useful instrument, the *Diet Readiness Test* (Brownell, 1985).

A second treatment protocol has been described by Fremoux and Heyneman (1984). This program is designed to last a total of ten sessions, in which the first session is an orientation, followed by six weekly sessions of active treatment and three monthly follow-up sessions. Each session lasts about 90 minutes. The group consists of three to six people, although the program has also been administered to individuals and to larger groups. Fremoux and Heyneman have found this protocol particularly useful in the community mental-health setting. The components of this program are described below on a session-by-session basis.

Session 1. The first session involves introducing the clients to one another and to the logistics of the program. The process of self-monitoring is described, and clients begin to work on their eating diaries.

Session 2. This session provides the rationale for the cognitive-behavioral approach, as the group learns to identify negative self-statements and problem situations. The group examines the eating diaries from the previous week and focuses on the negative self-statements, which generate considerable group discussion. Other aspects of eating diaries are also examined and discussed.

Session 3. Patients are weighed and diaries are checked for compliance, as are the self-monitoring instructions and other homework. This session focuses on the concept of coping statements and on alternate activities that can be used in conjunction with cognitive coping statements. A list of five activities is generated to serve as homework tasks.

Session 4. Previous assignments are reviewed and concepts are reviewed. A planned binge is prescribed, in which the clients intentionally overeat when they are not under stress.

Session 5. This session focuses on the abstinence-violation effect, and examples from each client are discussed. The group contracts for a second planned binge, choosing a situation that is slightly more difficult than the previous week's.

Session 6. This session concentrates on the effects of mood on eating. Negative self-statements relating to negative moods are discussed, specifically targeting depression, boredom, and anger. The group also contracts for a final planned binge.

Session 7. The focus of this session is on the general review of the program materials. The group makes new commitments to work on each of the areas that have been presented.

Follow-up Session. Three follow-up sessions are scheduled for four weeks, eight weeks, and twelve weeks following completion of treatment. These sessions focus on group discussion about shared problems, strategies, and troubleshooting individual concerns.

Relapse Prevention

One of the greatest challenges in treating obese clients is keeping them involved in treatment. The attrition in behaviorally and cognitive-behaviorally based weight-control programs is far lower than in other kinds of treatment programs, with dropout rates averaging 13.5 percent (Wilson & Brownell, 1980). Because relapse and noncompliance with treatment are such major issues in weight-control treatment, the health counselor is encouraged to become an expert in relapse prevention. Whether in the formal course of the weight-control program or in its maintenance phase, a client will inevitably lapse or slip. Clients will eat foods that they think they should have avoided; they will want to give up dieting at some point; or they will gain weight. Most initial relapses by dieters are the result of two high-risk factors: 50 percent of clients who slip do so when experiencing negative emotions, such as anxiety, boredom, and depression; the other 50 percent of clients who slip do so in interpersonal situations—often positive events, such as parties, when one's guard is down and the social pressure to eat is high. In many cases, the relapse of the slip itself is much less important than the thoughts and feelings that it engenders. Invariably, the patient believes that the relapse is a signal that more relapses will occur. This weakens restraint and increases the likelihood of further eating, which in turn weakens restraint even more, and the pattern continues.

Relapse prevention must be a component of any weight-control program. The patient is helped to prevent relapses by identifying high-risk situations, by developing coping skills for these high-risk situations, by practicing coping with potential relapses, by developing cognitive coping strategies to be used immediately after a relapse, and by developing a more balanced life-style (Marlatt & Gordon, 1985). The health counselor works with the client both to restructure the environment through stimulus-control techniques and to restructure the client's thoughts through cognitive-restructuring techniques. The client needs to anticipate troublesome negative thoughts or self-statements and learn to counter them with more positive ones. There are dozens of countering statements, and they must be matched to the client's needs. The key is to have clients prepare for relapses by rehearsing the negative statements and their positive counter-statements (Brownell & Foreyt, 1985).

Several studies have begun to test relapse-prevention methods with obese clients. Rosenthall and Marx (1979) studied the Marlatt and Gordon model of relapse prevention by identifying high-risk relapse situations. They found that situations involving the inability either to deal with depression, anger, or boredom or to cope with positive social events, such as celebrations or parties, were frequently involved in relapse episodes. In addition, Rosenthall and Marks designed a relapse-prevention program to teach obese clients to analyze high-risk situations and to use global problem-solving strategies to avoid relapse. Although the obese clients who received this training did not differ at the end of treatment from those who did not receive training, they did maintain their losses much better. Those who learned relapse-prevention techniques used more external attributions, in fact, they felt less guilty following a relapse and were less influenced by their "lack of willpower" than were those who did not receive relapse-prevention training. Peri and his associates (Peri, Shapiro, Ludwig et

al., 1984) studied relapse-prevention techniques utilized in conjunction with post-treatment contact with the counselor. These researchers found that the relapse-prevention program boosted long-term results only when teamed with continuing therapist contact.

Morton (1988) notes that, in addition to the relapse-prevention training system developed by Marlatt and Gordon, there are a number of other strategies that ensure weight maintenance. The first of these is exercise. Exercise may prevent relapse because it can serve as a positive replacement for a problem behavior, it can positively influence the client's self-concept, and it can remove the client to a safe setting. In addition, exercise becomes a constructive means for managing stress and other negative emotions while enabling the person to metabolize a greater number of calories than would otherwise be possible. A second strategy for maintenance is continued self-monitoring. Stuart (1980) found that those who maintain their weight more successfully continue many of the techniques they used to reach their weight goal, particularly self-monitoring. Another strategy is post-treatment support. As we noted before, continuing therapist contact has a role in successful weight maintenance. Finally, positive social support from significant others in the client's life has also been shown to foster long-term weight management.

Case Examples

The following are two case examples that illustrate many of the points made throughout this chapter. The first case involves a group format for weight control, and the second case illustrates weight-control counseling in the individual format.

Case 1

Mary Z. is a 42-year-old married female, employed as an insurance underwriter. She applied for treatment at the University Weight Management Clinic in late November, but requested that her treatment not begin until after the Christmas holiday so that she "could have one last food fling and really enjoy it." Holidays were difficult times for her, as she anticipated being embarrassed around her average-weight relatives whom she saw only once or twice a year.

Mary reported being overweight as a child, as was her mother, and having been on numerous diets since the age of 14. On these diets, she alternately lost and then gained back the weight "at least 15 to 20 times." She noted that while she was dieting as an adult, she seemed to add a few more pounds above her baseline after each attempt at weight control. She had joined TOPS but after three months, had left the program and gained back all the weight plus five pounds more. She had begun various exercise classes at local health clubs but found she was often the heaviest one in the class and would eventually drop out with the justification that "my arthritis started to act up anyway." The reason for seeking weight-loss treatment at this time was that she wanted to lose sufficient weight to look presentable at her daughter's wedding, which was scheduled for the following summer.

During the screening phase of treatment, it became clear that Mary had a

history of success at life-style change, having stopped smoking on her own two years earlier. This success "neutralized" some of her external motivation to lose weight to please her daughter and the wedding guests.

As part of the screening, Mary was asked to keep a food diary and self-monitoring records and to lose one pound per week for two weeks, as a condition for acceptance into the program. She lost three pounds during this time, but only kept a record for eight of the fourteen days. She was offered group treatment with six other moderately obese individuals. The group was to meet for 20 sessions, and she was to begin on a PSMF diet within a cognitive-behavioral format. She verbalized some skepticism about the program's goals, which she thought represented too little weight loss over too long a period of time, and she wanted to be prescribed a much-publicized appetite suppressant. As do many weight clients, Mary had applied magical attributions to weight-loss plans. Because her physician had previously discouraged the use of prescription appetite suppressants, the health counselor confirmed this action, but only after exploring Mary's beliefs and magical expectations for instant, dramatic change in her body image. Both Mary and the counselor jointly agreed to a target goal of a 35- to 40-pound weight loss over the course of the 20 weeks.

Mary had little difficulty adhering to the total life-style-change program, which included the diet, prescribed exercise, stimulus control, response prevention, and challenges to her dysfunctional self-talk. Initially, she took the role of devil's advocate in the group, questioning the intentions and behaviors of other group members. Yet, after other members confronted her on this, she ceased this role behavior. Since the group planned and scheduled food relapses and focused on the skills of relapse prevention, Mary reported only two minor, unplanned relapses during the 20 weeks.

After the fourth group session, the counselor met with Mary and her husband. Her husband's resistance to her weight loss was the focus of three individual sessions. As he became convinced that she would not leave him when she became more slim and attractive, he became more of an ally in the treatment process.

By the sixteenth session, Mary had lost 41 pounds, at which time she switched to a regular 1500-calorie diet. In the following weeks, she regained a few pounds but lost them by the time of her daughter's wedding, and she remained at that weight for approximately the next 12 months. Post-treatment follow-up sessions were scheduled for the group every four weeks for the first three months, and then at two-month intervals over the next year.

Case 2

The case of Eleanor S. was introduced in Chapter 2. As you'll recall, Eleanor was 50 pounds over her ideal weight and was referred for health counseling as an adjunct to the 1200-calorie diet she was prescribed, which was being monitored by her family physician.

A weight-loss plan was negotiated between the health counselor and Eleanor, in which she would meet for 20 weekly sessions for individual counseling and then for follow-up sessions at six-month intervals for the following two years. Her goal was to lose 45 pounds over the 20 sessions—approximately two

to three pounds per week—and to commit to a graduated exercise program, along with a behavioral and cognitive restructuring plan that included at least three conjoint sessions with Mr. S. Because she would continue to be monitored medically by her physician, Eleanor signed a consent form so that her counselor and her physician could consult regularly about her progress.

At the behavioral level, Eleanor was quick to learn. She applied a number of behavioral methods for changing her eating behaviors, and she learned and practiced some relapse prevention skills. Because lack of assertiveness was defined as a major issue, especially within the marriage, skill training was done in the third session. Environmental and stimulus control measures were stressed from the beginning. Eleanor agreed that she must avoid situations in which she would be "forced" by social convention to overeat, such as Sunday meals with her overeating relatives. She partially solved this problem by scheduling social activities with her children during that time and by inviting her relatives to her house for a light dinner that she prepared. She and a friend joined a beginner's aerobics class at a local YWCA.

At the cognitive level, Eleanor worked with the counselor to change and to restructure some of her personality-style convictions and health beliefs in a more socially useful direction. The counselor reframed her occasional relapses as slips rather than as failures.

At the social-support level, conjoint marital sessions were helpful in reducing Mr. S's fears about Eleanor leaving him should she slim down. And, after some communication training, he became more sensitive to her needs to assert independence. He also supported her when both sets of parents were upset about the change in their Sunday schedules. By the fifth session, Mr. S. agreed to go on the same diet plan as his wife, which helped her in complying with the program.

Eleanor's friend was of inestimable value in helping her stick to the weight-loss and maintenance on the job and to help her in menu planning. At the physiological level, Eleanor continued to be monitored weekly by her physician, who conferred regularly with the counselor. By the twentieth session, Eleanor had shed 55 pounds and 12 months later was within 8 pounds of her ideal weight.

Preventive Measures

Because helping clients achieve and maintain healthy weight is the most difficult and perplexing challenge for health promotion counselors, there is much to be said for primary prevention regarding nutrition and weight control. Streigel-Moore and Rodin (1985) provide an extensive review of the research on prevention of obesity. In their report, they emphasize primary prevention strategies that can be implemented throughout the course of human development and provide specific recommendations for prenatal health care and maternal nutrition during pregnancy, infancy, childhood, and adolescence. Their review of this research suggests that the best place to start the prevention of obesity is with the pregnant mother. In their recommendations for prevention

with adolescents, they note that considerable efforts should be directed toward helping adolescents accept the normal physical changes that accompany this stage of development. They believe that adolescents must be thoroughly apprised of the ill effects of crash dieting to control body weight.

Streigel-Moore and Rodin advocate that communities implement preventive efforts that are aimed at reducing the effects of social pressure for thinness. For example, a wider range in what is considered the female beauty ideal is needed, and the mass media can have a critical role in this change. They note that the sociocultural pressures to maintain a sylphlike body motivate thousands of girls to follow unhealthy diets that upset their biological balance and contribute to later obesity. Finally, they acknowledge the consequences of the extraordinary emphasis placed on weight by Western culture, which they believe is at the root of the enormous increase in eating disorders among groups most affected by this weight obsession—women, dancers, wrestlers, jockeys, and gymnasts.

There are a number of reasons for targeting obesity-prevention measures in the early years. First of all, obesity in childhood is likely to continue into adulthood. Whereas only 14 percent of obese infants become obese adults, 70 percent of obese 10- to 13-year-olds do. Few normal-weight children become obese adults. A second reason for beginning early is to prevent fat-cell hyperplasia, since fat-cell hyperplasia develops in childhood and adolescence. Obese adults who were fat in childhood must contend with both hypertrophic and hyperplastic fat cells. Third, those children who are in most need of preventive interventions are not likely to receive them at an early age. Efforts to help children to control their weight need to focus on both diet and physical activity. Therefore, health and physical education programs in schools can provide excellent opportunities to promote healthful eating and exercise habits in all schoolchildren. Streigel-Moore and Rodin (1985) note that primary preventive measures, such as receiving instruction on healthful diets, results in children's bringing healthier lunches to school and throwing fewer healthy foods away. Secondary preventive measures include identifying children who are at high risk of becoming obese on the basis of family history or current overweight. These children can then be given special attention and training in dietary and exercise behavior. Finally, since parents provide access to most of the food that their children eat, primary preventive interventions should be directed at ways that parents can help their children keep from becoming overly fat. The recommendations include encouraging regular physical activity and discouraging excessive TV watching; having fewer high-cholesterol and sugary foods in the home; using fruit, nuts, and other healthful foods as regular desserts, reserving rich, less healthful desserts for special occasions; ensuring that children eat a healthful breakfast each day; eliminating high-calorie snacks at night; and monitoring children's weight on a regular basis, comparing it against the chart of desirable weight.

In short, childhood is probably the ideal time to establish exercise and dietary habits to prevent people from becoming obese. Parents, schools, the mass media, and community agencies can and should play important roles in helping.

Summary

In this chapter we have presented a biopsychosocial view of normal weight and obesity. We have reviewed the etiology and theories of obesity, as well as a classification schema for types of obesity. We have also reviewed five principal factors in weight control: exercise, nutritional information, behavioral aspects of eating styles, cognitive aspects of weight control, and spousal and other social-support factors. We've described a comprehensive approach to the biopsychosocial assessment of weight problems and offered a number of general treatment guidelines and specific biopsychosocial interventions for both individual and group treatment of obesity. In addition, we've outlined clinically useful treatment protocols and two case histories that illustrate weight control in both the individual and the group format. Finally, we have stressed the need for the health counselor to emphasize relapse-prevention strategies within and during the course of treatment and listed primary and secondary prevention measures that can be employed in helping individuals control their weight. The chapter concludes with an annotated list of resources on weight-control materials.

Resources

Organizations

Overeaters Anonymous (OA) and Take Off Pound Sensibly (TOPS) have been described earlier in the chapter. Meetings of these two organizations take place in most cities. Consult the phone directory for the nearest meeting place or contact person.

Publications: Professional Rerferences

• Agras, W. S. (1987). *Eating Disorders: Management of Obesity, Bulimia and Anorexia Nervosa.* New York: Pergamon Press. This book is part of the popular and very practical Psychology Practitioner Guidebooks series. It contains both the useful eating questionnaire and the six-session protocol for obesity used at the Stanford Eating Disorders Clinic.

• Brownell, K. (1979). *Behavior Therapy for Obesity. A Treatment Manual.* Available from the author at the Department of Psychology, University of Pennsylvania, 133 South 36th Street, Philadelphia, PA 19104. This is "the" protocol for weight control from which all other cognitive-behavioral approaches derive. It contains 100 pages of step-by-step instructions for a 16-week program. It has also been used as a clinical guide for patients during the program.

• Brownell, K. (1985). *The LEARN Program for Weight Control.* Philadelphia, University of Pennsylvania Press. Available from the author at 133 S. 36th Street, Suite 507, Philadelphia, PA 19104. This excellent manual can be used by individuals and in small groups.

Publications: Patient Education

There are scores of brief, well-written tradebooks that offer an integrated diet- and cognitive-behavior-change approach to weight control. Each health coun-

selor would do well to search the mall bookstores for titles that are consistent with his or her treatment approach and that can be heartily recommended to patients. Because of the wide assortment of readily available titles, we mention only one, as an example.

• Mahoney, M. J., & Mahoney, B. K. (1976). *Permanent Weight Control: A Total Solution to the Dieter's Dilemma.* New York: Norton. This is one of the first and best of the popularly written accounts of the behavioral self-management approach to weight control. Available in hardcover and paperbook in libraries and from the publisher.·

References

AGRAS, S. (1987). *Eating disorders: Management of obesity, bulimia and anorexia nervosa.* New York: Pergamon Press.

ALLEN, R. (1981). *Lifegain.* New York: Appleton-Century-Crofts.

BECK, A. (1976). *Cognitive therapy and the emotional disorders.* New York: International Universities Press.

BJORNTORP, P. (1986). Fat cells and obesity. In K. D. Brownell & J. P. Foreyt (Eds.), *Handbook of eating disorders.* New York: Basic Books.

BLACKBURN, G. (1978). The liquid protein controversy: A closer look at the facts. *Obesity and Bariatric Medicine, 7,* 25–30.

BROWNELL, K. D. (1979). *Behavior therapy for weight control: A treatment manual.* Philadelphia: University of Pennsylvania Press.

BROWNELL, K. D. (1985). *The LEARN program for weight control.* Philadelphia: University of Pennsylvania Press.

BROWNELL, K. D., & Foreyt, J. P. (1985). Obesity. In D. Barlow (Ed.), *Clinical handbook of psychological disorders.* New York: Guilford Press.

BROWNELL, K. D., Greenwood, M., & Stellar, E. et al. (1986). The effects of repeated cycles of weight loss and regain in rats. *Physiological Behaviors, 38,* 459–464.

BRUCH, H. (1973). *Eating disorders.* New York: Basic Books.

BUCKMASTER, L., & Brownell, K. D. (1989). Behavior modification: The state of the art. In R. Frankle & M. Yang (Eds.), *Obesity and weight control.* Rockville, MD: Aspen.

CASPER, D., & Zachery, D. (1984). The eating disorder as a maladaptive conflict resolution. *Individual Psychology, 40,* 445–452.

COLLETTI, G., & Brownell, K. D. (1982). The physical and emotional benefits of social supports: Applications to obesity, smoking and alcoholism. In M. Herson, R. Eisler, & P. Miller (Eds.), *Progress in behavior modification.* New York: Academic Press.

DURIN, J., & Wormensley, J. (1974). Body fat assessed from total body density and its estimation from skinfold thickness. *British Journal of Nutrition, 21,* 681–689.

EPSTEIN, L., Wing, R., Roseke, R. et al. (1982). A comparison of lifestyle change and programmed aerobic exercise on weight and fitness changes in obese children. *Behavior Therapy, 13,* 651–665.

FAWZY, F., Wellisch, D., Pasnau, R. et al. (1984). Psychotherapy as an adjunct to supervised fasting for obesity. *Psychosomatics, 25,* 821–829.

FERSTER, C. B., Nurnberger, J., & Levitt, E. (1962). The control of eating. *Journal of Mathematics, 1,* 87–109.

FREMOUX, W., & Heyneman, N. (1984). Obesity. In M. Hersen (Ed.), *Outpatient behavior therapy: A clinical guide.* New York: Grune & Stratton.

GARNER, D. M., Garfinkel, P. E., Schwartz, D., & Thompson, M. (1980). Cultural expectations of thinness in women. *Psychological Reports, 47,* 483–491.

HALMI, K. A. (1980). Gastric bypass for massive obesity. In A. J. Stunkard (Ed.), *Obesity.* Philadelphia: Saunders.

JEFFREY, R., Wing, R., & Stunkard, A. (1978). Behavioral treatment of obesity: The state of the art in 1976. *Behavior Therapy, 6,* 189–199.

KANNEL, W. B., & Gordon, T. (1979). Physiological and medical concomitants of obesity: The Framingham study. In G. A. Bray (Ed.), *Obesity in America,* (Publication No. 79–359). Washington, DC: NIH.

KATCH, F., & McArdle, W. (1983). *Nutrition, weight control and exercise.* Philadelphia: Len & Febiger.

KEESEY, R. E. (1986). A set-point theory of obesity. In K. Brownell & J. P. Foreyt (Eds.), *Handbook of eating disorders.* New York: Basic Books.

KEESEY, R. E. & Corbett, S. (1984). Metabolic defense of the body weight set-point. In A. J. Stunkard & E. Stellar (Eds.), *Eating and its disorders.* New York: Raven Press.

KINGSLEY, R., & Wilson, G. (1977). Behavior therapy for obesity: a comparative investigation of long-term efficacy. *Journal of Consulting and Clinical Psychology, 53,* 43–48.

LAQUATERA, J., & Danish, S. J. (1988). A primer for nutritional counseling. In R. T. Frankle & M. Yang (Eds.), *Obesity and weight control.* Rockville, MD: Aspen.

LEVITZ, L., & Stunkard, A. (1974). A therapeutic coalition for obesity: Behavior modification and patient self-help. *American Journal of Psychiatry, 131,* 423–427.

LEW, E. A., & Garfinkel, L. (1979). Variations in mortality by weight among 750,000 men and women. *Journal of Chronic Disease, 32,* 563–567.

LINEHAN, M. (1987). Dialectical behavior therapy in groups: Treating borderline personality disorders and suicidal behavior. In C. Brady (Ed.), *Women's therapy groups.* New York: Springer.

MAHONEY, M., & Mahoney, K. (1976). *Permanent weight control: A total solution to the dieter's dilemma.* New York: Norton.

MARLATT, G., & Gordon, J. (Eds.). (1985). *Relapse prevention: Maintenance strategies in the treatment of addictive behaviors.* New York: Guilford Press.

McARDLE, W., Katch, F., & Katch, V. (1981). *Exercise physiology.* Philadelphia: Len & Febiger.

MILLER, W. J., & Stephens, T. (1987). The prevalence of overweight and obesity in Britian, Canada, and the United States. *American Journal of Public Health, 77,* 38–41.

MORTON, C. J. (1988). Weight loss maintenance and relapse prevention. In R. Frankle & M. Yang (Eds.), *Obesity and weight control.* Rockville, MD: Aspen.

NELSON, G. E. (1984). *Biological principles with human perspectives* (2nd ed.). New York: Wiley.

PERI, M., Shapiro, R., & Ludwig, W. et al. (1984). Maintenance strategies for the treatment of obesity. An evaluation of relapse prevention training and postreatment contact by mail and phone. *Journal of Clinical and Consulting Psychology, 52,* 404–413.

PI-SUNYER, F. X. (1989). Exercise in the treatment of obesity. In R. Frankle & M. Yang (Eds.), *Obesity and weight control.* Rockville, MD: Aspen.

RIMM, W., Weiner, L. H., Van Yserloo, B., & Berstein, R. (1975). Relationship of obesity and disease in 73,532 weight-conscious women. *Public Health Reports, 90,* 44–51.

ROSENTHALL, B., and Marx, R. (1979). A comparison of standard behavioral and relapse prevention weight reduction programs. Paper presented at the Associaton for Advancement of Behavior Therapy Convention, San Francisco, December, 1979.

SCHWARTZ, H. (1986). *Never satisfied: A cultural history of diets, fantasies and fads.* New York: Free Press.

STREIGEL-MOORE, R., & Rodin, J. (1985). Prevention of obesity. In J. Rosen and L. Solomon (Eds.), *Prevention in health psychology.* Hanover, VT: University Press of New England.

STUART, R. (1980). Weight loss and beyond: Are they taking it off and keeping it off? In P. Davidson & S. Davidson (Eds.), *Behavioral medicine: Changing health lifestyles.* New York: Brunnel/Mazel.

STUART, R. (1984). Indirection and promoting health behaviors. *The 1984 Polachek Lecture.* Mount Sinai Medical Center, Milwaukee, Wisconsin, October 9, 1984.

STUART, R., & Jacobson, B. (1987). *Sex, weight and marriage.* New York: Norton.

STUART, R., & Mitchell, C. (1980). Self-help groups in the control of body weight. In A. Stunkard (Ed.), *Obesity.* Philadelphia: Saunders.

STUNKARD, A. J. (1984). The current status of treatment for obesity in adults. In A. J. Stunkard & E. Stellar (Eds.), *Eating and its disorders.* New York: Raven Press.

SUITOR, C., & Hunter, M. (1980). *Nutrition: Principles and applications in health promotion.* Philadelphia: Lippincott.

UNITED STATES SENATE SELECT COMMITTEE ON NUTRITION AND HEALTH NEEDS. (1977). *Dietary Goals for the United States* (2nd ed.). Washington, DC: U.S. Government Printing Office.

VAN ITALLIE, T. V. (1979). Obesity. Adverse effects on health and longevity. *American Journal of Clinical Nutrition, 32,* 2723–2733.

VAN STRIEN, T., Frijters, J., Bergers, G., & Defares, P. (1986). The Dutch eating behavior questionnaire (DEBQ). *International Journal of Eating Disorders, 5,* 295–315.

WADDEN, T., Stunkard, A., Brownell, K. D., & Dey, S. (1984). The treatment of moderate obesity by behavior modification and very low-calorie diets. *Journal of Consulting and Clinical Psychology, 52,* 692–694.

WARDLE, J. (1989). The management of obesity. In S. Pearce and J. Wardle (Eds.), *The practice of behavioral medicine.* Oxford: British Psychological Society, Oxford University Press.

WILSON, G., & Brownell, K. D. (1980). Behavior therapy for adults. An evaluation of treatment outcomes. *Advances in Behavior Research and Therapy, 3,* 49–86.

4

Smoking Cessation

To cease smoking is the easiest thing I ever did: I ought to know because I've done it a thousand times.

Mark Twain

Cigarette smoking is a major public-health problem despite decreases over the past two decades in the number of people who smoke, and it remains the largest preventable cause of illness and premature death (Shiffman, 1985). Current estimates suggest that about 30 percent of the U.S. population smokes, with the age range of 30 to 44 disproportionately represented (Iverson, 1987). Additionally, a large number of children and adolescents begin smoking each year. It is interesting that most smokers report wanting to stop and having tried to do so unsuccessfully, with only approximately 25 percent experiencing lasting success.

Tobacco is probably the most dangerous substance commonly consumed by humans, and inhaling its burned by-products is an added health risk. A one-pack-a-day smoker inhales about 400 "doses" a day, or 150,000 doses per year. More than 300 known poisons are in the smoke, including substances such as nicotine, arsenic, cyanide, carbon monoxide, phenol, and formaldehyde. Smoking shortens a two-pack-a-day smoker's life expectancy by eight years, and even light smokers—those who smoke one to nine cigarettes per day—shorten their life expectancy by approximately four years. Smokers have a 22 percent higher rate of sickness and loss of job time and take 10 percent longer to recover from illness than do nonsmokers (Spence, 1987). The list of the diseases or conditions related to smoking resembles a medical encyclopedia: alcohol interaction, allergies, arterial sclerosis, bladder cancer, bronchitis, burns, cardiomyotomy, cavities, cerebral profusion deficiencies, child abuse, circulatory deficiencies, drug interferences, emphysema, cancer of the esophagus, fetal smoking syndrome, gingivitis, halitosis, headaches, heart attack, hypertension, infertility (male and female), influenza, cancer of the kidneys, cancer of the larynx, leukoplakia, lung cancer, menopause, oral cancer, osteoporosis, pancreatic cancer, PMS, radioactivity, strokes, ulcers, and wrinkles.

Traditional medical approaches have been relatively ineffective in dealing with this health problem. For example, medical and surgical interventions for lung cancer are still mostly ineffective yet, in theory, these smoking-related deaths and problems are 100 percent preventable.

Statements by the U.S. Surgeon General have underlined four general points: (1) smoking has adverse effects on several aspects of health; (2) secondary smoke affects the health of the nonsmoker; (3) nicotine meets the criteria for addiction in a way similar to that of other addictive behaviors; and (4) major and immediate health benefits are achieved by quitting smoking.

Researchers have traditionally focused on the physiological components of addiction rather than on its psychological or social aspects. When smoking is viewed as a total process, researchers begin to examine the client's participation in the process and the impact on society. Through this altered way of viewing smoking, a range of psychological, biological, and social interventions have been developed. In the research, as well as in this chapter, procedures are presented as separate approaches; however, in clinical practice, most procedures are used in combination.

Stages of Smoking

Smoking is a behavior that develops in a series of stages: preparation, initiation, and habituation. If this developmental progression is followed further, individuals may either quit and remain abstinent or quit unsuccessfully and relapse. Different variables (biological, psychological, and social) are important at different stages of the smoking process.

The preparation for smoking begins very early. By observing smokers, the young child is provided with information about the nature of smoking, its functions, and its acceptability. Thus, a more or less appealing, positive image is created early in the smoking process. Social pressure from peers is one of the prime initiators of experimentation. Smoking by family members and other important models may further promote experimentation.

After beginning smoking, it takes two to three years of continued use or

Table 4-1 Stages of Smoking

Stage 1. Preparation (Psychological factors before smoking)
  Modeling by significant others
  Attitudes concerning the function and desirability of smoking

Stage 2. Initiation (Psychosocial factors leading to experimentation)
  Peer pressure and reinforcement
  Availability
  Curiosity, rebelliousness, and impulsivity
  Viewing smoking as a sign of adulthood and independence

Stage 3. Habitual (Psychosocial and biological factors leading to continued smoking)
  Nicotine regulation
  Emotional regulation
  Cues in the environment
  Peer pressure and reinforcement
  Urges to smoke

Stage 4. Stopping (Psychosocial cues leading to attempts to stop)
  Health concerns
  Expense
  Aesthetic concerns
  Example to others, e.g., children
  Availability of social support for stopping
  Notions of self-mastery

Stage 5. Resuming (Psychosocial and biological factors leading to recidivism)
  Withdrawal symptoms
  Increased stress and other negative effects
  Social pressure
  Abstinence violation effects

Source: From *Health Psychology and Behavioral Medicine,* by J. J. Snyder, p. 287. Copyright © 1989 by Prentice-Hall.

practice to fully establish the habit. There is a gradual increase in the number of cigarettes smoked; more situations, activities, and experiences cue smoking, and more reinforcers accrue to the behavior until the person becomes a habitual smoker. Once the habit is well established, smoking becomes part of the daily routine. Smoking is evoked and reinforced by a wide variety of stimuli. At a biological level, nicotine is very addictive. With continued use, the smoker's body expects a certain level of nicotine and cues the individual to smoke if actual levels fall below those expected. Nicotine withdrawal symptoms are painful, and smoking is reinforced by a reduction in such symptoms. Smoking may be further reinforced by the stimulating and alerting effects of nicotine.

Smoking Maintenance

Smoking also plays a central role in the regulation of emotions. The experience of unpleasant emotions such as anxiety, anger, boredom, and depression may cue smoking. A consequent relaxation or reduction of these emotions then reinforces the smoking response. Smokers also report cravings for cigarettes or other tobacco products. These cravings may be cognitive correlates of low nicotine levels or of affective arousal, or they may be correlates of the positive consequences associated with smoking, including taste, relaxation, and stimulation. Cravings may also be cued by external stimuli, such as seeing others smoke, or by other behaviors, such as drinking a cup of coffee. Finally, a smoker may engage in self-reinforcement, such as seeing oneself as more adult or as having more machismo.

The social and physical environments, along with the smoker's own behavior through past associative learning, constantly bombard the habitual user with cues to smoke. Seeing others smoke, receiving invitations to smoke, seeing a pack of cigarettes, drinking coffee, finishing a meal, and watching TV are all capable of evoking tobacco use. That use may in turn be reinforced by social approval; peer affiliation; and the oral, manual, and respiratory actions involved in smoking.

Health counselors understand how behavior plays a central role in health and illness. Health-impairing habits and life-styles are important risk factors for chronic disease and death, whereas health-promoting habits and life-styles enhance biological and psychosocial functioning.

Maladaptive and adaptive health behaviors are acquired and maintained by the same processes. Their acquisition and shaping are a function of maturation and learning. Once established, their performance is evoked and maintained by the biological, cognitive-affective, social, environmental, and behavioral cues and consequences that define an individual's daily experience. The modification of health behaviors is therefore a complicated intervention that involves a collaborative, mutually active client/health provider relationship and the utilization of cognitive, behavioral, environmental, and biological change strategies.

Review of the Literature

Since 1968, the U.S. Department of Health and Human Services has issued an annual annotated bibliography of all published research studies on the topic of smoking and health. Each year, there are several thousand published research studies from around the world. Publications are divided into 16 different sections, including such topics as pharmacology and toxology, mortality and morbidity, neoplastic diseases, cardiovascular diseases, pregnancy and infant health, behavioral and psychological aspects, smoking prevention and intervention, smoking-cessation methods, tobacco product additives, tobacco manufacturing and processing, tobacco economics, and legislation. Because of the magnitude of the literature in this area, this section will be limited to the highlights of the biological, psychological, and social literature.

Basically, three theoretical models for understanding smoking behavior have been developed: a psychosocial, a psychological, and a biological or pharmacological one.

The *psychosocial model* views smoking behavior as a means of coping with stress and with stressful life events. Successful coping serves as the reinforcer for smoking behavior. Laboratory studies tend to support the hypothesis that smoking facilitates coping. Smoking has been found to reduce fluctuations or changes in mood during stress and to serve as a successful means for enduring a stressor, such as an electric shock. When compared to nonsmokers, people who smoke more than one pack of cigarettes per day have been found to have a lower tolerance for stress if they are not permitted to smoke and a greater tolerance for stress if they are permitted to smoke. Thus, people under high stress may have unusual difficulty in trying to quit smoking.

Another aspect of the psychosocial model is the concept of psychosocial assets—those personal attributes that may provide special strength in developing more satisfactory long-term coping mechanisms. Included in the concept of psychosocial assets are such attributes as self-efficacy (Bandura, 1977), internal locus of control (self-control), and a strong social-support network. These personal assets may make it easier for a person under high stress to quit smoking.

The *psychological model* focuses on needs, drives, and emotions. This model views smoking behavior as serving to minimize negative emotions such as distress, anger, fear, and shame; smoking is reinforcing and persistent because it is successful in warding off these feelings (Tomkins, 1966). This model has been elaborated and evaluated, and there is considerable evidence that an association exists between the amount of smoking and the extent to which cigarettes are used to ward off negative emotions. In addition, heavy smokers have been found to manifest more psychological disturbances than do light smokers.

The *pharmacological/biological model* seeks the specific chemical agent within the cigarette itself on which a smoker may become dependent or addicted. The most likely agent appears to be nicotine, and a number of studies support this hypothesis. Studies show that smokers smoke more when the

amount of nicotine in their cigarettes is reduced and that smoking is decreased when nicotine is provided in other ways, such as in nicotine gum, which is often part of a comprehensive smoking-cessation program.

In reviewing the large number of studies that have sought to evaluate the various smoking-cessation programs, psychologists have noted five methodological problems that they keep encountering. These problems are: (1) difficulties in verifying self-reports of smoking behavior; (2) lack of control groups in evaluating smoking-cessation programs; (3) difficulties in classifying levels of previous smoking or levels of smoking reduction; (4) lack of agreement regarding optimal length of follow-up; and (5) methodological differences in determining outcomes of smoking-cessation programs.

There does not appear to be agreement about how to classify smoking behavior and decreases in smoking behavior, and therefore it is impossible to compare and contrast the different outcomes of the smoking-control programs. When studying smoking behavior, most researchers assess the number of cigarettes smoked per day. It is clear, however, that one needs also to take into account such factors as how long people have smoked, how many puffs they take per cigarette, and how much they inhale when they smoke. To assess the degree of smoking reduction obtained, each study seems to use its own criteria: no cigarettes smoked in the previous week, no more than six cigarettes smoked in any given week, and so on.

Psychosocial Model

The social perspective involves understanding both how social and cultural forces affect the creation of smoking behavior and how influences can be used to prevent smoking and to help people stop smoking once they've started. When dealing with such a global problem that affects millions of people, taking a social perspective is often more useful than dealing with one smoker at a time. It is important to realize how the changes in public policy could be the most effective route to smoking cessation. For example, high prices of or lack of access to cigarettes could well have a far greater impact on the smoking habit than could the results of any psychological research into smoking motivation or smoking cessation. In a sense, the researchers could themselves be accused of helping to sustain the habit, since the focus of their concern is typically on the nature of the smoker, rather than on the larger social and economic structures that support the tobacco industry. Tobacco companies are multinational, multi-product corporations that benefit society through a wide range of diversified manufacturing and commercial enterprises. Tobacco companies provide employment and stimulation to the local economy. They also have considerable power to act as pressure groups to influence government policy as well as potential customers. Their advertising budgets far exceed those allocated to health-promotion organizations. Even where traditional advertising routes are closed, tobacco companies are willing to sponsor sports and the arts and to fund basic research.

There appears to be considerable evidence that some social groups consistently smoke more than others. Research indicates that men smoke more than women and that both men and women in the 30 to 44 age group smoke more

than those in any other group. Certain ethnic groups, such as blacks, tend to smoke more than whites, regardless of gender. People with less education smoke more than those with more education, and blue-collar workers smoke more than white-collar workers. Divorced and separated people tend to smoke far more than people who have intact marriages. Only a social perspective can help us to understand and to focus intervention programs on these group differences.

Two major social influences on the establishment of smoking behavior have been noted: the influence of others and the influence of media advertising. During adolescence, when most smoking starts, smoking plays a symbolic role in the three great issues that teenagers face: the deemphasis of parental influence; the establishment of bonds with peers; and the establishment of an independent self-identity. Teenagers who have parents, older siblings, and friends who smoke are more likely to smoke themselves. In fact, those who have two parents who smoke are twice as likely to smoke as those who have no parents who smoke. Smoking is thought of by teenagers as adult behavior that is normally off-limits to children. Thus, by smoking, teenagers are showing signs of emerging adulthood and are probably defying their parents as well. On the other hand, fewer teenagers smoke today than they did a few years ago, partly because of an increased concern with health and partly because smoking does not have the peer approval that it once had.

Today our society—including the mass media—continues to encourage smoking, although there is considerable evidence that societal values are changing and that cigarette advertising is having a less persuasive impact on smoking behavior. Educational efforts have been fairly successful in discouraging smoking. Further advances will need to include the social perspective—that is, the examination of the context within which smoking occurs.

Scientists who emphasize the importance of a social perspective in considering smoking cessation stress four general points (Bloom, 1988):

1. Efforts to inform the public about the dangerous effects of smoking on health will probably need to continue indefinitely.
2. In terms of its prevalence, smoking must be presented for what it is—the atypical behavior of a minority of the population. The increasing constraints on smoking behavior and the increasing attention being accorded to the rights of nonsmokers help keep smoking in its proper demographic perspective.
3. Constant attention needs to be devoted to the influence that public policy and public policymakers have for counteracting the tobacco industry's efforts to encourage smoking.
4. In spite of their high cost and the enormous effort involved, antismoking advertisements must be revived, maintained, and increased.

Perhaps the best antismoking advertisement is the nonsmoker, and as the number and proportion of nonsmokers continue to increase, smoking will be increasingly seen as deviant and unacceptable. It will become more and more difficult to smoke when a larger and larger proportion of the population think of smoking not only as unhealthy and unpleasant but also as stupid (Syme & Alcalay, 1982).

The list of potential antismoking strategies is remarkably long, and many of them can be used in combination. In addition to prohibiting smoking in general (a strategy that few, if any, people believe will be effective), other strategies that have been suggested include:

1. restricting where people may smoke (and, in some cases, who may smoke)
2. identifying and reducing the hazardous substances in cigarette smoke
3. restricting advertising of tobacco products
4. increasing knowledge of the harmful effects of smoking, particularly among such groups as preadolescents and pregnant women, through consumer health education
5. incorporating information about the dangers of smoking in the public school curriculum
6. expanding smoking-cessation programs for people who want to quit smoking
7. increasing taxation on tobacco products
8. finding other uses for tobacco, such as in animal feed or in the manufacture of pesticides and medicinal products
9. retraining tobacco farmers for other ways of earning a living (Bloom, 1988).

Smoking is an integral part of common social situations. Bars and parties are the most frequently encountered social situations, and they are doubly troubling. They provide potent smoking cues, and the disinhibitory effects of alcohol can easily overcome the smoker's resolve. Counselors often warn clients about these effects and suggest that clients avoid such situations immediately after quitting.

The importance of interpersonal relationships in facilitating as well as impeding a smoker's abstinence from cigarettes is well documented in the research literature, but the mechanism by which this influence is exerted is not clear. Perceived support of others helps the smoker maintain abstinence. McIntyre, Mermelstein, and Lichtenstein (1982) suggest that partner behaviors can be categorized as either helpful or detrimental. These investigators acknowledge that the exact form that helpful behaviors take depends in part on the couple. However, the research has shown that helpful behaviors include providing rewards, giving compliments for the decision to quit as well as for the actual quitting, expressing both interest in being involved and confidence in the partner, and not smoking in the quitter's presence. Detrimental behaviors include nagging, shunning, and policing. Expounding on these findings, these investigators have prepared a manual for partners of smokers (Lichtenstein & Mermelstein, 1982).

Psychological Model

Psychologists have emphasized the role that specific knowledge of the health consequences of smoking, beliefs about personal susceptibility, attitudes toward smoking, and expectations of the benefits of quitting play, both in the decision to quit smoking and in the long-term success or failure of that decision. Most smoking-intervention programs focus on the participants' attitudes and beliefs as well as on their behavior during smoking and during the quitting process. For example, a review of the health consequences of smoking is often used as a

motivational boost for quitting. Programs may also emphasize clients' self-defeating thoughts, particularly when the focus is on the maintenance of treatment gains or on relapse prevention.

One particular set of cognitions has been given a good deal of attention recently in the literature on smoking. The concept of perceived self-efficacy (Bandura, 1977) appears to be a very useful tool in the cessation process. Self-efficacy is defined as an individual's belief in his or her ability to perform a given behavior. Information from past behaviors, modeling, affective states, and instruction all combine to produce a performance expectation that predicts future behavior. It is likely that these self-efficacy expectations are better predictors of behavior than are previous behaviors alone. These beliefs in self-efficacy often reflect an individual's perceived ability to refrain from smoking in various situations or for designated periods of time. Just as personality factors are likely to affect one's ability to refrain from smoking, these factors further underlie the origins of smoking behavior. Research (Marlatt & Gordon, 1985; Baer & Lichtenstein, 1985) has shown that certain personality factors, such as the ability to delay gratification, predispose individuals to substance abuse. When these predisposing factors are paired with certain situational factors, such as the availability of substances and positive reinforcing stimuli, a common response is often substance use.

There appear to be at least three stages in the process of quitting: preparing to quit, quitting itself, and maintaining cessation. Researchers have demonstrated that individuals who are quitting smoking tend to use different types of coping strategies at different stages of the quitting process. For example, during the course of a cessation program, especially after initial quitting, ambivalence about nonsmoking and rationalizations for resuming smoking may become critical concerns. As clients strive to maintain their newly achieved nonsmoking status, they are often beset with thoughts that can undermine their efforts. Clinicians have found that the measurement of such thoughts or rationalizations can provide a useful stimulus for treatment planning and coping. Danaher and Lichtenstein (1978) have outlined a number of potentially self-defeating thoughts or rationalizations.

1. *Nostalgia:* "I sure did like to smoke with coffee after dinner. I wonder how a cigarette would taste now."
2. *Testing:* "I wonder if I could smoke just one cigarette, and then not have any more."
3. *Crisis:* "I could handle the situation much better if I only had a cigarette." Or alternatively, "I've been under such pressure that I deserve a cigarette."
4. *Avoiding unwanted side effects:* "Quitting smoking is causing me to become overweight."
5. *Self-doubts:* "I'm still getting strong urges to smoke. I must be one of those addicted people."

Labeling such rationalizations helps clients recognize how they can undermine their efforts to quit smoking. Clients can then be trained and encouraged to combat or rebut these self-defeating thoughts.

Biological Model

A number of theorists in the late 1970s conceptualized smoking as primarily an escape/avoidance response to the aversive consequences of nicotine withdrawal (Schachter, 1978). This formulation is essentially an addiction model, which states that a minimal amount of nicotine must be provided because withdrawal symptoms will occur. Nicotine-withdrawal symptoms, however, have been somewhat difficult to document and generally have been found to vary from smoker to smoker, as well as from environment to environment. Several investigators have observed that smokers are able to undergo extended periods of deprivation under certain conditions without experiencing much discomfort (Ashton & Stepney, 1982). Only recently have investigators agreed that there is a physiological addiction to nicotine.

Although addiction is clearly a factor in the maintenance of smoking, the theories seem inadequate to provide a comprehensive explanation or to account satisfactorily for the difficulties most smokers experience in quitting. Researchers, however, indicate that stimuli independent of the nicotine-addiction cycle—that is, unrelated to the time since the last cigarette—reliably increase the probability of smoking. Such stimuli include the end of a meal, the consumption of coffee, feeling upset or unhappy, and cognitive and intellectual pressures. Consistent with these observations are reports that many cigarettes are smoked because the smoker perceives improvement in performance, enhancement of pleasure or relaxation, and relief of anxiety (Pomerleau & Pomerleau, 1989). Thus, with the exception of the first cigarette of the day or after an extended period of deprivation, many cigarettes smoked have no clear connection with nicotine deprivation or time since the last cigarette.

Schachter, a prominent proponent of the addiction model, attempted to resolve this apparent difficulty. He and his colleagues demonstrated that smokers smoke more when anxious or when subjected to painful stimulation. The researchers also found that these stressors decreased urinary pH, which led them to hypothesize that acidification of the urine by stress caused nicotine withdrawal. Schachter (1978) concluded from these and related studies that the principal consequence of smoking is simply relief from the painful and anxiety-provoking state of nicotine withdrawal.

There is now considerable evidence to suggest that the tenacity of the cigarette-smoking habit is based on different reinforcing effects that are appropriate to a variety of circumstances (Pomerleau & Pomerleau, 1989). In fact, most behavioral strategies for treating smoking have been based on the assumption that both escape from withdrawal and disruption of other reinforcing consequences of smoking must occur in order to break the habit. This perspective is derived from behavior modification theory and ultimately from operant conditioning concepts that emphasize the contribution of antecedent and consequent environmental stimuli in determining behavior. Implicitly or explicitly, however, these formulations ascribe the rewarding aspects of smoking to conditioning and have little to say about the biological basis for the reinforcement of smoking or for the mediation of environment/behavior interactions. What is called for at this time is an integrative formulation of smoking that takes into

account the complexity of the pharmacological actions of nicotine and the contributions of social, psychological, and biological factors.

Table 4-2 gives an idea of the range and diversity of the subjective and behavioral consequences that have been reported or demonstrated for smoking. The congruence of these consequences with the psychological effects of the endogenous neuroregulators known to be stimulated by nicotine is striking, as can be seen in Table 4-3.

In addition, the number of affective states or performance demands that might cue smoking, independent of nicotine withdrawal, is potentially very large and provides a plausible explanation for the thorough interweaving of the smoking habit into the fabric of daily life. The fact that nicotine does not produce a dramatic intoxication or withdrawal may even add to its reinforcing value, in that the benefits of smoking may be achieved without disrupting ongoing activities.

The withdrawal symptoms that occur immediately after cessation of drug use are collectively called acute withdrawal syndrome. It is not clear whether there is a specific acute syndrome that can be ascribed to tobacco dependency. Most smokers report some symptoms, but the nature of the symptoms varies greatly from smoker to smoker. Generally, symptoms are most acute during the first seven to ten days of quitting. The most common complaints are heightened anxiety, irritability, inability to concentrate, fatigue, increased mucus production, and headache. Occasionally, smokers report mouth sores and mild gastrointestinal upset. A nearly universal symptom is tobacco craving. At first, the ex-smoker may experience constant withdrawal symptoms but, with the exception of craving, most symptoms usually subside after the first seven to ten days.

Table 4-2 Commonly Reported Behavioral and Subjective Effects of Smoking

---

Consequences of Smoking in Habitual Smokers

↑ concentration/ability to tune out irrelevant stimuli

↑ memory (recall)

↑ psychomotor performance

↑ alertness/arousal

↓ anxiety/tension

↑ pleasure/facilitation of pleasure

↓ body weight (↓ consumption of sweet-tasting substances?)

Consequences of Not Smoking in Habitual Smokers

↓ concentration/ability to tune out irrelevant stimuli

↑ memory impairment

↓ psychomotor performance

↑ dullness/anhedonia

↑ anxiety/tension

↑ irritability/dysphoria

↑ craving for cigarettes

↑ body weight (↑ consumption of sweet-tasting substances?)

Source: From *Smoking and Human Behavior,* by T. Ney and E. Gale (Eds.). Copyright © 1989 by Wiley. (Adapted from Pomerleau & Pomerleau, 1984.)

Table 4-3 Reinforcement Consequences of Smoking and Putative Neuroregulatory Mechanisms

Positive Reinforcement	*Negative Reinforcement*
Pleasure/enhancement of pleasure	Reduction of anxiety and tension
↑ dopamine	↑ acetylcholine
↑ norepinephrine	↑ beta-endorphin
↑ beta-endorphin	Antinociception
Facilitation of task performance	↑ acetylcholine
↑ acetylcholine	↑ beta-endorphin
↑ norepinephrine	Avoidance of weight gain
Improvement of memory	↑ dopamine
↑ acetylcholine	↑ norepinephrine
↑ norepinephrine	Relief from nicotine withdrawal
↑ vasopressin	↑ acetylcholine
	(↑ noncholinergic
	nicotinic activity)

Source: From *Smoking and Human Behavior,* by T. Ney and E. Gale (Eds.). Copyright © 1989 by Wiley. (Adapted from Pomerleau & Pomerleau, 1984.)

Counselors may find it helpful to have the client rank the intensity of the tobacco craving on a scale from 1 to 10, with 1 being nonexistent and 10 being severe. Most clients find that they are able to get some control over the cravings and are able to see some moderate changes.

From a physiological perspective, the occurrence of such symptoms is puzzling. Nicotine has a half-life of four to five hours. Its most active metabolite, cotinine, has a half-life of 24 to 48 hours. Therefore, the symptoms continue to occur long after nicotine and its major active metabolite are cleared from the body. Similar phenomena have been described with opiates. Theorists suggest that chronic withdrawal symptoms are classically conditioned reactions to internal and environmental stimuli associated either with smoking or with changes in nicotine blood levels. For example, within minutes after smoking, the nicotine blood level rises to a peak and then begins to fall. The fall in the level of nicotine in the blood may result in mild withdrawal symptoms, which become conditioned to the environment in which they occur (Leventhal & Cleary, 1980).

From the preceding review of the literature, we find that the interactions among the biological, psychological, and social factors are great. We now turn our attention to assessing how these factors fit people who are looking for relief from their smoking habit.

Assessment

Assessment is an ongoing process that is tied to the course of treatment. Some assessments occur prior to or early in treatment, whereas others are possible only once smoking has stopped, and still others are most relevant in long-term follow-up. Generally, assessment begins with a smoking history that leads up to the current cessation attempt. Self-reports of smoking patterns and motives are

best obtained early in treatment, because responses change as treatment proceeds. Assessment then progresses to a more detailed evaluation of the client's current smoking behavior. Self-reports and self-monitoring are used to measure the amount and distribution of smoking. This type of information can help provide the counselor with a client's self-reported baseline of smoking behavior.

Assessment procedures vary in their clinical utility. Many valid assessments yield information that is primarily of prognostic value—that is, predicting the client's probability of success. Although this information may be intellectually interesting, it is of little clinical value because it provides little implication for action. Knowing that a particular person is a poor risk for treatment is of little use unless the information provides action that improves the outcome. We believe that, to be clinically useful, an assessment should have immediate implications for the conduct of treatment. Assessment is most valuable when it is linked to a set of clinical procedures that are differentially applied, each dependent on the results of the assessment. Also, we find that assessment may also increase the client's motivational level by changing their way of thinking. For example, we often ask clients to list the benefits that they plan to receive from quitting. A handout sheet with the following list is provided that asks, "Does your list include these?"

- overall improved health
- lower pulse rate
- easier breathing
- no more smoker's cough
- no more angina pain in the chest
- improved taste and smell
- cleaner, fresher-smelling clothes
- more energy
- less tension
- less need for sleep
- more-refreshing sleep
- increased physical endurance level
- monetary savings
- pride of accomplishment
- improved self-confidence and esteem
- personal satisfaction of a job well done

Clients are then asked to carry this list with them at all times and to agree to look at the list before putting another cigarette in their mouth.

A variation of this technique comes from Judy Perlmutter (1986). In her strategy, clients are asked to go through a list of smoking consequences and quitting benefits and check off the items that apply to them. The questionnaire focuses on the emotional, health, social, and financial consequences of smoking and benefits of quitting. In this process of assessment, clients are learning the consequences of smoking and the benefits of quitting. Clients understand what they're willing to give up as well as the benefits and payoffs that they expect to obtain once they've quit. This helps them understand that they are not stopping,

quitting, or losing something, but rather are gaining and benefiting from not smoking.

Lederman and Scheiderman (1986) have developed a smoker's self-assessment profile that helps smokers understand what motivates them to smoke. The simple, 18-item questionnaire provides a useful way of categorizing smoking motivation. The six motivational categories are: (1) stimulation by nicotine; (2) handling or touching things; (3) pleasure/accentuation of pleasure; (4) tension reduction/relaxation; (5) psychological dependency; and (6) habit.

Additionally, we have found it helpful during the assessment phase to develop an assessment of the client's current level of physical and psychological stress and to identify what coping skills the client has or needs to develop to cope effectively with this stress and meet his or her goal (Donovan & Marlatt, 1988; Davis & Glaros, 1986; Shiffman; 1985).

The level of stress in the smoker's life influences the treatment process. Lower levels of stress can be a motivational factor that stimulates clients to seek change, whereas clients who experience high levels of stress are less likely to see themselves as capable of effecting a change until some tension is reduced. Clinical instruments are available to assess the client's current level of stress and anxiety. However, we have found it useful to ask a simple question: "On a scale of 1 to 100, with 1 being low and 100 being high, what would you estimate your current level of stress?" This simple question can help the client assess the present stress, predict the likelihood that this stress is going to change in the future, and better understand whether this is the best time to be considering smoking cessation.

Donovan and Marlatt (1988) feel that social contagion (that is, external cues) is an important factor in the assessment phase of the treatment process. By determining the external cues that impact on the client, the counselor can help identify possible pitfalls in the cessation program. The client can consciously choose which coping behaviors have the greatest likelihood of being effective. Once the client has identified external cues and situations that increase the likelihood of smoking, he or she can develop preventive self-adaptive responses to modify the environment or to cope more effectively with the situation. It is important for the client to realize that these external cues change and often require revision throughout the cessation process. Although it is desirable to continue to monitor changes, we have found that noncompliance with instructions to monitor oneself is a common difficulty. Rather than develop a power conflict with the client regarding self-monitoring, we have found it helpful to shift the focus, keep the client busy with other activities such as exercise and diet, and repeat positive affirmations.

It is also important during the assessment process to help the client understand and develop his or her coping skills—that is, how to take direct action to prevent or resist temptation. According to Shiffman (1985), coping is easily assessed through self-reports. Clients can be asked open-ended questions about what they have been doing or saying to themselves to prevent, resist, or recover from temptation. This process not only assesses the coping strategies but also helps educate the client about other possibilities. The Coping With Temptation Inventory (CWTI) is organized by categories of responses, with

specific examples for each type of response. The questionnaire highlights both behavioral and cognitive coping responses, and it provides many helpful suggestions derived from reports of coping by ex-smokers.

Coping strategies are diverse and, when they are assessed, both cognitive and behavioral aspects should be examined. Many clients will favor either a cognitive or a behavioral approach and will utilize it almost exclusively. Helping the client determine his or her dominant coping orientation is helpful because it can be employed throughout the smoking-cessation process, especially during relapse prevention (Donovan & Marlatt, 1988). The counselor can help the client develop his or her repertoire of coping strategies. Through this assessment process, the client can develop a repertoire of possible responses to what are perceived to be difficult or challenging situations.

Interventions

Virtually every procedure imaginable—from talk therapies to behavioral therapies to drug treatments—has been used to beat the smoking habit. Regardless of the strategy, all interventions need to address at least two separate underlying mechanisms: (1) motivation to avoid smoking and (2) coping skills to maintain avoidance. It is also important that successful interventions build on a thorough knowledge of the underlying behavioral, social, and biological mechanisms involved in the development and maintenance of smoking as well as how these mechanisms will interface with interventions. Effective interventions usually involve a combination of approaches, including counseling, psychoeducation, and pharmacological agents. Counselors need to be familiar with each process and able to tailor the treatment process to match the client's needs (Beutler & Clarkin, 1990). The recognition that there needs to be an integrated approach to the cessation process is a recent theme in the literature on this subject (Miller & Heather, 1986). This section describes each of the processes and then provides an integrated case example.

Counseling

In smoking-cessation programs, two separate counseling goals can be identified: (1) attempts to persuade people to quit smoking and (2) attempts to persuade people who have quit smoking to stick to their decision. Shiffman (1985) views the therapeutic task as one of strengthening the client's motivation to change. This process is achieved through a series of steps. The first step is to educate the client about the risks of smoking behavior. Once educated, the client becomes an ally in the cessation process. The actual therapeutic task involves hooking into the client's ambivalent attitude about quitting and heightening his or her desire to stop smoking. Shiffman (1985) believes that the motivational resources that the client utilizes originate in the interactive relationship that develops between counselor and client. The counselor can create an atmosphere in which the client experiences the discomfort of cognitive dissonance (Festinger, 1957) between smoking behavior and pro-health values. Once dissonance is experienced, the client can move forward from contemplating change to com-

mitting to acting. Once the counselor determines that the client has moved into the commitment stage, the next task is to match the client with the appropriate treatment and adequate supports.

Five different smoking-intervention strategies designed to encourage people to quit smoking have been identified in the literature: (1) aversion, (2) self-control, (3) a combination of aversion and self-control, (4) pharmacological approaches, and (5) health education (Bloom, 1988).

Aversion strategies can be grouped into four categories: electric shock, rapid smoking, satiation, and cognitive sensitization. None of these methods has been found to be remarkably effective.

Self-control methods include (1) environmental planning, (2) behavioral programming, and (3) cognitive control. Environmental planning involves helping the client change smoking behaviors, either by altering the circumstances in which smoking occurs or by working with others to reinforce each other's smoking-cessation efforts. In the case of behavioral programming, the smoker institutes a self-directed system of rewards and punishments to facilitate smoking cessation. In the case of cognitive control, the smoker attempts to limit smoking behavior by changing his or her way of thinking about smoking.

The counselor's real work seems to begin after smoking stops. Research indicates that the majority of relapse occurs within the first three months following cessation. Clients need to learn cognitive vigilance as an asset in the cessation process. By learning to recognize the thought processes at work, the client can successfully intervene when faulty thinking occurs. Through psychoeducation, the client can effectively program new cognitive responses.

Counselors need to have an array of skills to help the client. During the assessment phase of the cessation process, the counselor identifies the client's strengths and develops strategies for how these strengths can best be utilized. Additionally, the client's weaknesses and skill deficits are assessed, and remediations are prescribed. In addition to cognitive and behavioral components, some counselors use hypnosis, with good results. Crasilneck (1990) reports a cessation rate of 81 percent through the use of hypnotic techniques after a one-year follow-up. His treatment plan utilizes psychoeducation, hypnosis, and reinforcers meted out by the counselor and by mutual-aid groups.

Pharmacological approaches to smoking cessation are based on the premise that the smoker has become addicted to nicotine. One approach is to provide nicotine to the smoker, mainly in the form of special chewing gum. There is considerable evidence that chewing gum is an effective adjunct in the smoking-cessation program. An aspect of this program that defies logic is that, although cigarettes that contain considerable nicotine are freely available to the public, a physician's prescription is currently needed to purchase nicotine gum. Nicotine supplements have been used to lessen the physical symptoms of withdrawal. Gottlieb, Killen, Marlatt, and Taylor (1987) identified the client's expectations as the determinant factor in the effectiveness of nicotine supplements. Their study questions the effectiveness of nicotine supplements and looks at how the client's expectations actually alter the supplements' perceived effects. Other researchers have been experimenting with transdermal clonidine and transdermal nicotine patches. Although these patches have limited applicability, they have

been shown to be effective in reducing the physical discomforts associated with nicotine withdrawal.

The Food and Drug Administration in 1992 approved several different brands of skin or transdermal nicotine patches. These adhesive pads, about 2 inches square and available by prescription, release a trickle of nicotine through the skin into the bloodstream, thus satisfying the smoker's craving for nicotine. Studies submitted to the FDA indicate that smokers who used nicotine patches for 8 to 12 weeks were about twice as likely to have quit at the end of that period (that is, not to have smoked since the second week of the study) as were those who used dummy patches without nicotine. Quitting rates in different studies ranged from 8 percent to 92 percent for the nicotine-patch users, as compared with 3 percent to 46 percent for those who got dummy patches (Weiss, 1992). Unfortunately, quitting smoking is often the easy part. The more difficult problem is not starting again. Many smokers wonder whether the nicotine patch will conquer smoking permanently. So far, research suggests that those who quit with the help of patches relapse at about the same rate as anyone else. The quitting rates for those who use patches seem to be roughly similar to the rates of those who use nicotine gum. The severity of the side effects in both products is comparable: hiccups, sore throat, and jaw aches for gum; minor skin irritation, insomnia, and occasional nightmares for patches. It is important to note that the patches are relatively ineffective unless they are used in conjunction with a smoking-cessation program that includes counseling, relaxation training, hypnosis, or some other form of behavioral therapy. All manufacturers offer forms of psychological support, such as a toll-free hotline, day-by-day motivational suggestions, audiotapes, and a pamphlet to be given to a friend or spouse that contains hints about how to provide support to the quitter.

Edwards, Murphy, Downs, Ackerman, and Rosenthal (1989) studied the use of antidepressants. In their research, Doxepin was identified as an effective agent both in the precessation process and in the active quitting. Researchers have noticed that, since the symptoms of depression and withdrawal are very similar, treatments for depression are likely to be very helpful during the withdrawal process. More comprehensive research should indicate how antidepressants and other medications can be utilized effectively.

Other Treatment Considerations

Group versus individual treatment.   Most smoking-cessation treatment is provided in small groups of five to ten people. However, there appears to be no evidence that groups are superior to individual treatment. However, many clients who have participated in groups report that the group support was central in achieving and maintaining abstinence. Groups are also more cost-effective than individual sessions. However, there are certain pitfalls in group treatment. First, relapse can sometimes be contagious, especially if those who relapse are vocal or have achieved high informal status in the group. Second, group members sometimes give each other permission to fail. Last, if group members are poorly matched or antagonistic to one another, attendance rates can be poorer than in individual sessions.

Abrupt versus gradual quitting.   We recommend abrupt cessation because it is most congenial with the methods that we have found helpful. We ask smokers to set a quit date and to stop smoking completely on that day. Many smokers will cut down gradually before that day, and some will continue to smoke right up until the last moment. We haven't noticed any difference in outcome as a function of which strategy was used.

Psychoeducation

A psychoeducation model for smoking cessation represents an attempt to encourage smokers to stop smoking and keep from relapsing by using traditional educational approaches, such as curricula that point out the harmful effects of smoking.

Marlatt and Gordon (1985) view smoking cessation as one part of the holistic life-style approach. In their book, they urge both the client and the counselor to view the smoking behavior as part of the individual's total life-style. The program includes four main components.

1. *Learning self-observational skills.*   When clients have a clear understanding of the successive steps that lead to their smoking behavior, two things happen. First, clients are able to ascertain what stressors or external cues precipitate smoking behaviors. By identifying these stressors, clients can then learn which interventions would best alleviate or dissipate their effects, thus enabling the clients to effectively avoid relapse. The individual would also learn to predict what triggers a potential slip. These client self-observation skills are a valuable tool in relapse prevention.

2. *Learning self-efficacy.*   As a learned behavior, self-efficacy is an essential feature of a psychoeducational approach. Brod and Hall (1984) list four components of self-efficacy that are necessary for its successful application.

   a. *Past performance:* What past accomplishments can the client recall that would lead to the assumption that this effort will also succeed? When the client remembers past efficacious behaviors, she or he can then begin to visualize success in the cessation process.

   b. *Vicarious experience:* Does the client know someone who has completed a program and successfully quit? If so, the individual can then affirm that his or her goal can be accomplished and can visualize him- or herself as having achieved it.

   c. *Verbal persuasions:* When the individual is able to recall personal past achievements and can see that others have achieved successful cessation, she or he can better put into service the information presented in the psychoeducational process.

   d. *Recognition of internal cues:* Within the context of a greater sense of one's efficacy, the individual can better recognize his or her own physiologic cues and can then respond accordingly. For example, once the client believes that she or he has the capacity to counter a challenge, there is considerably less resistance to identifying the negative physiologic reactions from smoking.

3. *Understanding coping strategies.*   Another important part of the psychoeducational model is a clear understanding of coping strategies: what they

are and how they can be most effectively utilized. The smoker can also identify which reinforcers are most helpful in situations that call for an immediate coping behavior.

One direct way in which the counselor can utilize the clients' newly acquired coping skills is by providing an interactive format. When the counselor models his or her belief in the clients' ability to successfully reach their goal, clients can then introject the counselor's perception that they can be efficacious in their newly acquired behaviors.

4. *Understanding the cessation process.* Part of the educational process includes the client's developing an understanding of the entire cessation process, including the maintenance of the newly acquired behaviors.

In general, recent studies of smoking-cessation programs suggest that their impact is related to (1) the level of motivation to stop smoking, (2) the development of better physical and psychological well-being, and (3) the achievement of milder smoking habits. People who have better problem-solving skills and who make greater use of self-reward in controlling their own behavior appear to be most successful in smoking cessation.

Systemic Interventions

Economic factors, continuing emphasis on the rights of nonsmokers, and the growth of Employee Assistance Programs (EAPs) have contributed to increased interest in workplace smoking-control programs. The economic factors are apparent. Smokers use significantly more health services, have higher absenteeism rates, and have more accidents at work than do their nonsmoking colleagues. The greatest concentration of programs is to enforce policies that either restrict smoking to certain areas or ban it altogether. Whether these programs actually affect smoking behavior outside the workplace has yet to be studied.

Workplace smoking-control programs usually utilize one or a combination of the following approaches:

1. company policies that restrict or prohibit smoking
2. economic incentives that encourage smokers to quit or provide rewards for nonsmokers
3. sponsorship of smoking-cessation programs, including educational campaigns, self-help programs, referral to community agencies, counseling by staff medical personnel, and smoking-cessation programs

School-Based Smoking Control Programs

The purpose of these programs is to prevent or delay the onset of smoking and decrease the number of students who smoke. These prevention programs have the following primary goals: (1) to educate the students and modify their attitudes about smoking through traditional health-education approaches; (2) to alter social pressures to smoke by increasing skills to resist pressures; (3) to modify the decision-making process of experimental smokers through the development of personal and interpersonal skills; and (4) to modify the con-

sequences of smoking; and (5) to stop smoking via behavioral approaches (Elder & Stern, 1986). Even though programs based on the modification of social factors and those based on dissemination of information on the harmful effects of smoking (including the addictive properties of tobacco) both seem to be effective, programs based on the acquisition of skills are the most effective.

Community-Based Smoking Control Programs

Community programs often use varying combinations of mass media, environmental modifications, group interventions, and one-to-one interventions. The mass-media programs hope to increase the public's awareness of the smoking problem, increase the smokers' desire to make changes in their smoking behaviors, and provide smokers with guidance in quitting, which includes detailed suggestions on how to quit. Many media-based programs have depended on public-service announcements. Recent trends are to use a much broader array of available media, including special television programs, news programs, radio programs, newspapers, billboards, and educational materials, such as pamphlets.

A review of the available literature on smoking indicates that the encouraging effect that smoking advertisements have on smoking behavior is significant and, if it is not countered, is likely to result in continued increases in the number of people who take up smoking and in reinforcement for those who are current smokers. The literature also indicates that community-based smoking-control programs that utilize the media in combination with other approaches are effective in reducing the smoking prevalence and incident rates within a community. If the programs are sustained over time, it is likely that the cessation rate will increase and that fewer people will become smokers.

Physician-Based Smoking-Control Programs

Physicians are in an excellent position to assess a significant portion of the population, and they are also considered to be credible sources of health information. Physician-based smoking-control programs ideally should include: (1) an office environment that supports the delivery of a nonsmoking message to smoking patients, (2) counseling of patients on strategies of quitting, (3) inclusion of smoking on the patient's problem list, (4) distribution of self-help materials, and (5) involvement of office staff in some aspect of the program.

Policy-Based Smoking Control Programs

As mentioned earlier, smoking-prevention and control interventions that are founded on public policy are likely to have the greatest effect because they are population-based and their enforcement is often the responsibility of one or more government agencies. Breslow (1982) identified ten action alternatives that governments could consider as they strive to control the smoking problem. The alternatives are prohibition of cigarettes; restriction of cigarette smoking; reduction in hazardous substances in cigarette smoke; restrictions on advertising cigarettes; public information, education, aid to persons who want to quit smoking; taxation and other economic measures; international cooperation; and

research. When these policy interventions are combined with specific smoking-prevention and cessation interventions, the effect on smoking behavior is significant.

Economy-Based Smoking Control Programs
Although economic interventions are clearly part of policy-based interventions, they are considered separately because of their popularity and use as a means of influencing smoking behavior (Iverson, 1987). Smoking costs the economy billions of dollars each year in health costs.

Treatment Adherence and Relapse Prevention

It is easy for some people to stop smoking. However, it is not these people who usually seek the help of formal treatment programs. The clients of smoking clinics and private practitioners usually represent the more physically and psychologically dependent smokers. For these clients, quitting smoking is often a difficult process that involves readjustment in physical, intrapsychic, and social domains. If smokers fail to acknowledge these potential problems when quitting smoking, they are poorly prepared for the difficulties involved and are at higher risk for relapse. Relapse may occur because: (1) ex-smokers are not aware that the acute discomfort they are experiencing is time limited and fear that they must endure it indefinitely; (2) they believe that the problems they are experiencing are uncommon, and so they relapse because they feel alone and helpless to deal with the problems; and (c) they do not develop appropriate cognitive and behavioral coping strategies (Hall & Hall, 1987).

The difficulties that occur after quitting smoking are many and varied. It is not possible to predict with any certainty who will experience problems or how difficult the course of quitting will be for a given smoker. We do not discuss all the problems with potential quitters before they begin treatment. However, the client should understand the following points: (1) cigarette smoking is an ingrained habit that may have become intertwined in many aspects of his or her life; (2) the client may have become addicted to nicotine; (3) the client can expect that quitting smoking will be a difficult task that may require readjustment in social, emotional, and physical demands; (4) others with the same problems have succeeded; (5) the difficulties that the client experiences are time limited; and (6) effective tools are available to help the client through this period.

Counselors and other health professionals have been effective in helping smokers quit. However, as we said earlier, the problem is that most who quit smoking relapse and break their abstinence. The key is not to help an individual to simply quit but, rather, to maintain long-term abstinence. Many of the same factors that are involved in the cessation phase are involved in the maintenance phase. Social support, for example, can sustain commitment in the face of withdrawal symptoms and assist individuals through potential relapse situations long after cessation is achieved. Mermelstein, Cohen, Lichtenstein, Baer, and Kamarck (1986) conducted research that supported the relationship between

perceived level of support—especially from significant others—and long-term maintenance. McGovern (1984) discovered that the likelihood of relapse is significantly increased if individuals live with family members who smoke. Additional data indicate that high proportions of smokers in social and occupational networks are associated with less successful outcomes.

It is also likely that self-reward strategies that are initially important during early stages of treatment need to continue in some form later in the maintenance process. Individuals might be encouraged to contract formally for tangible self-rewards. These rewards should be realistic and quickly accessible. The rewards have the advantage of increasing commitment to abstinence as well as reducing subjective feelings of deprivation. Self-rewards also allow the individual recognition without depending on social support. Coping skills, as well as biological/pharmacological agents, are also helpful in the prevention of relapse.

Marlatt and Gordon (1980) developed the following list of situations that can result in relapse. It is important for the counselor to prepare the client for alternative responses in each of these situations.

1. Eating is a frequent stimulus for smoking and a prominent antecedent of relapse (Shiffman, 1982). Smoking after meals or with coffee is so common that these occasions must be considered high risks for all smokers.
2. Times of stress or upset are also frequently associated with smoking and relapse. In these situations, the smoker seems to use cigarettes to blunt unpleasant emotions.
3. Alcohol consumption is strongly associated with smoking. Smokers are almost always drinkers, and laboratory experiments have demonstrated that smoking facilitates drinking.
4. Social situations are also common triggers for smoking. In addition to being cued by other smokers, many smokers seem to use smoking to manage feelings of awkwardness in social situations.
5. Boredom is also associated with smoking. Smokers who are bored may see it "as something to do" or may seek the stimulating pharmacological action of nicotine. In our experience, boredom is often used to describe a condition of mild depression.
6. Positive-affect situations are also conducive to smoking. Although smoking is more common when one is in the grip of negative emotions, some smokers are especially likely to smoke when they feel good, claiming that smoking accentuates their positive feeling.
7. Food substitution is another function that cigarettes often serve. Smokers sometimes have a cigarette instead of food. Fear, sometimes justified, of weight gain after quitting often undermines clients' motivations to stay abstinent.

Danaher and Lichtenstein (1978) have also identified the following common problem thoughts that tend to encourage smoking: (1) feeling nostalgic about the old pleasures of smoking; (2) keeping cigarettes around to test oneself; (3) believing that a crisis is an acceptable excuse for a cigarette;

(4) believing that not smoking brings about unwanted changes, such as weight gain, that can be ameliorated only by returning to smoking; and (5) believing that one is unable to quit.

Research seems to support the idea that it is important to help the client plan what he or she is going to do. This proactive versus reactive stance will decrease the likelihood of relapse. Very clear, first-line strategies need to be developed to cope with the temptation to smoke. These should include avoidance, escape, distraction, and delay (Shiffman, Read, Maltese, Rapkin, & Garvik, 1985). Shiffman and colleagues also suggest that clients develop cognitive and behavioral coping responses to counter very specific high-risk situations. Some cognitive procedures are imagery, cognitive restructuring, and self-talk, and some behavioral procedures are physical activity, relaxation, and other substitute behaviors. These suggestions are utilized later in the case example.

Dealing with Slips

If clients do experience a slip, it is important that they do not fall victims to the so-called abstinence violation effect. In this all too common pattern of self-defeatist thinking, a single slip triggers a period of intense self-castigation, depression, and negativity. Thoughts such as "I'm no good; I have no willpower; I wasn't really cured anyway" lead to a decreased sense of self-control, a drop in self-esteem, and further slips until the person abandons all efforts to quit (Marlatt, 1985b).

A slip is basically a two-step process: a smoking-risk situation plus an inadequate coping response. A slip or two on the way to eventual success do not make you a failure. Actually, some psychologists recommend planned slips, or programmed relapse (Marlatt, 1985b). The only real failure that clients can experience is giving up their efforts to quit. It is important to teach them that, if they find themselves slipping, they can catch themselves and then take control again. It is important to have clients accept the fact that they have slipped and allow themselves to return to a nonsmoking state without self-blame. A no-fault approach will increase their chances of ultimate success. We find it helpful to point out to clients that many people who eventually succeed experience many slips on their way to reaching their goal. Slips seldom occur because of physical withdrawal symptoms but, rather because of anxiety, anger, frustration, or depression. This is one of the reasons that we use self-hypnosis and relaxation procedures to help clients gain more self-control and therefore minimize the likelihood of relapse.

In summary, we tend to know more about how to help people quit smoking than we do about preventing relapse. In the future, it will be important to learn more about smoking relapse and how to prevent it, with specific attention to the variables that contribute to relapse and the mechanisms of relapse. It is important again to stress that whatever makes the avoidance of relapse possible must be included in the cessation process, and specific strategies that individuals can rely on during periods in which they experience the urge to resume addictive behavior need to be developed.

Case Example

The following case presents a biopsychosocial approach that tailors treatment to the specific individual involved.*

Jilian is a 42-year-old divorced female with a 25-year history of smoking one and a half packs of cigarettes a day. A detailed assessment, which included background information, a smoking history, a health assessment, and life-style data including early recollections (ER), yielded the following profile. The client was a relatively healthy woman with no concurrent medical problems except for chronic neck pain sustained as a result of a car accident about 12 years before her consultation. Her smoking history was quite unique in that the majority of her smoking occurred at only three times throughout the day: on arising in the morning, on retiring at night, and while engaged in her livelihood as a portrait artist. Furthermore, her smoking was strictly a solitary activity that gave her a feeling of safety and a sense of satisfaction. Unlike the typical smoker, Jilian would absent herself from social situations to smoke and never smoked in the presence of others. None of her friends smoked, and her decision to quit smoking was primarily for health reasons. She reported that smoking seemed to exacerbate her neck pain. In fact, she noted that she had nearly no neck pain during two previous attempts to quit. She had a family history of heart attacks and stroke among both male and female smokers. Her father had been a three-pack-per-day smoker who had died suddenly at 43 of a heart attack. Her mother was a nonsmoker and did not permit smoking inside the house. Jilian recalls that during her parents' marital quarrels, her father would stop fighting abruptly and go outside to smoke. Further inquiry showed that Jilian had learned to "solve" conflicts by "walking out" of a difficult situation and lighting up a cigarette.

Smoking appeared to serve at least two functions for Jilian: first, as a stress reducer and second, as a "trigger" for creative productivity—her painting and artistic efforts. Psychologically, she was an only child and "Daddy's girl." Father was a hard-working and successful businessman with strong perfectionist strivings. He was described as intense, nice, and fun to be around. Mother was described as serious, artistic, and a loner. On the *Kern Lifestyle Scale* (Kern, 1986), Jilian scored highest on perfectionism and lowest on the need to please. Her early recollections suggested that she was guarded and aloof and cordoned herself off from others following conflicts. It also seemed that she utilized withdrawal as a means of controlling others' feelings, as well as her own. She viewed the world as hostile, unpredictable, and unsatisfying.

It is interesting to note that Jilian's smoking behavior occurred in places and situations in which she was withdrawn from others—such as in her art studio—just as it was a general theme throughout her early recollections. She appeared to use smoking as a socially acceptable way of absenting herself from a social group when she became anxious and uncomfortable. And when it was

*From "Hypnosis, Tailoring, and Multimodal Treatment," by L. Sperry and J. Carlson. In *Individual Psychology, 45*(4). Copyright © 1990 by The North American Society of Adlerian Psychology and the University of Texas Press.

suggested that perhaps she feared that she might not be able to control herself or others if she was successful in quitting smoking, a recognition reflex was elicited.

On the basis of this information, a treatment program was tailored to her needs. The program consisted of four interventions: education, diet and exercise, behavioral change strategies, and hypnosis. The reader is referred to Carlson (1989) for a detailed description of this treatment program. A handout (see the Appendix at the end of this chapter) provided Jilian with information on smoking cessation. It was recommended that Jilian make diet changes to influence the acid-alkaline balance in her body. Nicotine is a very strong alkaline substance, and if Jilian's acidity levels rose, her alkaline levels would need to be changed to maintain a pH, or acid/alkaline balance. (If her acidity levels rose, her alkaline level would drop and she would crave cigarettes.) By making dietary changes, it was possible to minimize changes in the pH balance. This was done by getting her to eat more fruits and vegetables; stay away from meat, eggs, and alcohol; eliminate refined-sugar products; and decrease the use of stimulants. It was further suggested that she increase her intake of juices and water.

On the behavioral level, it was suggested that Jilian practice deep diaphragmatic breathing and muscle relaxation each hour. A daily exercise program was developed to improve her health, burn off calories, and give her something to occupy her time. She decided that walking and biking would be good for her and that she would rotate these activities on a daily basis. It was further suggested that she make an appointment to get her teeth cleaned in order to get rid of any residual tobacco stain or taste so she would have a fresh, clean mouth. This was to be followed by regular brushing.

She was advised to break up the routines in the places where she smoked and to plan other ways to use her time when rising, retiring, and while engaged in painting. It was further suggested that she plan to keep very busy during the following few weeks and that she increase her daily activity patterns. She should take walks, shower, go to church, bicycle, pray, swim, make love, play tennis, and engage in activities that would keep her hands busy. She was asked to think of times when it was going to be difficult for her not to smoke and to schedule things that she could do instead. Since Jilian used smoking primarily to reduce stress—particularly interpersonal stress—and to induce creativity and productivity, an important behavioral change strategy was to find more effective substitutes for stress reduction and creativity. She recalled that taking a walk through a small horticultural park or looking through a particular art portfolio seemed to have a similar effect of inducing a creative mood. She also decided to join two of her friends for an aerobics class and lunch, thinking that these activities would be interpersonal stress reducers. An assertiveness class was also suggested, as was chewing sugarless gum as further means of reducing her discomfort when she was with people.

A mainstay of this two-session treatment program was the hypnotic suggestions. These were of two types: positive affirmations and self-hypnosis. Jilian was given a sheet with six affirmations tailored to her underlying motivations. She was asked to write out each of these affirmations five times in the morning and then to repeat them aloud to herself. The affirmations were:

"Taking care of myself physically is important to me. I know I will live a longer and a more satisfying life."

"I have more energy and less pain than I ever had before. I enjoy life and I'm glad to be here."

"I have no habits that control or influence me in any harmful way. I am in control of myself and everything I do. I always do what is best for me, myself, and my future."

"All of my senses are clear and alive. I am more productive and creative than when I was a smoker."

"I give myself permission to relax, feel good, breathe deeply and fully, and enjoy being a healthy nonsmoker at all times and in all circumstances."

"People enjoy being around me, and I like being around others. I have self-confidence and self-respect. I like myself, and it shows!"

The self-hypnosis component began near the end of the first session. Standard breathing, relaxation, and guided-imagery techniques were utilized, along with directives for smoking cessation. The induction was audiotaped, and Jilian was given a copy of the tape for personal use outside the session. She was told to listen to the tape at least once a day for at least the next two weeks, at a time when she could be without interruptions. This was used to reinforce what she had learned during the sessions. The following is the script of the self-hypnosis tailored to Jilian's situation.

Hypnosis Script

Begin to become aware of your breathing . . . breathe slowly and deeply . . . breathe freely and easily . . . sit back comfortably in your chair, close your eyes, and let yourself begin to relax . . . feel your muscles relaxing and your mind relaxing . . . sitting quietly and peacefully, more at ease . . . your body is slowing down . . . time is slowing down . . . there is lots and lots of time . . . lots and lots of time . . . we're in no hurry . . . you feel more at ease, at peace with your surroundings, at peace with yourself . . . so peaceful, relaxed, calm, and tranquil . . . as you breathe easily and gently, you feel yourself relaxing more and more . . . calmness is present throughout your body and your mind . . . calmness, peace, and relaxation are spreading throughout every part of your body and your mind as you feel more and more relaxed . . . you feel as if you're floating along on a soft, soft cloud . . . floating gently and easily . . . so relaxed and calm and comfortable . . . soft, gentle, quiet, peaceful, and restful relaxation . . . as your mind and your body are relaxing more and more . . . your thoughts are fading away . . . a feeling of well-being now exists, as though all of your cares have been rolled away . . . breathe peacefully and comfortably and imagine your worries, uncomfortable thoughts, and problems being carried away with each breath . . . stop worrying, being anxious, being afraid, being tense, being upset and frustrated . . . instead you feel calm, free, at ease, confident, and peaceful . . . allow any distractions, whether thoughts or outside noises to drift away . . . imagine clouds drifting smoothly across the sky, carrying with them all distractions, all worries, all uncomfortable thoughts and problems . . . allow stress, tension, worry, and anxiety to float away as clouds with each breath you take . . . allow them to drift easily and effortlessly away . . . feel your pressures disappearing,

drifting easily and effortlessly away . . . now imagine yourself at the top of a large hill . . . I'm going to count backwards from 10, and I want you to imagine yourself going down the hill . . . as you ease down, you will move further and further into a deeper, more comfortable state . . . when you reach the bottom you will find yourself in a special place . . . that's the place, whether it's real or imaginary, where you are peaceful and comfortable . . . whether it's by the sea, on a mountain top, near a brook, in a meadow . . . wherever it is that you are peaceful and comfortable . . . breathe in slowly and deeply as I begin to count: 10, deeper and deeper; 9, 8, feel yourself easing into deeper and deeper relaxation; 7, 6, a deeper relaxed state; 5, 4, breathe in the clean, fresh air as you feel a healthier, happier person; 3, 2, you are deeper and deeper . . . feel yourself fully relaxed as if a cloud of relaxation has covered you; 1 . . . now imagine yourself deeply relaxed and deeply alive and aware in your special place . . . breathe in the clean and fresh air . . . notice the colors, scenery, noises, smells, your good feelings . . . imagine them on a canvas now in front of you . . . feel how warm you feel. Warmth has spread throughout your body . . . such a pleasant experience . . . notice how good you feel and how good your body can feel . . . you can be calm, relaxed, and feel good like this whenever you want . . . whenever you feel tense, you will hear the words "calm and relaxed and peaceful . . . calm and relaxed and peaceful" and they will trigger this good feeling for you . . . the quality of your life depends on what you do and think . . . smoking is a poison to your physical health and to your creativity . . . therefore, make a private commitment to be healthier and more creative . . . smoking is a poison to your body and to your mind . . . therefore make a private commitment to be healthy and more creative . . . raise your finger once you've made this commitment . . . each day this commitment becomes stronger . . . every day, in every way, your commitment is stronger and stronger . . . you don't ever want to say to yourself when you die that you didn't live your life well, that you wished that you would have quit smoking . . . when you learned to smoke you had to train your body to really take it and then want it and then need it . . . feel how it was . . . really experience it . . . you learned that smoking gave you a way to get away from other people when conflict and bad feelings came up . . . experience that now . . . feel how it was . . . starting today you are going to live your life fully . . . you are going to be comfortable and charming around other people . . . let the beautiful person you are fully emerge . . . the message now is going through all your mind and all throughout your body, on down into your smoking arm and your smoking hand, programming all of you: no smoking . . . your whole system is now programmed . . . you are now a nonsmoker . . . you are now a nonsmoker . . . you are now a nonsmoker . . . you want to live and will choose to live well . . . when you have the urge to smoke, breathe deeply and say to yourself, "I have a commitment with myself to be a nonsmoker and live well . . . I have a commitment with myself to be a nonsmoker and live well . . . I have a commitment with myself to be a nonsmoker and live well" . . . let these words go deep . . . deep . . . deep . . . into your unconscious mind . . . so they will be there when you need them . . . breathe in now and breathe out . . . nothing will get in your way . . . you are free from tension, worry, disruption, and smoking . . . you are free in your life works . . . and you are in control.

Summary

Smoking cessation is a process, not a discrete event as previously assumed. When the client is aware of the steps involved in the process, she or he can be a more effective agent of change. This awareness also predisposes the client to be more efficacious in the cessation program.

Once the client seeks out a cessation program, the counselor makes a thorough assessment of the client's current level of stress and of the coping skills the client has within his or her repertoire. This allows the counselor to understand how to better assist the client.

A number of treatment modalities were examined in this chapter. Counseling, when paired with other interventions, has been an effective treatment option. Psychoeducation plays a very broad part in the cessation process, since one prerequisite for successful cessation is the understanding of the health aspects of the addiction process.

It is important to note that although virtually anyone can and at some point does quit, the maintenance of cessation is the heart of success in the smoker's efforts to stop. Relapse prevention therefore is the essential component in achieving this end. Relapse prevention requires a thorough initial assessment, a solid understanding of the psychoeducational process, and a tailored treatment plan based on the initial assessment. A counselor's careful work in the relapse prevention stage of treatment ensures that the maintenance of cessation has a solid chance.

Another important aspect of relapse prevention is the clients' understanding of their role in the smoking process and their ability to be effective agents of change. Current thinking has shifted away from an acceptance of the smoker as a victim of the habit and toward an understanding of the smoker as capable of learning and incorporating self-management skills. With this new perspective on the cessation process and the client's awareness of and active participation in it, we remain hopeful that future "stop smoking" programs will enjoy a high level of success.

Resources

Organizations
- *Action on Smoking and Health (ASH), 2013 H Street, NW, Washington, DC 20006. (202) 659-4310.* This is the leading antismoking consumer group in the United States. The organization provides support for antismoking activists and seeks to promote legal changes that will protect the nonsmoker's right to breathe fresh air. ASH also sells buttons and bumperstrips with antismoking messages and a variety of NO SMOKING signs. The ASH newsletter is one of the best available sources of current news on smoking and health and antismoking activism.
- *American Cancer Society, 4 West 35th Street, New York, NY 10001. (212) 736-3030.* Local affiliates of the American Cancer Society sponsor a four-session stop-smoking program called Fresh Start. Sessions last one hour each

and extend over a two-week period. Sessions focus on behavior modification, goal setting, mastering of obstacles, and social support. The American Cancer Society also publishes a free handbook for potential quitters, the *I Quit Kit,* which is available from your local chapter (consult your telephone directory for the address and phone number) or from their national headquarters at the address above.

- *American Heart Association, 7320 Greenville Avenue, Dallas, TX 75231.* The AHA offers a wide and varied range of services, which include educational modules, on-site workshops, and the coordination of self-help cessation programs.

- *American Lung Association, 1740 Broadway, New York, NY 10019. (212) 315-8700.* The ALA offers workplace smoking-cessation programs and a family-oriented program that emphasizes prevention, psychoeducation, and cessation. The ALA offers a variety of literature designed to educate the individual as well as provide a useful adjunct to smoking-cessation programs. The American Lung Association sponsors stop-smoking groups in most cities. It also publishes an excellent guide to quitting, *Freedom from Smoking for You and Your Family.* This book guides readers through a step-by-step, 20-day program that leads to quitting and provides guidelines for remaining a nonsmoker. The book is available from your local chapter of the American Lung Association (consult your telephone directory for the address and phone number) or from their national headquarters at the address above.

- *The Breathe-Free Plan to Stop Smoking, Narcotics Education, Inc., 6830 Laurel Street, NW, Washington, DC 20012.* Many local affiliates of the Seventh-Day Adventist Church run a highly recommended program that is usually led by a pastor-physician team. The Breathe-Free Plan to Stop Smoking is based on motivation, life-style modification, values clarification, modeling, visualization, affirmation, positive thinking, and self-rewards. There is also an optional nondenominational spiritual component. The plan consists of eight sessions that take place over three weeks, with periodic phone contacts for one year thereafter. Prospective group members are invited to attend the first two sessions before making the decision to register for the remainder of the course. During the third week, a graduation ceremony is held. Successful quitters receive a BNS (Bachelor of Nonsmoking) degree during the third week. MNS (Master of Nonsmoking) degrees are awarded at six months, and DNS (Doctor of Nonsmoking) degrees at twelve months.

- *Center for Disease Control, Office of Smoking and Health, Park Building, Room 1-10, 5600 Fisher's Lane, Rockville, MD 20857.* This federal agency offers both scientific and technical information about smoking. With an extensive data base of resources that is quite comprehensive, the CEC is an excellent resource center.

- *National Cancer Institute, Smoking, Tobacco and Cancer Program, Executive Plaza North Room 320, 9000 Rockville Plaza, Bethesda, MD 20892.* STCP offers various intervention strategies (workplace, self-help, psychoeducation, and one-on-one cessation) as well as preventive efforts.

- *National Clearinghouse on Alcohol and Drug Information, P.O. Box 2345, Rockville, MD 20852.* This is a resource service for the clinician. This group

pioneered behavioral/cognitive research on cessation, and its current research focuses on relapse prevention.

- *National Institute on Drug Abuse.* The National Institute on Drug Abuse has published excellent resource materials on cigarette smoking. Titles, editors or authors, and addresses at which to obtain these materials are given in the "Publications" section that follows. Descriptions of monograph content in quotation marks are taken from National Institute on Drug Abuse publications. While supplies last, copies of NIDA monographs may be obtained free from the National Clearinghouse for Drug Abuse Information (NCDAI) at Room 10A-43, 5600 Fishers Lane, Rockville, MD 20857. Copies may also be purchased from the U.S. Government Printing Office (GPO), Washington, DC, or the National Technical Information Service (NTIS), Dept. of Commerce, 5285 Port Royal Rd., Springfield, VA 22161. (703) 487-4650.

- *Smokers Anonymous, P.O. Box 25335, West Los Angeles, CA 90025. (212) 474-8997.* This group provides information on starting your own support group. They will also let you know if there is a Smokers Anonymous group in your area. Write to them at the above address, enclosing a self-addressed stamped envelope.

Publications

- Grabowski, J., & Bell, C. S. (Eds.). (1984). *Measurement in the Analysis and Treatment of Smoking Behavior.* GPO Stock No. 017-0240-01181-9, NTIS Publication No. 84-145-184. "An attempt to delineate measures for analysis of smoking behavior in research and treatment settings." The chapter by Benowitz on biochemical verification of abstinence and smoking is excellent.

- Grabowski, J., & Hall, S. M. (Eds.). (1985). *Pharmacological Adjuncts in Smoking Cessation.* NIDA Research Monograph No. 64, DHHS, Washington, DC. This is a review of smoking treatment and related research issues, using pharmacological adjuncts to smoking treatment. Focus is on nicotine replacement therapy.

- Jarvik, M. E., Cullen, J. W., Gritz, E. R., Vogt, T. M., & West, L. J. (Eds.). (1977). *Research on Smoking Behavior.* GPO Stock No. 017-024-00694, NTIS Publication No. 276 353/AS. "Includes epidemiology, etiology, consequences of use, and approaches to behavioral change." This publication contains useful chapters on smoking and disease (Van Lancker) and sociocultural factors in smoking (Reeder). The treatment section is now a bit outdated.

- Krasnegor, N. A. (Ed.). (1979). *Cigarette Smoking as a Dependence Process.* GPO Stock No. 017-024-00895-8, NTIS Publication No. 297 721/AS. "Discusses factors involved in the onset, maintenance, and cessation of the cigarette smoking habit." The publication discusses tobacco use from a psychopharmacologic perspective.

- The Surgeon General's Report. Each year, the Office on Smoking and Health produces *The Health Consequences of Smoking: A Report of the Surgeon General.* The content depends on the theme of the report for that year. Topics in recent years have been the health consequences of smoking for women (1980); health consequences related to changes in cigarette constituents, with emphasis on low-tar, low-nicotine cigarettes (1981); the relationship between

cigarette smoking and cancer (1982); and cigarette smoking and cardiovascular disease (1983). The 1980 report is noteworthy for its excellent summary of the etiology, demographics, and descriptive data on smoking in women. It is also a good review of treatment methods to that time. Sound reviews of treatment outcome are also found in the 1982 and 1983 reports. These latter two reports are especially good sources for preparing materials on the health consequences of smoking. These reports are usually out of print within a year or so of their publication. However, most university libraries should be able to obtain back copies.

Publications: Pamphlets

Several government agencies have produced pamphlets that contain information about the effects of smoking and quitting or describe self-managed quitting programs. A list of them follows. Those published by the American Cancer Society, the American Heart Association, and the American Lung Association can be obtained from the local offices of these organizations. The NIH publication can be ordered either from the U.S. Government Printing Office in Washington, DC, or from the address listed.

- *Cigarette Smoking: The Facts about Your Lungs.* (1975). American Lung Association.
- *Clearing the Air. A Guide to Quitting Smoking.* (1982). (NIH Publication No. 82-1647). Office of Cancer Communications, National Cancer Institute, Bethesda, MD 20205.
- *How to Stop Smoking!* (1969). American Heart Association.
- *It's a Matter of Life and Breath.* (undated). American Lung Association.
- *Me Quit Smoking? How?* (1970). American Lung Association.
- *Quitter's Guide: 7 Day Plan to Help You Stop Smoking Cigarettes.* (1978). American Cancer Society.
- *What Everyone Should Know about Smoking and Heart Disease.* (1976). American Heart Association, Communications Division.

References

ABELIN, T., Buehler, A., Muller, P., Vesanen, K., & Imhof, P. R. (1989). Controlled trial of transdermal nicotine patch in tobacco withdrawal. *Lancet*, 7–9.

ASHTON, H., & Stepney, R. (1982). *Smoking psychology and pharmacology*. London: Tavistock.

BAER, J. S., & Lichtenstein, E. (1985). Classification and prediction of smoking relapse episodes: An exploration of individual differences. In G. A. Marlatt & J. Gordon (Eds.), *Relapse prevention: Maintenance strategies in the treatment of addictive behaviors*. New York: Guilford Press, pp. 189–213.

BANDURA, A. (1977). Self-efficacy: Towards a unifying theory of behavioral change. *Psychological Review, 84,* 191–215.

BECONA, E., Frojan, M. J., & Lista, M. J. (1988). Comparison between two self-efficacy scales in maintenance of smoking cessation. *Psychological Reports, 62,* 359–362.

BEUTLER, L. E., & Clarkin, J. F. (1990). *Systematic treatment selection*. New York: Brunner/Mazel.

BLOOM, B. L. (1988). Health psychology: A psychosocial perspective. Englewood Cliffs, NJ: Prentice-Hall.

BRESLOW, L. (1982). Control of cigarette smoking from a public policy perspective. *Annual Review of Public Health, 3,* 129–151.

BROD, M., & Hall, S. M. (1984). Joiners and non-joiners in smoking treatment: A comparison of psycho-social variables. *Addictive Behaviors, 9,* 217–221.

CARLSON, J. (1989). Brief therapy for health promotion. *Individual Psychology, 45* (1 & 2), 220–229.

COHEN, S., Kamarck, T., & Mermelstein, R. (1983). A global measure of perceived stress. *Journal of Health and Social Behavior, 24,* 384–396.

CRASILNECK, H. B. (1990). Hypnotic techniques for smoking control and psychogenic impotence. *American Journal of Clinical Hypnosis, 32,* 147–153.

DANAHER, B. G., & Lichtenstein, E. (1978). *Become an ex-smoker.* Engelwood Cliffs, NJ: Prentice-Hall.

DAVIS, J. R., & Glaros, A. G. (1986). Relapse prevention and smoking cessation. *Addictive Behaviors, 11,* 105–114.

DONOVAN, D. M., & Marlatt, G. A. (1988). *Assessment of addictive behaviors.* New York: Guilford Press.

EDWARDS, N. B., Murphy, J. K., Downs, A. D., Ackerman, B. J., & Rosenthal, T. L. (1989). Doxepin as an adjunct to smoking cessation: A double blind pilot study. *American Journal of Psychiatry, 146* (3), 373–376.

ELDER, J., & Stern, R. (1986). The ABCs of adolescent smoking prevention: An environment and skills model. *Health Education Quarterly, 13* (2), 181–192.

FESTINGER, L. (1957). *A theory of cognitive dissonance.* Stanford, CA: Stanford University Press.

GOTTLIEB, A. M., Killen, J. D., Marlatt, G. A., & Taylor, C. B. (1987). Psychological and pharmacological influences in cigarette smoking. *Journal of Consulting and Clinical Psychology, 55,* 606–608.

HALL, S. M., and Hall, R. G. (1987). Treatment of cigarette smoking. In J. A. Blumenthal & D. C. McKee (Eds.), *Applications in behavioral medicine and health psychology: A clinician's sourcebook.* Sarasota, FL: Professional Resource Exchange, pp. 301–323.

IVERSON, D. C. (1987). Smoking control programs: Premises and promises. *American Journal of Health Promotion, 1* (3), 16–30.

KERN, R. M. (1986). *Lifestyle scale.* Coral Springs, FL: CMTI Press.

LEDERMAN, S., & Scheiderman, P. (1986). *If you smoke, please try quitting.* National City, CA: Learning Process Center, San Diego.

LEVENTHAL, H., & Cleary, P. D. (1980). The smoking problem: A review of the research and theory in behavioral role modification. *Psychological Bulletin, 88,* 370–405.

LICHTENSTEIN, E., & Mermelstein, R. (1982). Helping your partner quit smoking: A manual for the Oregon Smoking Control Program. Unpublished manuscript. University of Oregon Psychology Department, Eugene, Oregon.

McGOVERN, P. (1984). Two statistical analysis procedures applied to multivariate smoking cessation data. Unpublished doctoral dissertation. Iowa State University, Ames.

McINTYRE, K., Mermelstein, R., & Lichtenstein, E. (1982). Counselor manual for the Oregon Smoking Control Program. Unpublished manuscript. University of Oregon Psychology Department, Eugene, Oregon.

MARLATT, G. A. (1985a). Cognitive factors in the relapse process. In G. A. Marlatt, & J. R. Gordon (Eds.), *Relapse prevention: Maintenance strategies in the treatment of addictive behaviors.* New York: Guilford Press.

MARLATT, G. A. (1985b). Cognitive assessment and intervention procedures for relapse prevention. In G. A. Marlatt, & J. R. Gordon (Eds.), *Relapse prevention: Maintenance strategies in the treatment of addictive behaviors.* New York: Guilford Press.

MARLATT, G. A., & Gordon, J. R. (1980). Determinants of relapse: Implications for the maintenance of behavior change. In P. O. Davidson, & S. M. Davidson (Eds.), *Behavioral medicine: Changing health lifestyles.* New York: Brunner/Mazel.

MARLATT, G. A., & Gordon, J. R. (1985). *Relapse prevention: Maintenance strategies in the treatment of addictive behaviors.* New York: Guilford Press.

MERMELSTEIN, R., Cohen, S., Lichtenstein, E., Baer, J. S., & Kamarck, T. (1986). Social support and smoking cessation and maintenance. *Journal of Counseling and Clinical Psychology, 54,* 447–453.

MILLER, W. R., & Heather, N. (1986). *Treating addictive behaviors.* New York: Guilford Press.

NEY, T., & Gale, E. (Eds.). (1989). *Smoking and human behavior.* New York: Wiley.

PERLMUTTER, J. (1986). *Kick it! Stop smoking in five days.* Los Angeles: H. P. Books.

POMERLEAU, O. F., & Pomerleau, C. S. (1989). A biobehavioral perspective on smoking. In T. Ney & A. Gale (Eds.), *Smoking and human behavior.* New York: Wiley.

SCHACHTER, S. (1978). Pharmacological and psychological determinants of smoking. In R. E. Thornton (Ed.), *Smoking behaviour: Physiological and psychological influences.* Edinburgh: Churchill Livingstone.

SHIFFMAN, S. (1982). Relapse following smoking cessation: A situational analysis. *Journal of Consulting and Clinical Psychology, 50,* 71–86.

SHIFFMAN, S. (1985). Behavioral assessment. In G. A. Marlatt & J. R. Gordon (Eds.), *Relapse prevention: Maintenance strategies in the treatment of addictive behaviors.* New York: Guilford Press, pp. 139–187.

SHIFFMAN, S., Read, L., Maltese, J., Rapkin, D., & Garvik, M. E. (1985). Preventing relapse in ex-smokers: A self-management approach. In G. A. Marlatt, & J. R. Gordon (Eds.), *Relapse prevention: Maintenance strategies in the treatment of addictive behaviors.* New York: Guilford Press, pp. 472–520.

SHUMAKER, S. A., & Grunberg, N. E. (Eds.). (1986). Proceedings of the National Working Conference on Smoking Relapse. *Health Psychology, 5,* 1–2.

SNYDER, J. J. (1989). *Health psychology and behavioral medicine.* Englewood Cliffs, NJ: Prentice-Hall.

SPENCE, W. R. (1987). *The ABC's of smoking.* Waco, TX: Health Edco Inc.

SPERRY, L., & Carlson, J. (1990). Hypnosis, tailoring and multimodal treatment. *Individual Psychology, 46* (4), 459–465.

SYME, S. L., & Alcalay, R. (1982). Control of cigarette smoking from a social perspective. *Annual Review of Public Health, 3,* 179–199.

TOMKINS, S. (1966). Psychological model for smoking behavior. *American Journal of Public Health* (supplement), *56,* 17–20.

WEISS, R. (1992). Update on nicotine patches: For some it may help. *New York Times,* April 8, p. B9.

WOJCIK, J. V. (1988). Social learning predictors of the avoidance of smoking relapse. *Addictive Behaviors, 13,* 177–180.

Appendix to Chapter 4: Smoking-Cessation Prescriptions

1. Physical Dimension (for two weeks minimum)

Diet modification:	More sunflower seeds
	More fruits and vegetables
	Less meats, eggs, alcohol
	Less refined-sugar products
	Less stimulant usage
Fluids:	Eight glasses of water or juice each day
Vitamin C:	
(sodium ascorbate)	One 500-mg capsule every 3 to 4 hours, i.e., 2000 mg per day. (*Note:* Do not follow this prescription if you have a problem with sodium intake—e.g., cardiovascular disease or edema). An alternative: 100 or 300 mg of Acerola Plus (chewable)
Vitamin B complex:	One high potency per day
Deep breathing:	Once every hour and as needed
Muscle relaxation:	Once every hour and as needed
Meditative/self-hypnotic exercise:	Once per day and as needed
Walking:	One to two times per day. Vigorous exercise (if medically indicated) once per day

2. Behavioral Dimension

• Brush your teeth and use mouthwash at least three times per day—after awakening, after every meal, and as the last thing before retiring. Make an appointment to have your teeth cleaned to get rid of any residual tobacco stain and taste.

• Avoid sitting in chairs where you customarily would smoke. Get rid of reminders! Ashtrays, lighters, and certainly all cigarettes!

- Change your daily routine, being certain to be busy at those times when you would ordinarily light up. Substitute a healthy activity, such as exercise, relaxation, and so on, for those time periods previously occupied with smoking.
- If necessary, avoid as much as possible the presence of people who smoke, especially those who disapprove of quitting or who are likely to tempt and tease you. Try to increase your time with nonsmokers if possible.
- Increase your daily-activity pattern. Take a lot of walks, showers, go to church, bicycle, pray, swim, make love, play tennis. Engage in activities that keep your hands busy, if necessary.
- Write down at the end of the day (and during the day if you can) about how it was for you today—on your job, at home, at the office or school—and how it was for your hands, your lungs, and mouth to be breaking the association with cigarettes. Record any "withdrawal side effects" *if* they occur and how you dealt with them. Watch out for overeating in particular. Record associations that might remind you of smoking.
- If you feel it would be helpful, set up a program of intermediate rewards (e.g., after one week, three weeks, six weeks, three months) and a big reward to be received at the end of six months and/or one year.

3. *Psychological Dimension*
- Read and reread information about smoking cessation and healthful living daily—at least 15 minutes per day.
- Estimate the number of cigarettes you have smoked in your life, the amount of money you have spent thus far, and project how many cigarettes you will smoke and how much money you will spend if you live to be 70 years old and continue to smoke at your present rate. Share this information at the next meeting.
- On a *daily* basis, remind yourself of your motives with regard to "giving up" smoking. *Remember*—it is *your decision.* Take responsibility for yourself! YOU ARE NOT SO MUCH QUITTING BUT CHOOSING NOT TO SMOKE. Your choice is not out of fear but out of love—love of those who love you and a healthy love of yourself. Your doctor or family is not making you quit. You are the one who has decided not to smoke for your own self-motivated reasons.
- Also, remember: you are not taking something away from your life (e.g., smoking). Rather, you are adding something to your life—a new dimension of self-control. Positive motivation (e.g., an attitude of self-mastery) will be much more effective than negative motivation (e.g., an attitude of self-denial or quitting out of fear of disease).
- Pick out at least one or two friends or family members whom you feel you can count on to be supportive and encouraging in your decision to quit. Ask them if you can call them if you feel you need support.
- ANTICIPATE STRESS PERIODS by having stress-reduction strategies ready for implementation at all times. Do not undertake any additional stress load during the next few weeks if you don't have to. Do not use stress as an excuse to go back to smoking. That is a game!
- Remember, each stress period will pass. Wait it out. It will subside. Each time

you persist through such a stress period, it will leave you stronger, so that you can handle any future stress periods that may arise. Eventually, the stress periods will become farther and farther apart.

- Focus on the quality of your life. Clarify your values and priorities, attitudes, and beliefs. Your decision to not smoke will ideally be made and reinforced in the context of an awareness of self-worth and meaning and purpose in your life.

- Choose positive attitudes—not only about freedom from cigarettes but about all aspects of your life. Let yourself experience a sense of vitality and zest with everything that you do, think, and say. Do not allow yourself to experience negativity for any prolonged period of time. Generate high amounts of positive energy doing things you enjoy—provided they do not entail health risk. Increase your enjoyment of life as much as possible. *Your attitude is the most important and the most powerful tool you have to effectively give up smoking for all time.*

5

Drug and Alcohol Abuse

Reality is a crutch for people who can't cope with drugs.
Lily Tomlin

Excessive use of alcohol or other drugs can be considered a health-compromising behavior, even when the pattern of use falls short of physical addiction. In today's society, millions of people exhibit problems related to substance use. These people need and deserve assistance, whether or not they are willing to describe themselves as "alcoholics" or "addicts." When a drug or alcohol issue becomes part of the health-counseling process, the important questions to be asked involve what effects the substance is having on the person's life and what can be done to resolve the problems at hand. Obviously, the answers to these questions will vary widely from person to person. No two individuals can possibly display the same collection of problems and life experiences, so no two people can possibly have identical treatment needs. The generalized, lock-step treatment programs that are frequently offered to substance-abusing clients need to be replaced by approaches that focus on individual needs and recognize the degree to which substance abuse is multivariate in nature.

A Biopsychosocial Approach to Substance Abuse

A biopsychosocial approach recognizes the complexity of the issue of substance abuse. Each client who develops a problem related to drugs or alcohol does so because of a combination of biological, social, and psychological factors. There is strong evidence that genetic factors may increase an individual's degree of susceptibility to alcohol problems (Department of Health and Human Services, 1987; Goodwin, 1984; Goodwin et al., 1973) and weaker evidence of a genetic role in the abuse of other drugs (Crabbe, McSwigan, & Belknap, 1985), but substance use behaviors are also affected by cultural, environmental, interpersonal, and intrapersonal factors (Leigh, 1985). Consider, for example, the array of psychosocial factors that add to the risk of substance abuse among young people. Newcomb, Maddahian, and Bentler (1986) identified a number of risk factors associated with drug use or abuse among adolescents, including low grades, lack of religiosity, early alcohol use, low self-esteem, psychopathology, poor relationships with parents, lack of social conformity, a tendency toward sensation seeking, and perceptions that drugs are used widely by peers and adults. Jessor and Jessor (1977) found that adolescents who exhibited a proneness toward substance abuse and other problem behaviors were identifiable by the following factors: a low value placed on academic recognition, a high value placed on independence, low expectations for academic recognition, a high tolerance for deviance, a perception of being more strongly influenced by peers than by parents, and actual participation in other problem behaviors. Similarly, Hawkins and Catalano (1987) stated that the factors increasing the likelihood that adolescents will abuse drugs include a family history of alcoholism or drug use; poor family-management practices; early antisocial behavior; academic failure beginning in the late elementary school grades; a low degree of commitment to education; and general alienation, rebelliousness, and association with drug-using peers. Vaillant (1983) found that, among adult males with alcohol problems, the most predictive factors were family history of alcoholism and

ethnicity (being members of cultures that encouraged intoxication). A sub-stance-abuse problem exhibited by any one individual is clearly affected by the interaction among biological, social, and psychological risk factors.

> It may be that cultural factors exert their greatest influence on the initial decision to experiment with a particular substance. Biological factors may be seen to account for relatively more variance in determining continuation of use and in the transition from use to abuse. Here is where genetic differences in drug sensitivity and metabolism, the development of tolerance, conditioned or otherwise, abstinence phenomena, and the reinforcing properties of the drug may play a critical role. Finally, psychosocial and environmental factors may be most critical in the determination of cessation and relapse (Galizio & Maisto, 1985, p. 428).

If the etiology of substance-abuse problems is complex and highly individualized, treatment approaches must take this variability into account. Lewis, Dana, and Blevins (1988, p. 4) present the following general guidelines for an individualized counseling process:

1. View substance-abuse problems on a continuum from nonproblematic to problematic use, rather than as an either/or situation.
2. Provide treatment that is individualized, both in goals and in methods.
3. Use methods and approaches that enhance each client's sense of self-efficacy.
4. Provide multidimensional treatment that focuses on the social and environmental aspects of long-term recovery.
5. Support selection of the least intrusive treatment possible for each client.
6. Remain open to new methods and goals as research findings become available.
7. Be sensitive to the varying needs of diverse client populations.

The health-counseling model suggests that health and illness should be considered along a continuum between optimal health and serious illness. In a similar fashion, substance-abuse problems should also be considered in terms of a continuum rather than in terms of a dichotomous classification. An attempt to make an either/or diagnosis of alcoholism or addiction risks oversimplification and makes appropriate treatment planning difficult. Regarding alcoholism, for instance:

> Most scientific authorities in the field of alcoholism now concur that the construct of alcoholism is most accurately construed as a multivariate syndrome. That is, there are multiple patterns of dysfunctional alcohol use that occur in multiple types of personalities, with multiple combinations of adverse consequences, with multiple prognoses, that may require different types of treatment interventions (Pattison & Kaufman, 1982, p. 13).

Abuse of other drugs presents an equally complex picture. "It is now generally accepted that nonmedical drug users comprise a great diversity of individuals who are drug dependent in different ways and degrees, use drugs to meet different needs, have different socioeconomic backgrounds, are of both sexes, and represent a wide range of ages, races, and ethnic groups" (Brill, 1981, pp. 5–6).

Dependence on a dichotomous classification tends to disguise individual

differences and has led many clinicians to believe that one course of treatment could be appropriate for the large number of people who share the same diagnosis. This disease-focused approach assumes a commonality that may not in fact exist and that makes early intervention at the level of risk reduction difficult to accomplish. Traditional treatments were designed for people who were clustered toward the extreme end of the continuum: those with obvious drug or alcohol dependence. With few alternatives available, people with minor or moderate problems have often been left unserved. Viewing substance-abuse problems along a continuum between the poles of nonproblematic use and life-threatening addiction makes it possible to respond to a specific client's needs at the time of contact rather than wait until problems have become sufficiently severe to warrant heroic interventions. Thus, a college student who has been disciplined for marijuana use in the dormitory may need help with decision-making or other life skills. An individual who has lost his or her driver's license because of driving under the influence of alcohol may need to learn impulse control, planning processes, or methods for discriminating blood-alcohol level. A person who has used alcohol or other drugs to cope with anxiety may need assistance in developing healthier relaxation techniques. These people should be able to receive counseling without having to accept diagnostic labels that might be inappropriate.

When counselors base their work on the recognition that their clients are complex human beings affected by a variety of factors, they are more likely to develop multidimensional treatments that are tailored to their clients' individual needs. Although the goals of substance-abuse counseling, by definition, should always include the reduction or elimination of drug or alcohol use, the treatment plan also needs to address other areas of life functioning. Depending on the issues that affect an individual client, the general life areas that might be addressed include the following (Lewis, Dana, & Blevins, 1988, p. 11):

- resolving or avoiding legal problems
- attaining financial stability
- attaining marital or family stability
- setting and meeting career development goals
- setting and meeting educational goals
- improving interpersonal or social skills
- improving assertion skills
- enhancing physical health and fitness
- learning more effective methods for coping with stress
- developing more effective problem-solving and decision-making skills
- learning relaxation skills
- learning to recognize and express feelings
- adapting more effectively to work or school situations
- developing social-support systems
- increasing involvement in recreational and other social pursuits
- dealing with psychological issues such as depression or anxiety
- increasing general feelings of self-esteem . . .

The specific goals of counseling, as well as the methods used, depend on the client's own strengths, deficits, and values.

Involving the client actively in his or her treatment planning helps to individualize the process and, at the same time, enhances the individual's sense of self-efficacy. Miller (1985) suggests that the traditional confrontation methods used to force problem drinkers to own the label of "alcoholic" and to accept externally imposed treatments may engender feelings of helplessness that can become self-fulfilling prophecies. In contrast, treating clients as people who are capable of making responsible and independent decisions about their own drinking improves their self-esteem and self-efficacy and makes positive, self-directed change more likely. Once clients have begun the process of behavior change, their self-efficacy is enhanced as they learn to recognize situations that pose risks for problem drinking and as they acquire skills that they can use to cope with these situations (Curry & Marlatt, 1987). Self-efficacy is improved further and behavior change is maintained as the client achieves success in coping with difficult situations in the natural environment (Annis, 1986).

Such opportunities for successful coping are obviously more likely to be available for clients who are being seen on an outpatient basis than for clients who are hospitalized. At the same time, outpatient treatment allows clients to maintain social ties and helps them avoid the sense of powerlessness and dependence that often comes with hospitalization. Research conducted by Longabough, McCrady, Fink, Stout, McAuley, Doyle, and McNeill (1983) supports this view. Longabough et al. compared alcoholics who were treated in an inpatient setting with a group who lived at home and commuted to the same hospital for day or evening sessions. They found no difference between the two groups in terms of drinking behavior, but they did note differences in psychological well-being and interpersonal functioning. The fact that the partial-hospitalization group showed more improvement in these areas than the hospitalized group did led the researchers to believe that the stigmatization and dependency of institutionalization might have negative influences on long-term recovery. Moreover, such life-disrupting treatment fails to provide benefits that can balance its shortcomings. "The absolutely consistent testimony of . . . controlled studies . . . is that heroic interventions—that is, longer, more intensive residential settings—produce no more favorable outcomes overall than treatment in much simpler, shorter, and less expensive settings" (Miller, 1985, p. 2).

The preferability of outpatient over inpatient treatment holds true for other drugs as well as for alcohol. Regarding cocaine addiction, for example, Washton emphasizes the advantages of outpatient treatment, both because it is less disruptive and less stigmatizing than hospitalization and because of its clinical advantages.

> While inpatient treatment temporarily removes the cocaine addict from ready access to drugs, it may not adequately prepare the patient for remaining abstinent after hospital discharge—as evidenced by the fact that relapse rates after inpatient treatment remain extraordinarily high. Outpatient treatment teaches the cocaine addict to manage his/her drug compulsion within the "real world" rather than the artificially safe environment of an inpatient facility. Treatment can focus immediately on the inevitable task of learning how to manage daily life without drugs—despite the availability of cocaine and the presence of environmental cues that trigger cocaine cravings (Washton, 1989, p. 75).

Of course, clients with serious medical problems or highly unstable living conditions may need a period of time under the close supervision that a hospital or residential facility can offer. For many clients, however, less disruptive options would be far more appropriate.

> Traditionally, patients have been slotted into treatment modalities and programs based on preconceived assumptions concerning what "all alcoholics" or "all heroin addicts" needed. Frequently, alcoholics have been hospitalized in 21- or 28-day programs with some form of "aftercare" following inpatient treatment. "Drug addicts" have either been channeled into long-term (6 months to 2 years or more) residential treatment (therapeutic communities) or into outpatient methadone treatment (withdrawal or maintenance) for opiate addicts and outpatient "drug-free" counseling for polydrug abusers. . . . As patients are more carefully assessed based on specific characteristics, it becomes apparent that not all patients require the same level of care (Giuliani & Schnoll, 1985, pp. 204–205).

As Giuliani and Schnoll make clear, the intensity of treatment required by any one client can be determined only through careful assessment. Providing the same generalized treatment package to each client overlooks individual differences and fails to lead to positive outcomes. In fact, many of the methods most widely used in substance-abuse treatment have failed to demonstrate their effectiveness with any group of clients. When Miller and Hester (1985) reviewed the literature regarding alcoholism treatment, they listed the methods that controlled research studies had shown to be more promising. Among the methods supported by research were aversion therapies, behavioral self-control training, community reinforcement, marital and family therapy, social-skills training, and stress management. Miller and Hester also listed the components of the standard treatments available to alcohol-abusing clients: Alcoholics Anonymous, alcoholism education, confrontation, disulfiram (a substance that causes nausea when alcohol is consumed), group therapy, and individual counseling. The point made by Miller and Hester was not that the standard methods were necessarily ineffective, but that they were largely untested. In contrast, the methods that had been most thoroughly researched were not widely available. No method appeared on both lists. This finding becomes even more striking when we consider the fact that most alcoholism treatment programs have, in recent years, broadened their clientele and now offer similar treatment to a combined group of alcoholics and other drug abusers. Thus, programs that have not shown evidence of effectiveness with alcoholics now offer the same untested treatments to additional populations.

The appropriate response to this situation is not to develop a new standard program but to offer more differentiated treatments.

> As research warrants, clients should be matched to optimal interventions based on predictors of differential outcome. Clients should be informed participants in their own treatment planning process, and should be offered a range of plausible alternatives along with fair and accurate information upon which to base a choice (Miller & Hester, 1985, p. 562).

Such differentiation would make substance-abuse treatment more responsive both to individual differences and to sociocultural diversity. Effective treatment

can be possible only when counselors and researchers show sensitivity to the individual, social, and cultural differences among substance-abusing clients.

Assessment

Individualized treatment planning requires that the counselor develop an understanding of his or her client that goes beyond the narrow limits of information about substance-use behavior. A broad-ranging initial interview can address issues concerning the client's history of drug and alcohol use, while eliciting data concerning more general life functioning. This general interview can lay the groundwork for the treatment-planning process and help in the decision-making process as instruments for more specific information are selected.

Instruments to Assess Drug and Alcohol Problems

Before developing a treatment plan with a substance-abusing client, the counselor needs to add to the initial interview by assessing in more depth the nature and seriousness of the alcohol or drug problem. A number of easily administered instruments that focus directly on substance-abuse problems are available for use by counselors.

Comprehensive drinker profile.   The Comprehensive Drinker Profile (Miller & Marlatt, 1984) is one of the most well-researched instruments currently available. The CDP uses a structured interview format that covers a wide range of issues. An unusual aspect of this instrument is that the counselor who uses it as directed can obtain an exceptionally accurate picture of the amount and pattern of the client's alcohol use. The counselor can also learn a great deal about such alcohol-related factors as range of drinking situations, beverage preferences, reasons for drinking, effects of drinking, and client perceptions of alcohol problems. The instrument also yields several quantitative scores, including a score for physiological dependence on alcohol and a score for general alcohol problems that is based on incorporation of the Michigan Alcoholism Screening Test (Selzer, 1971) within the CDP.

Michigan alcoholism screening test.   The MAST is a widely used instrument designed to give a general estimate of the seriousness of an individual's problems related to alcohol. Twenty-four questions with yes-or-no answers focus on drinking habits and related problems. Points are scored as follows: 0–4, nonalcoholic; 5–6, suggestive of alcohol problem; greater than 7, alcoholism; 10–20, moderate alcoholism; 20–55, severe alcoholism.

Substance abuse problem checklist.   The Substance Abuse Problem Checklist (Carroll, 1984) examines problems in eight categories: (1) motivation for treatment, (2) health problems, (3) personality problems, (4) problems in social relationships, (5) job-related problems, (6) problems associated with leisure time, (7) religious or spiritual problems, and (8) legal problems. The instrument is a self-administered checklist, allowing clients to participate actively in the assessment process.

Alcohol dependence scale. The ADS (Horn, Skinner, Wanberg, & Foster, 1984) is a brief, self-administered instrument. Its 25 multiple-choice items focus on such aspects of alcohol dependence as withdrawal symptoms, obsessive/compulsive drinking style, tolerance, and drink-seeking behavior.

Addiction severity index. This index (McLellan, Luborsky, Woody, & O'Brien, 1980) assesses seven areas: medical status, employment status, drug use, alcohol use, legal status, family/social relationships, and psychological status. It is one of the few well-tested instruments that addresses drugs other than alcohol. Using a structured interview format, the instrument yields severity ratings for each area, from 0 (no treatment necessary) to 9 (treatment needed to intervene in life-threatening situation).

Time-line follow-back assessment method. This assessment method, designed by Sobell et al. (1980), gathers information concerning the client's drinking behaviors over time, making it an especially useful tool for considering drinking behaviors as continuous rather than dichotomous variables. Clients are interviewed to solicit reports of their daily drinking as they remember its having occurred over a specific period of time. The client fills in a blank calendar using codes to identify the amount consumed and the setting in which drinking occurs on each day. Similar mechanisms can be used to gather information concerning the use of other drugs.

DSM-III-R

The *Diagnostic and Statistical Manual of Mental Disorders* (DSM-III-R) (American Psychiatric Association, 1987) provides a significant addition to the assessment process through its diagnostic guidelines for substance-use disorders. The DSM-III-R is especially helpful because of the clear distinction it makes between substance use and substance abuse or dependence. Psychoactive substance use is considered a disorder only (1) when the individual demonstrates an inability to control his or her use despite cognitive, behavioral, or physiological symptoms; and (2) when the symptoms have persisted for at least one month or have occurred repeatedly over a longer period of time.

A client is diagnosed as being *dependent* on the substance only if at least three of the following nine symptoms are present (American Psychiatric Association, 1987*):

1. Substance often taken in larger amounts or over a longer period than the person intended.
2. Persistent desire or one or more unsuccessful efforts to cut down or control substance use.
3. A great deal of time spent in activities necessary to get the substance (e.g., theft), taking the substance (e.g., chain smoking), or recovering from its effects.
4. Frequent intoxication or withdrawal symptoms when expected to fulfill major role obligations at work, school, or home (e.g., does not go to work because

hung over, goes to school or work "high," intoxicated while taking care of his or her children), or when substance use is physically hazardous (e.g., drives when intoxicated).

5. Important social, occupational, or recreational activities given up or reduced because of substance use.

6. Continued substance use despite knowledge of having a persistent or recurrent social, psychological, or physical problem that is caused or exacerbated by the use of the substance (e.g., keeps using heroin despite family arguments about it, cocaine-induced depression, or having an ulcer made worse by drinking).

7. Marked tolerance: need for markedly increased amounts of the substance (i.e., at least a 50% increase) in order to achieve intoxication or desired effect, or markedly diminished effect with continued use of the same amount. . . .

8. Characteristic withdrawal symptoms. . . .

9. Substance often taken to relieve or avoid withdrawal symptoms.

Psychoactive Substance *Abuse* is the diagnosis given to people who have shown maladaptive patterns of use but who have not met the criteria for dependence. The maladaptive pattern is defined by "(1) continued use of the psychoactive substance despite knowledge of having a persistent or recurrent social, occupational, psychological, or physical problem that is caused or exacerbated by use of the substance, or (2) recurrent use of the substance in situations when use is physically hazardous (e.g., driving while intoxicated)" (American Psychiatric Association, 1987, p. 169). Nine classes of psychoactive substances are associated with both abuse and dependence: alcohol; amphetamines or similarly acting sympathomimetics; cannabis; cocaine; hallucinogens; inhalants; opioids; phencyclidine or similarly acting arylcyclohexylamines; and sedatives, hypnotics, or anxiolytics. Nicotine has a dependence diagnosis but not an abuse diagnosis. Each class of substance has its own code number, but the general criteria for abuse and dependence are consistent across categories. Categories of severity are also consistent across substance categories and include: (1) mild, (2) moderate, (3) severe, (4) in partial remission, and (5) in full remission.

The DSM-III-R provides diagnostic criteria without attaching them to a specific instrument. If the assessment process has been carefully implemented, however, the applicability of the criteria to the specific client will be clear. A combination of interviewing, history taking, and administration of assessment instruments should provide both a reasonably accurate picture of the degree to which substance use has interfered with the client's life and an overview of the life problems that should be addressed.

Instruments to Assess Cognitive/Behavioral Factors

Once the client has made the decision to take action toward behavior change, he or she needs to identify the situations and cognitions that affect drug or alcohol use. Annis (1986) emphasizes the need to work with each client both to identify high-risk situations and to analyze his or her cognitive appraisals of these situations. Toward this end, Annis developed three very practical assessment instruments: The Inventory of Drinking Situations (Annis, 1982b), the Situational Confidence Questionnaire (Annis, 1982c), and the Cognitive Appraisal Questionnaire (Annis, 1982a).

Inventory of drinking situations (IDS).   The IDS is used to identify situations that the individual client associates with heavy drinking. Drinking situations are divided into eight categories—five associated with personal states and three associated with other people. The five types of situations categorized as relating to personal states involve negative emotional states, negative physical states, positive emotional states, testing of personal control, and urges and temptations. The situations associated with other people involve interpersonal conflict, social pressure to drink, and pleasant times with others. The inventory provides a profile that shows the individual client's high- and low-risk situations. The profile then forms the basis for the client's efforts to understand the antecedents of his or her drinking and develop mechanisms for behavior change. He or she is encouraged to begin by handling easy tasks and to progress gradually to more difficult situations.

Situational confidence questionnaire.   This instrument is based on self-efficacy theory. Clients are asked to react to drinking situations (the same situations that are addressed in the IDS). They are asked to imagine themselves in each of these situations and to indicate their degree of confidence in their ability to handle the situation without drinking. This instrument, like the IDS, helps in the design of a hierarchy of drinking situations, and clients are encouraged to work gradually toward involvement in situations about which they feel less confident.

Cognitive appraisal questionnaire.   The Cognitive Appraisal Questionnaire helps clients identify cognitive factors that might interfere with their self-efficacy. Based on a structured interview, the CAQ explores what cognitions are working to influence the individual's appraisal of his or her success. Treatment can then be adjusted so that self-efficacy is enhanced. According to Annis (1986, pp. 417–418), "unless a client's experiences in drinking situations can be arranged so as to foster gains in self-efficacy, it is unlikely that the changes brought about in drinking behavior during treatment will be maintained after discharge."

Treatment Strategies

Because self-efficacy is an important component of long-term recovery, treatment strategies for substance abuse should include interventions that enhance the client's self-management abilities and encourage the perception that change is possible. Behavioral self-control training and skill-development programs, along with efforts to help social systems become more reinforcing, are among the promising approaches that tend to lead in this direction.

Behavioral Self-Control Training

Behavioral self-control training is an educational intervention designed to teach clients how to initiate and maintain changes in their own behavior. Clients learn to analyze their own drinking or drug use behavior, to monitor their consump-

tion, and to use self-reinforcement and stimulus-control methods to bring use down to desired levels. The training, which can be provided in either individual or group settings, helps clients work toward their self-selected goals.

This behavior change technology can be used by clients who are working toward either abstinence or moderation outcomes. One of the most important factors affecting success is the appropriateness of the goal for the individual client. Among clients whose drug of choice is alcohol, controlled drinking may be a good option for some. The client for whom a moderation outcome is most realistic is one who is young and healthy, who has not shown symptoms of physical addiction to alcohol, whose problem is of short duration, who has not yet developed a large number of life problems associated with alcohol, and who objects to abstinence. In contrast, people whose problems are chronic and severe or who have health problems that are exacerbated by drinking tend to be poor candidates for controlled drinking. The key to setting appropriate goals involves the recognition of what constitutes nonproblematic use for a particular client. General guidelines about the problems associated with various levels of consumption can help clients make these decisions. For instance, Sanchez-Craig, Wilkinson, and Walker, based on the results of a program for early-stage problem drinkers, make the following recommendations:

> (1) We discourage clients from adopting goals where quantity exceeds 4 drinks per day. . . . (2) We discourage clients from drinking daily, even if they wish to restrict their consumption to one or two drinks per day. . . . (3) We recommend that consumption be limited to no more than 20 drinks per week. . . . (4) We strongly advise clients to avoid drinking before noon, to avoid drinking in situations where drinking has caused problems, and to avoid using alcohol for coping (Sanchez-Craig, Wilkinson, & Walker, 1987, p. 310).

Although Sanchez-Craig and her colleagues set twenty drinks per week as their recommended consumption limit, they noted that, at these levels, some clients continued to have problems. There were no problems reported by clients who drank less than twelve drinks per week. Of course, some clients who believed that they could moderate their drinking changed their goals once they learned about these recommended limits. "Some heavy drinkers (i.e., usually people who have been consuming 10 or more drinks per day) who present to treatment with a goal of moderation in mind, reappraise this goal when they are informed that it usually involves very conservative levels of drinking" (Sanchez-Craig, Wilkinson, & Walker, 1987, p. 310).

Regardless of whether individual clients are working toward long-term outcomes of abstinence or of moderation, Sanchez-Craig and her colleagues suggest an initial three-week period of total abstinence. Clients who accept this recommendation benefit in several ways: improvement in their cognitive functioning, opportunities to identify situations associated with urges or temptations to drink, early recognition of the coping mechanisms that are most helpful for them, and—perhaps most important—an experience of early success that enhances self-efficacy and increases the likelihood of long-term adherence. Attempting abstinence for this period of time is challenging enough to lead to a sense of accomplishment but less daunting than the notion of lifelong abstinence.

Clients who are attempting to make changes in their substance use be-haviors need to monitor their substance use and identify the situations that are most problematic for them. Instruments like the Inventory of Drinking Situa-tions (Annis, 1982b) can help in this process, but high-risk situations can also be recognized through clients' day-to-day monitoring of their experiences and recollections of past challenges. When clients are asked to specify incidents of problematic drinking or drug use, whether in the past or in their current lives, they can begin to recognize the cues that tend to trigger problems for them. These situations can vary widely from client to client and may be associated with positive or negative affect, with positive or negative social situations, or with specific times or places.

Once clients have identified the situations that pose risks for them, they need to learn coping strategies. At the most basic level, clients can learn how to anticipate and plan for challenging situations.

> Clients should be trained to anticipate impending high-risk situations and to take preventive action at the earliest possible point. Once trained, clients are better equipped to make a relatively simple decision either to avoid a particular situation or to make advance plans about how they will deal with it when it occurs (Curry & Marlatt, 1987, p. 129).

Clients may choose to avoid certain situations until they have successfully met less difficult challenges; they can work their way up a hierarchy of situations from those that are perceived as only moderately difficult to those that are seen as more formidable (Annis, 1986). A client can anticipate situations that are likely to occur in the following week—a party, a wedding, an invitation to drink with colleagues after work on Friday—and plan strategies that may involve either avoidance or active coping.

The active coping strategies that might be used by clients can generally be categorized as either cognitive or behavioral (Sanchez-Craig et al., 1987). Cogni-tive coping methods involve self-statements that clients use to remind them-selves of their commitment or to reappraise the situation. Behavioral methods can include alternative behaviors or the application of such coping skills as assertion or relaxation. An important component of behavioral self-control training is helping clients increase the repertoire of coping skills available to them, using such methods as instruction, modeling, behavioral rehearsal, and homework assignments. Counselors also need to recognize that clients differ widely in terms of coping styles. Each client's coping skills and deficits should be carefully assessed, with attention being paid to the client's recollections of what strategies have worked most effectively for him or her in the past.

Clients' new coping behaviors can be enhanced through self-reinforce-ment strategies. "The concept of self-control implies that an individual can be taught to rearrange powerful contingencies that influence behavior in such a way that he experiences long-range benefits" (Kanfer, 1980, p. 344). Clients can control these contingencies both by trying to eliminate environ-mental cues (such as avoiding parties where drugs are likely to be in use) and by arranging their own rewards for positive performance (such as purchasing new clothes with the money saved through nonpurchase of drugs or alcohol).

Positive reinforcement for successful performance should be part of each client's self-management strategy.

In addition to helping clients cope with high-risk situations, behavioral self-control training should also include attention to the kinds of behaviors that are directly associated with nonproblematic use. If the drug being used is alcohol, clients can learn how to limit their consumption by mixing and diluting their drinks, learning to sip slowly, spacing drinks either by keeping track of the time between them or by alternating with nonalcoholic beverages, consuming food along with alcoholic beverages, and making purposeful attempts to engage in alternative activities. Use of such moderation strategies, which are based on information about nonproblematic, social use of alcohol, are obviously less applicable to other drugs, but all of the other aspects of behavioral self-control training—functional analyses of substance-use behavior, identification of high-risk situations, and development and reinforcement of appropriate coping behaviors—clearly apply to the whole gamut of substance-use disorders.

Skill-Development Programs

Self-management and long-term recovery can also be enhanced through training in a number of intrapersonal and social skills. The focus of such skill training depends, of course, on the individual client's needs.

Some clients can benefit by attention to stress management, especially training in relaxation methods. Many substance-abusing clients have learned to use drugs as their only response to stress or anxiety. Their years of drug or alcohol abuse have masked anxiety, making it unlikely that they have learned to deal effectively with physiological responses to stress. Their efforts to maintain behavior changes are likely to be jeopardized if they become overwhelmed by stressful situations or internal states of anxiety. Relaxation training can be helpful, as long as it is joined by efforts to help clients deal directly with stressful life situations. Clients can gain control over their physical tension through such mechanisms as progressive muscle relaxation, biofeedback, or meditation. If relaxation methods are in their skill repertoires, anxiety is less likely to precipitate impulsive drug or alcohol use.

Many clients also need social-skills training, especially in the area of assertiveness. One frequent concomitant of drug or alcohol problems is social pressure to use. Although clients may have strong motivation to remain abstinent, they frequently find themselves engaging in unwanted behaviors because of deficits in assertion. Nonassertive clients may also have general feelings of self-pity, despair, and low self-esteem—all strongly associated with substance abuse. If clients have problems in any of these areas, they can learn to make assertive statements that protect their own decision-making rights and self-esteem. Short-term assertiveness training based on coaching, modeling, behavior rehearsal, and feedback can have an impact on the client's recovery that strongly outweighs its costs.

Another skill that has special relevance for substance-abusing clients is problem solving. Clients frequently report a history of having avoided problems by escaping into intoxication. Thus, they need to learn the kind of general problem-solving skills that are needed to function effectively. Training in this

area can also help clients solve problems associated more directly with drug or alcohol use. For example, clients may need to learn how to avoid getting into situations that involve drinking and driving or how to plan ahead for dealing with the absence of nonalcoholic drinks at a party. Clients can work on problem-solving strategies in either individual or group-counseling settings, developing and judging alternative solutions to a broad range of real and hypothetical problem situations.

Enhancing the Responsiveness of Social Systems

The individual client's recovery depends not just on his or her internal changes but also on the degree to which new behaviors are reinforced in the environment.

> Newly acquired social skills are subject to multiple environmental influences. For example, the physical environment (mass media, advertising, sensory cues for drinking) is structured to increase likelihood of drinking, and drinking is associated with such social activities as conversation, recreation and dating. Under these environmental influences, recovering alcoholics may not only lose existing support, but receive negative sanctions from former drinking associates. Finally, many recovering alcoholics do not have the personal resources (e.g., transportation, family, friends, employment) necessary to engage in new social situations. . . . An alternative approach is to create a new social system in the alcoholics' natural environment that provides wide varieties of social and recreational activities and reinforces the acquisition of appropriate social behaviors (Mallams, Godley, Hall, & Meyers, 1982, p. 1116).

If it is difficult for a recovering alcoholic to gain social support for his or her attempts at abstinence, it may be even more problematic for clients whose life-style was previously based on use of illicit drugs. Many drug-abusing clients become increasingly isolated from mainstream society over the years of drug use, and their only associates may be other users. Their sole hope for recovery lies in an attempt to restructure the social systems that affect them.

Community reinforcement program.   Miller and Hester (1985), in their review of promising treatment approaches for alcoholics, cited the Community Reinforcement Program as one of the approaches best supported by research. This program (Azrin, 1976), designed for inpatient male alcoholics in a state hospital, was unusual in its comprehensiveness. It included the following components:

- *job counseling:* helping clients find permanent, full-time, well-paying jobs that would interfere with a return to drinking
- *marital counseling:* providing counseling for all married couples and arranging "synthetic families" for unmarried alcoholics
- *resocialization and recreation:* arranging alcohol-free social and recreational activities in addition to making Alcoholics Anonymous referrals
- *problem-prevention rehearsal:* teaching clients how to handle situations that might otherwise lead to drinking
- *early warning system:* providing a mail-in "Happiness Scale" to be used daily by clients

- *disulfiram:* developing positive, supportive mechanisms for clients to use Antabuse for impulse control
- *group counseling:* providing supportive group sessions that can develop into social or recreational groups after release
- *buddy procedure:* selecting recovering peer advisers to work closely with each client
- *contracting:* using written contracts to formalize the agreements between counselors and clients regarding the program's procedures and the client's responsibilities

One of the things that made the Community Reinforcement Program unique was its emphasis on the individual's reentry into the community. Clients were prepared to cope with the demands of the environment. At the same time, the program tried to make the community itself more reinforcing to clients' recovery through family counseling, group situations, social and recreational activities, and the buddy procedure. Such efforts can work even more effectively for clients whose health allows them to be treated on an outpatient basis from the beginning. It is unreasonable to expect that clients can be so changed as a result of treatment that they will be able to withstand whatever social pressures are imposed on them. The social systems that affect clients most strongly must change if recovery is to be made permanent. Of all of these social systems, the family is most important.

Family counseling. If one family member has a substance-abuse-related problem, the entire family is affected to the degree that the problem may become the system's primary organizing factor. In many cases, the family's interactions are built around the substance use, so that predictable patterns develop. In a discussion of alcoholism, Kaufman (1985) stated:

> Drinking behavior interrupts normal family tasks, causes conflict, shifts roles, and demands adjustment and adaptive responses from family members who do not know how to appropriately respond. A converse dynamic also occurs: marital and family styles, rules, and conflict may evoke, support, and maintain alcoholism as a symptom of family system dysfunction or as a coping mechanism to deal with family anxiety (Kaufman, 1985, pp. 30–31).

Thus, the drinking behavior of one family member and the responses of others can allow the family to maintain an unhealthy equilibrium and avoid change. Because family members play their part in this ongoing pattern of behavior, the alcohol abuse not only may be allowed to continue but may actually be encouraged.

If family members choose to remove themselves from the established pattern of interaction—if they fail to play their customary roles—the system can be transformed. In fact, individual recovery may depend to a large part on whether such a transformation takes place. Family-counseling interventions should aim toward the long-range goal of systemic change. Such changes, however, take place slowly, through a step-by-step process. The three general stages of change include the following (Lewis, 1992):

Stage 1: Interrupting ongoing patterns
Stage 2: Facing the reality of change
Stage 3: Deepening and maintaining change

In the first stage of counseling a substance-abuse-affected family, the counselor's focus should be placed on helping family members interrupt the patterns that have helped maintain the problem. In some cases, change may involve confronting the substance-abusing client and pressing him or her into treatment. If this option is unworkable in a particular situation, family members may interrupt ongoing patterns by disengaging, by withdrawing from the performance of roles that have enabled the substance abuser to avoid negative consequences, and by taking better care of themselves. The purpose of this strategy is not to stop the individual's drinking or drug use but to help the family "decenter" itself from its singular focus on the alcohol or drug use (Ackerman, 1983) and achieve an improved level of health.

When an alcohol- or drug-abusing family member does achieve abstinence, the family is frequently thrown into crisis. Facing the reality of change (Stage 2) involves developing new transactional patterns that are more adaptive to a new reality. It also means recognizing the limitations of change. Family members may be disappointed when they realize that not all of their problems magically disappear with the onset of abstinence. They may be fearful concerning the possibility of relapse or angry about years of abuse. Expectations may conflict if the former substance abuser expects to regain power and trust that had been relinquished in the past and if other family members are unable to make sudden changes in their roles and responsibilities. Bepko and Krestan (1985) suggest that the most appropriate goals to help families weather this crisis include keeping the system calm, helping individual family members focus on their own issues, anticipating extreme reactions, addressing concerns about relapse, and teaching new skills that can be used to cope with stress. At this point, structural changes need to be limited to minor adaptations for the purpose of ensuring adequate parenting.

Once these basic steps have been taken and individual family members feel that their own needs are being addressed, the family as a whole can learn to reframe issues in systems terms. At Stage 3, the counselor can help the family develop deep structural changes that make the system as a whole more functional for each of its members. The family as a whole—not just the identified substance-abusing client—is seen as the appropriate target of intervention.

Participation in self-help organizations.   "In self-help organizations, people with common bonds are able to make contact with one another, mutually support one another, request or offer active assistance, and deal with common problems in an understanding but realistic group" (Lewis & Lewis, 1989, p. 175). For people with substance-abuse problems, participation in such groups offers a dual reward: the chance to enter a helpful, supportive social system and the chance to help others. If people can enter such equal partnerships, they have the advantage of feeling useful and valuable to others. This sense of accomplishment can enhance self-efficacy in a way that playing the role of patient or client cannot.

For many years, the fellowship of Alcoholics Anonymous has provided the kind of social support that enhances the recovery process. More recently, the basic AA model has been adapted to the needs of people who are dealing with related issues. Organizations such as Al-Anon, Alateen, and Families Anonymous give the family members of alcoholics or addicts a chance to help themselves and one another. Narcotics Anonymous, Cocaine Anonymous, and numerous other groups help people maintain abstinence from mood-altering substances. Although the self-help phenomenon should not be considered a form of "treatment," these groups can play a vital role in supporting the individual's long-term recovery.

Relapse Prevention

Because relapse rates for substance-abusing clients have always been high, substance-abuse treatment providers have begun to integrate relapse prevention training into the treatment process for each client as quickly as possible. As clients begin, early in treatment, to identify high-risk situations and develop methods for coping with them, they are, in effect, initiating their relapse prevention efforts.

The work of Marlatt and Gordon (1985) has been especially helpful in this effort. Their model is, in effect, a strategy of preparedness that is based on the notion that clients can develop effective coping responses and plan in advance for their implementation. Each time the client is successful in coping with a high-risk situation, his or her self-efficacy is enhanced, and the likelihood that positive behaviors will be maintained is increased.

Relapse prevention efforts also address the question of how clients can deal with the times when their coping efforts do not succeed. It is possible for a minor slip to evolve into a full-scale relapse if clients believe that they have failed in their efforts or believe that they have lost control. Clients who believe that abstinence must be total and absolute may experience the abstinence violation effect (AVE) following initial use of the substance. The slip is interpreted as a loss of control, and this interpretation may become a self-fulfilling prophecy. The relapse prevention model encourages clients to think differently about the process, "to realize that lapses are not irreversible, but that instead they can be the occasion for growth, understanding, and learning—a prolapse rather than a relapse" (Curry & Marlatt, 1987, p. 133). Even at this point, preparedness is the key, with each client being armed with concrete plans for coping with substance use. Reminder cards (Curry & Marlatt, 1987) help clients deal with initial lapses by reminding them to keep calm, to be aware of what is happening, to renew their commitment, to think about the situation leading to the lapse, to make a plan for immediate steps to be taken, and to ask for help.

Case Example

Mary Smith presented herself as a self-referral to a mental-health center counselor specializing in substance-abuse issues. In her mid-thirties, married, childless,

and employed in a high-powered corporate job, Mary was uncertain whether she had a problem at all. Her husband had been complaining about her drinking, but she felt that this was simply his way of blaming everything that went wrong on one issue. The incident that made her decide to seek an assessment involved a friend, Jane, who refused to ride with her to a company picnic because of her fear that Mary would drink too much. Mary drove on her own and was stopped by a police officer on the way home. She was not charged with driving under the influence of alcohol, but the incident frightened her.

Mary agreed to participate in an assessment process and was given the Comprehensive Drinker Profile. The results showed that, in an average week, she consumed between fifty and sixty drinks, which was well over the norm. The fact that she seldom felt intoxicated indicated a high tolerance level. The CDP also showed that Mary scored in the significant-problem range on the measure of general alcohol problems. On the measure of physical dependence on alcohol, she showed definite and significant symptoms of dependence. Mary believed that her father, who died young, might have been an alcoholic.

Mary was surprised at the level of her problem that was indicated by the counselor's interpretation of the test results. She decided that she should attempt to make some changes in her drinking behaviors. Because she showed some signs of physical addiction to alcohol and because of the possibility that alcoholism might be present in her family, the counselor encouraged her to consider a goal of abstinence, at least for a few months. It was agreed that, after this period of time, she could reconsider her goal and decide whether to maintain abstinence or attempt moderate drinking. Behavioral self-control training was used to help Mary make immediate changes in her drinking behaviors. Among the situations that she found difficult were work-related drinking occasions and evenings when she arrived home exhausted from a stressful workday. She was especially concerned about the work situation, stating that there was very real pressure to drink with clients and that, as a woman, it was hard enough for her to be accepted without also going against the social norm. At the same time, she knew that too much drinking would jeopardize her career. Her work organization was, in a sense, giving her mixed messages.

Mary worked with the counselor to make some life-style changes that were very helpful to her. In job-related drinking situations, she decided to substitute soft drinks for alcohol, and she practiced ways to assert herself so that alternative beverages could be substituted without calling undue attention to herself. Her friend and colleague, Jane, provided support for Mary's efforts. Mary and Jane decided to join a health club and got into the habit of working out several evenings a week after work. This practice helped Mary arrive home refreshed rather than exhausted. Mary's husband agreed to participate in marriage counseling sessions that helped him to become more supportive of her efforts at abstinence.

Mary used several methods to cope with cravings for alcohol. She wrote down her reasons for making the commitment to address her drinking problem and carried the card with her as a reminder in difficult situations. She had several sessions of relaxation training that, in combination with her exercise regimen, helped her cope more effectively with work-related stressors. She set

up a reinforcement schedule for herself, rewarding herself with a small luxury item after each week of abstinence.

Mary was strongly encouraged to make her own decisions concerning the goals and methods of the counseling process. It is likely that, if she had been confronted actively and pushed to admit to an "alcoholic" label, she might have denied the problem, citing her effectiveness in her work situation and her general good health. The counseling process helped Mary gain a better balance in her life between work and pleasure, independence and social connectedness. These changes supported her successful efforts at changing her drinking behaviors.

Preventive Measures

DiCicco et al. (1984), disseminating the results of an evaluation of a major alcohol-education curriculum at the junior high school level, noted an interesting phenomenon. In junior high schools where alcohol education was implemented intensively and continuously, alcohol misuse did not rise as sharply as it did among adolescents in a comparison school. But this effect did not persist if a child moved to a new school.

> These data do not show that early instruction can prevent later alcohol misuse. Any impact on drinking behavior that does occur is noted during the period in which the student is still a member of the group with whom he participates in alcohol education activities. . . . Changing youthful drinking behavior is tantamount to changing a culture (DiCicco et al., 1984, p. 168).

This finding provides support for the notion that prevention cannot depend solely on direct educational interventions, but must also take into account the effects of the social environment. As Bandura (1989, p. 137) points out:

> People effect self-directed change when they understand how personal habits threaten their well-being, are taught how to modify them, and believe in their capabilities to marshal the effort and resources needed to exercise control. However, personal change occurs within a network of social influences. Depending on their nature, social factors can aid, retard, or undermine efforts at personal change.

Substance-abuse prevention involves an effort to help people avoid such health-jeopardizing behaviors as overuse of alcohol or other drugs. The only way such behavior changes can occur, however, is when individual knowledge and skill are combined with an environment that supports healthy behaviors. Programs aimed toward prevention must be comprehensive efforts that include skill development, self-efficacy enhancement, and social change along with the provision of information. Bandura (1989) suggests that programs designed to lessen detrimental life-style practices should include four components:

> The first is informational, designed to increase people's awareness and knowledge of health risks. The second component is concerned with development of the social and self-regulatory skills needed to translate informed concerns into effective preventive action. The third component is aimed at skill enhancement and

building resilient self-efficacy by providing opportunities for guided practice and corrective feedback in applying the skills in high-risk situations. The final component involves enlisting social supports for desired personal changes (p. 130).

If we think of substance-abuse problems on a continuum, we can see that there is no possibility of a clear dichotomy between the methods that we use for prevention and the techniques that we use for treatment. Whether the program being implemented is a primary prevention effort in a school or a treatment program for severely addicted individuals, our interventions need to teach self-management skills, enhance self-efficacy, and build strong networks of social support.

Summary

A biopsychosocial approach to substance abuse is built on the recognition that each client who develops a program with alcohol or other drugs does so because of a complex and highly individualized combination of factors. Substance abuse counselors can adapt their practice to this conceptualization by using the following general guidelines: (1) view substance abuse on a continuum, rather than as a dichotomy; (2) provide treatment that is individualized in goals and methods; (3) use methods that enhance each client's sense of self-efficacy; (4) provide multidimensional treatment that focuses on social and environmental factors; (5) support selection of the least intrusive treatment alternative for each client; (6) remain open to new methods and goals as research findings become available; and (7) be sensitive to the needs of diverse client populations.

Such individualized treatment depends on careful assessment linked to comprehensive treatment plans. Treatment strategies should be based on the kinds of interventions that are most likely to enhance the client's self-management skills and self-efficacy. Such interventions include behavioral self-control training and skill-development programs. Strategies should also help make social systems more conducive to the client's recovery. Examples of efforts to enhance the responsiveness of social systems include community reinforcement programs, family counseling, and referrals to self-help organizations.

Resources

Organizations

Several sources provide information that may be useful either to professionals or to clients. A list of some of them follows.

- National Clearinghouse for Alcohol Information
  Box 2345
  Rockville, MD 20852 (301/468-2600)

- National Institute on Alcohol Abuse and Alcoholism
  5600 Fishers Lane
  Rockville, MD 20857

- National Institute on Drug Abuse
  5600 Fishers Lane
  Rockville, MD 20857

- Office of Substance Abuse Prevention
  5600 Fishers Land
  Rockville, MD 20857

- Addiction Research Foundation of Ontario
  Toronto, ONT M55 251
  Canada

- National Council on Alcoholism
  12 West 21st St.
  New York, NY 10010

Self-help organizations.   The following self-help organizations provide personal help and support as well as extensive written materials.

- Alcoholics Anonymous
  World Service Center
  Madison Square Station
  New York, NY 10010

- Al-Anon Family Group Headquarters
  PO Box 182
  Madison Square Station
  New York, NY 10010

- Children of Alcoholics Foundation, Inc.
  200 Park Avenue
  New York, NY 10166

- National Association for Children of Alcoholics
  31706 Coast Highway, Suite 201
  South Laguna, CA 92677

Alcoholics Anonymous has been in existence since 1935, and meetings can be found in most cities. The fellowship of Alcoholics Anonymous is based on Twelve Steps and Twelve Traditions, which have been adapted for use in such other groups as Narcotics Anonymous, Cocaine Anonymous, and others. Clients can check their local directories for appropriate meetings, but counselors working with substance-abusing clients should become familiar with these resources so that prompt referrals can be made.

References

ACKERMAN, R. J. (1983). *Children of alcoholics: A guidebook for educators.* Holmes Beach, FL: Learning Publications.

AMERICAN PSYCHIATRIC ASSOCIATION. (1987). *Diagnostic and statistical manual of mental disorders* (3rd ed., rev.). Washington, DC: Author.

ANNIS, H. M. (1982a). *Cognitive Appraisal Questionnaire.* Toronto: Addiction Research Foundation of Ontario.

ANNIS, H. M. (1982b). *Inventory of Drinking Situations.* Toronto: Addiction Research Foundation of Ontario.

ANNIS, H. M. (1982c). *Situational Confidence Questionnaire.* Toronto: Addiction Research Foundation of Ontario.

ANNIS, H. M. (1986). A relapse prevention model for treatment of alcoholics. In W. R. Miller & N. Heather (Eds.), *Treating addictive behaviors: Processes of change* (pp. 407–434). New York: Plenum.

AZRIN, H. (1976). Improvements in the community-reinforcement approach to alcoholism. *Behavior Research and Therapy, 14,* 339–348.

BANDURA, A. (1989). Perceived self-efficacy in the exercise of control over AIDS infection. In V. M. Mays, G. W. Albee, & S. F. Schneider (Eds.), *Primary prevention of AIDS: Psychological approaches* (pp. 128–141). Newbury Park: Sage.

BEPKO, C., & Krestan, J. A. (1985). *The responsibility trap: A blueprint for treating the alcoholic family.* New York: Free Press.

BRILL, L. (1981). *The clinical treatment of substance abusers.* New York: Free Press.

CARROLL, J. F. X. (1984). Substance Abuse Problem Checklist: A new clinical aid for drug and/or alcohol treatment dependency. *Journal of Substance Abuse Treatment, 1,* 31–36.

CRABBE, J. C., McSwigan, J. D., & Belknap, J. K. (1985). The role of genetics in substance abuse. In M. Galizio & S. A. Maisto (Eds.), *Determinants of substance abuse: Biological, psychological, and environmental factors* (pp. 13–64). New York: Plenum.

CURRY, S. G., & Marlatt, G. A. (1987). Building self-confidence, self-efficacy and self-control. In W. M. Cox (Ed.), *Treatment and prevention of alcohol problems: A resource manual* (pp. 117–136). New York: Academic Press.

DEPARTMENT OF HEALTH AND HUMAN SERVICES (1987). *Sixth special report to the U.S. Congress on alcohol and health* (DHHS Publication No. ADM 87-1519). Washington, DC: U.S. Government Printing Office.

DiCICCO, L., Biron, R., Carifio, J., Deutsch, C., Mills, D. J., Orenstein, A., Re, A., Untenberger, H., & White, R. E. (1984). Evaluation of the CASPAR alcohol education curriculum. *Journal of Studies on Alcohol, 45,* 160–169.

GALIZIO, M., & Maisto, S. A. (1985). Toward a biopsychosocial theory of substance abuse. In M. Galizio & S. A. Maisto (Eds.), *Determinants of substance abuse: Biological, psychological, and environmental factors* (pp. 425–429). New York: Plenum.

GIULIANI, D., & Schnoll, S. H. (1985). Clinical decision making in chemical dependence treatment: A programmatic model. *Journal of Substance Abuse Treatment, 2,* 203–208.

GOODWIN, D. W. (1984). Biological predictors of problem drinking. In P. M. Miller & T. D. Nirenberg (Eds.), *Prevention of alcohol abuse* (pp. 97–118). New York: Plenum.

GOODWIN, D. W., Schulsinger, F., Hermansen, L., Guze, S. B., & Winokur, G. (1973). Alcohol problems in adoptees raised apart from alcoholic biological parents. *Archives of General Psychiatry, 28,* 238–243.

HAWKINS, J. D., & Catalano, R. F. (1987, March). *The Seattle social development project: Progress report on a longitudinal prevention study.* Paper presented at the National Institute on Drug Abuse Science Press Seminar, Chicago.

HORN, J. L., Skinner, H. A., Wanberg, K., & Foster, F. M. (1984). *Alcohol Dependence Scale.* Toronto: Addiction Research Foundation of Ontario.

JESSOR, S. J., & Jessor, R. (1977). *Problem behavior and psychosocial development: A longitudinal study of youth.* New York: Academic Press.

KANFER, F. H. (1980). Self-management methods. In F. H. Kanfer & A. P. Goldstein (Eds.), *Helping people change* (pp. 334–389). New York: Pergamon Press.

KAUFMAN, E. (1985). *Substance abuse and family therapy.* Orlando, FL: Grune & Stratton.

LEIGH, G. (1985). Psychosocial factors in the development of substance abuse and alcoholism. In. T. E. Bratter & G. G. Forrest (Eds.), *Alcoholism and substance abuse: Strategies for clinical intervention* (pp. 3–48). New York: Free Press.

LEWIS, J. A. (1992). Treating the alcohol-affected family. In L. L'Abate, J. Farrar, & D. Serritella (Eds.), *Handbook of differential treatment for addictions.* Boston: Allyn & Bacon.

LEWIS, J. A., Dana, R. Q., & Blevins, G. A. (1988). *Substance abuse counseling: An individualized approach.* Pacific Grove, CA: Brooks/Cole.

LEWIS, J. A., & Lewis, M. D. (1989). *Community counseling.* Pacific Grove, CA: Brooks/Cole.

LONGABOUGH, R., McCrady, B., Fink, E., Stout, R., McAuley, T., Doyle, C., & McNeill, D. (1983). Cost-effectiveness of alcohol treatment in partial versus inpatient setting. *Journal of Studies on Alcohol, 44,* 1049–1071.

MALLAMS, J. H., Godley, M. D., Hall, G. M., & Meyers, R. J. (1982). A social-systems approach to resocializing alcoholics in the community. *Journal of Studies on Alcohol, 43,* 1115–1123.

MARLATT, G. A., & Gordon, J. R. (1985). *Relapse prevention: Maintenance strategies in the treatment of addictive behaviors.* New York: Guilford Press.

McLELLAN, A. T., Luborsky, L., Woody, G. E., & O'Brien, C. P. (1980). An improved diagnostic instrument for substance abuse patients: The Addiction Severity Index. *Journal of Nervous and Mental Disorders, 168,* 26–33.

MILLER, W. R. (1985). Motivational interviewing with problem drinkers. In W. R. Miller (Ed.), *Alcoholism: Theory, research, and treatment* (pp. 484–503). Lexington, MA: Ginn Press.

MILLER, W. R., & Hester, R. K. (1985). The effectiveness of treatment techniques: What works and what doesn't. In W. R. Miller (Ed.), *Alcoholism: Theory, research, and treatment* (pp. 526–574). Lexington, MA: Ginn Press.

MILLER, W. R., & Marlatt, G. A. (1984). *Manual for the Comprehensive Drinker Profile.* Odessa, FL: Psychological Assessment Resources.

NEWCOMB, M. D., Maddahian, E., & Bentler, P. M. (1986). Risk factors for drug use among adolescents: Concurrent and longitudinal analyses. *American Journal of Public Health, 76,* 525–531.

PATTISON, E. M., & Kaufman, E. (1982). The alcoholism syndrome: Definitions and models. In E. M. Pattison & E. Kaufman (Eds.), *Encyclopedic handbook of alcoholism* (pp. 3 30). New York: Gardner Press.

SANCHEZ-CRAIG, M., Wilkinson, D. A., & Walker, K. (1987). Theory and methods for secondary prevention of alcohol problems: A cognitively based approach. In C. W. Cox (Ed.), *Treatment and prevention of alcohol problems: A resource manual* (pp. 287–331). New York: Academic Press.

SELZER, M. L. (1971). The Michigan Alcoholism Screening Test: The quest for a new diagnostic instrument. *American Journal of Psychiatry, 127,* 1653–1658.

SOBELL, M. B., Maisto, S. A., Sobell, L. C., Cooper, A. M., Cooper, T., & Sanders, B. (1980). Developing a prototype for evaluating alcohol treatment effectiveness. In L. C. Sobell, M. B. Sobell, & E. Ward (Eds.), *Evaluating alcohol and drug abuse treatment effectiveness: Recent advances* (pp. 129–150). New York: Pergamon Press.

VAILLANT, G. E. (1983). *The natural history of alcoholism.* Cambridge, MA: Harvard University Press.

WASHTON, A. M. (1989). *Cocaine addiction: Treatment, recovery, and relapse prevention.* New York: Norton.

6

Exercise

The labor of the human body is rapidly being engineered out of working life.

John F. Kennedy

The nature of human activity has changed radically since the Industrial Revolution. Most people do not have to chop wood, plow fields, or carry water; instead they are required to sit at a desk or in a vehicle for long hours or stand on the assembly line or behind a store counter. With few exceptions, life today calls on us to move physically very little. Cars, buses, planes, and trains seem to do all the work for us.

Despite a growth of interest in physical fitness and exercise in the past decade, the contemporary life-style is still sedentary. Recent data consistently estimate that only about one-third of the population exercises regularly, and most of these people do not exercise in such a way as to achieve maximum benefits.

The cardiovascular system, muscles, ligaments, tendons, and bones were made to be used. Throughout most of human history, people weren't really aware of that fact, but they used their bodies anyway. Today, regular participation in physical activity is frequently cited by the general public as a very important habit in maintaining good health, but relatively few people do it.

Success seems to be measured by lack of physical exertion. Pushing paper affords a person more status than hammering a nail into a board. Machines are designed with an eye toward lessening or altogether alleviating manual output. As more and more goods and services are readily available without the need for physical activity, people experience a loss in the capacity to perform them. A clear case of the proverbial axiom "use it or lose it" seems to be occurring.

Very few research studies have been conducted that have adequately investigated the impact of an increase in physical activity on the primary or secondary prevention of any specific disease. Therefore, current data on the relationship between increased physical activity and the primary prevention of disorders such as diabetes, hypertension, and stroke are taken from observation rather than from experimental studies (Heyward, 1984). These data make the interpretation of the cause-and-effect relationship between physical activity and disease prevention impossible. However, we seem to accept the notion that physically active people of all ages generally tend to be healthier than their sedentary counterparts. The health benefits attributed to regular physical activity are diverse and include the enhancement of both psychological and social functions.

The documentation of the mental and physical benefits of a regular program of exercise also show the difficulties in establishing and maintaining such programs (Martin & Dubbert, 1982). In order to receive the benefits, exercise must be done properly and on a regular basis. Yet, according to Martin and Dubbert (1982; 1985), one-half of those enrolled in some of the best equipped and staffed programs drop out within the first few months, and the majority of participants cease to exercise within one to two years. The picture is probably much worse for those who undertake fitness programs on their own. Surveys suggest that, in spite of the so-called fitness boom, two-thirds of Americans still do not exercise on a regular basis and between 28 percent and 45 percent do not exercise at all (Martin & Dubbert, 1985).

The role of exercise in health promotion and disease prevention has become very important. Counselors are beginning to be asked to develop and

conduct programs that emphasize the behavioral and motivational aspects of initiating and maintaining a physically active and healthful life-style. Although there is a great deal of knowledge about why one should exercise regularly, little information is available about how best to start and continue such a program.

The Goals and Benefits of Exercise

There are many possible goals for exercise. In health-related settings, however, research supports the following objectives:

1. cardiovascular research/improvement
2. caloric expenditure/weight management
3. cardiovascular risk-factor modification
4. cardiac rehabilitation
5. adjunctive treatment for blood pressure and diabetes control
6. reduction of anxiety and depression
7. rehabilitation of specific joint and muscle functions that are limited by disease or injury

Various forms of exercise affect the body differently. Therefore, programs must be tailored to each client's needs. For example, walking and swimming improve cardiovascular fitness, endurance, and muscle strength. However, weight lifting will improve only muscle strength. For further discussion of the physiology of exercise, interested readers are referred to texts such as McArdle, Katch, and Katch (1981) and Montoye (1978). Most exercise programs are developed by physicians, exercise physiologists, or physical therapists. However, counselors are being consulted to ensure that the program is properly tailored and to create optimal adherence to the prescribed program.

The Body's Response to Exercise

When an individual engages in an exercise such as walking, running, cycling, or swimming, the contraction of skeletal muscles that produces movement requires an immediate increase in energy. To supply the energy, the muscle cells begin to increase their rate of metabolism through the use of available metabolic substrates, which include muscle glycogen and fat, blood glucose, and free fatty acids that are transported to the blood from fat stores to the working muscles. In order to maintain this increase in metabolic activity, oxygen also has to be provided to the working muscles, or fatigue will develop rapidly. This increase in metabolic rate by the muscles, the need to transport substrates and oxygen to the muscle tissue, and the need to rapidly remove the metabolic waste products all produce a variety of adaptive responses by the body.

To meet these demands, the central nervous system also changes. There is a reduction in the parasympathetic tone and a rapid rise in the sympathetic nervous system drive. These two component systems act in opposition to each

other in order to keep balance. The magnitude of these responses is directly proportional to the intensity of the exercise. To facilitate the delivery of extra oxygen and remove carbon dioxide, the rate and depth of breathing increase. When a person feels short of breath during exercise, this has nothing to do with the lung function; rather, it is the result of the inability of the heart and the blood vessels to transport sufficient oxygen to the working muscles. During vigorous exercise, the metabolic demands rise rapidly, and the blood flow to the working muscles must rise to meet these demands; this produces an increase in cardiac performance. Blood pressure rises during exercise; the result is a greater driving pressure, which increases blood flow. Heart rate reflects (more or less) the amount of effort being expended in the exercise. The body's responses to low-resistance, dynamic exercise—running, swimming, cycling—are usually considered to place a high load on the heart and vascular system. More static or heavy resistance exercise, such as weight lifting, creates a pressure load that exerts a relatively small increase in cardiac output but a large rise in blood pressure (Asmussen, 1981). This type of exercise will increase the strength of the muscle being contracted but has very few, if any, health-related benefits. Thus, it is usually not included in a health-oriented exercise program.

Exercise and Mental Health

It has been claimed that mental health in both clinical and nonclinical populations is positively affected by regular vigorous physical activity (Carlson & Ardell, 1981). Some of the proposed psychological benefits are improved confidence, a feeling of well-being, sexual satisfaction, anxiety reduction, the moderation of symptoms of depression, and improved intellectual functioning. The important preventive role of exercise in making people less susceptible to factors that might produce mental illness seems apparent. Sime (1984) notes that avid exercisers frequently report improved quality of life; increased sense of accomplishment, worth, and well-being; and feelings of relaxation, euphoria, and elation during and after exercising.

Research studies on anxiety tend to support the hypothesis that state anxiety (anxiety related to specific life events) is more responsive to exercise than trait anxiety (persistent anxiety that appears to be related to one's personality). Exercise programs of moderate intensity, frequency, and duration appear to be far more effective in reducing anxiety and tension than does a single episode of exercise. Other researchers (Taylor, Sallis, & Needle, 1985; Sime, 1984) also provide evidence of the effectiveness of exercise in reducing mild to moderate depression. Physical activity and exercise appear to alleviate some of the symptoms of depression, particularly for people whose level of depression is higher than normal before the start of the exercise program. The research also suggests that physical exercise may provide a beneficial adjunct for alcoholism and substance-abuse programs; improve self-image, social skills, and cognitive functioning; and reduce the symptoms of anxiety and stress.

The Effect of Exercise on the Aging Process

The human body was designed for the enjoyment of physical activity. If the body is not utilized, the individual is denied the enjoyment and can expect that the body will degenerate more quickly. The signs of physical degeneration are what we usually call aging. The effects of aging include slumped shoulders, sagging skin, loss of vitality, stiff joints, weakness, fatigue, and decreased libido. Of course, these changes are inevitable, but exercise seems to serve to mitigate the effects of the aging process. A major determinant of the rapidity of the aging process is the individual and the way he or she takes care of him- or herself.

One important consideration about exercise is the effect that it has on the circulatory system as well as on the aging process. The maintenance of optimal health requires that tissues both receive fresh nutrients and excrete waste sufficiently. When an individual remains sedentary, the circulatory system maintains a level of efficiency that will sustain the current level of activity (inactivity) but nothing extra. The end result is that when an extra burst of energy is needed, it just isn't there. There are no reserves of energy, because there isn't a higher degree of circulatory efficiency.

Assessment

Exercise Program Screening

Once an exercise program has been prescribed for an individual, it is necessary to consider safety precautions related to the client's capacities and limitations. For example, people with high blood pressure should not be involved in strenuous weight-lifting activity because it increases blood pressure. Counselors who supervise exercise programs need to be aware of methods to determine high-risk candidates who need medical screening and assessments and decide which clients would not be good candidates for unsupervised exercise programs.

Although research and experience have indicated that exercise programs are not very dangerous, we still recommend some initial medical screening for the safety and protection of the client, as well as for the counselor. The following statements, which require the client to answer yes or no, have been taken from a variety of sources. Counselors need to ask these questions before clients go through exercise assessment, prescription, or programming.

____ You are over 35 years old and have been physically inactive.

____ You have been told that you have heart trouble, heart disease, a heart murmur, or that you have had a heart attack.

____ You frequently have pains or pressure in the left or midchest area or in the neck.

____ You often feel faint or have spells of severe dizziness.

____ You experience extreme breathlessness after mild exertion.

____ Your doctor said your blood pressure is too high and is not under control, or you do not know whether your blood pressure is normal.

—   You have bone or joint problems, such as arthritis.
—   Your family has a history of early heart attacks or strokes.
—   You have another medical condition, such as diabetes or asthma, that may need special attention in an exercise program.
—   You are significantly overweight.
—   You have an old, serious injury (knee, back) that might warrant special precautions or a special exercise evaluation or prescription or that might be worsened by a strenuous exercise program.

If a "yes" answer occurs to any of the questions, a physician's opinion and often a medical evaluation is warranted. It is the physician who must decide whether a complete physical and/or exercise "stress" test is warranted. We feel that physician consultation is strongly recommended before any strenuous exercise or fitness testing or whenever there is any doubt about the appropriateness of a particular client's beginning an exercise program.

In addition to the medical doctor, exercise physiologists specialize in screening and assessing individuals at various risk levels. Exercise physiologists often represent an important resource for the health counselor as a source of information or consultation. More and more exercise physiologists are interested in using counselors to help them construct effective exercise motivation packages that make use of modern behavioral technology to increase exercise adherence and compliance.

Exercise Assessment

Assessment is a complicated process that includes an evaluation of the individual's current state of physical health and a projection of future potential, as well as an appraisal of which interventions would be most beneficial. It is also necessary to assess the level of cooperation that can be expected from the client.

Measuring an individual's habitual exercise pattern is difficult. It is very hard, if not impossible, to obtain a "gold standard" measurement, because it is difficult to ascertain the truth about a person's exercise habits. It is also hard to utilize paper-and-pencil instruments or other self-report devices to estimate exercise. As was indicated in the previous section, it is essential to first assess the client's current state of physical fitness before an exercise program can be employed. Without an adequate assessment of the client's current physical condition, the counselor runs the risk of actually creating more problems for the client. It is germane to note at this point that the most effective counselors work in tandem with a physician or a physician's assistant. The components that the physician will most often assess are cardiovascular fitness, muscular fitness, and flexibility.

Cardiovascular fitness.   When cells in the human body combine oxygen with nutrients, they produce energy. The body can store some nutrients, but it must replenish others with each new breath inhaled. An efficient cardiovascular system will supply each cell with an optimal amount of oxygen and will remove the maximum amount of waste possible each time the lungs are used. Exercise that develops an efficient cardiovascular respiratory system is

known as aerobic. This type of exercise is an excellent source of stimulation for the lungs and the heart. Not surprisingly, many physicians suggest an aerobic activity for patients who have recently suffered from heart attacks or who currently have high blood pressure. Clinical studies have shown that aerobic exercise such as running, walking, cycling, or swimming helps the entire cardiovascular system work more efficiently. This in turn builds up the heart muscles, and changes can be measured in the heart rate of the heart at rest. Those who engage in regular aerobic activity, for example, can expect to have a lowered resting heart rate. In assessing cardiovascular fitness, the physician must get an accurate reading of the patient's heart rate, blood pressure, and a stress electrocardiogram to determine the current condition of the heart (Heyward, 1984).

Muscular fitness.   Muscular fitness refers to the strength, endurance, and power of the muscle, and physicians often test this area as well. Muscle strength refers to the amount of force that the muscle produces when it contracts. Development of strength is directly related to the number of trials that the muscle endures against resistance; that is, we become stronger as we keep lifing heavier objects. Another component of muscular fitness is endurance, which refers to the ability of the muscle to work overtime. Specifically, endurance is the ability to repeat an activity or to continue one for a long span of time. Muscular endurance is something that increases with concentrated use of the muscles (Dishman, Sallis, & Orenstein, 1985). Power is the speed at which the muscle can contract and apply a measure of strength. Different exercises will provide very different benefits for muscular development. If an individual is involved in only one sport or one activity, he or she is likely to gain benefits from it but not develop the overall fitness that may be needed to ensure the maintenance of good health.

Flexibility.   The assessment of flexibility is concerned with the range of movement of a joint. Inactivity will reduce the flexibility of a joint. Many people make the mistake of assuming that elderly people have lost some mobility of their joints as part of the aging process, whereas in reality their loss has more to do with their level of activity than with the aging process. Lack of flexibility is usually preceded by a decline in physical activity. It is well documented that less active people have a more limited range of motion than do those who exercise regularly (Heyward, 1984; Ardell, 1986). Even regular use of the muscles, if restricted to one pattern because of limited activity or a sedentary life-style, often results in a restricted range of movement.

In addition to determining one's fitness level and exercise capacity, a thorough initial assessment with regular follow-up sessions can document changes in health status for the clients who do not feel that they are changing. We have often found clients who report no change in weight but whose physical measurements indicate that they have lost inches and whose clothes no longer fit the same way. Additionally, clients may notice a decrease in resting and exercise heart rates.

Failure to show change after a reasonable time can cue the counselor to explore the following possibilities.

1. The client is not adhering well enough to the exercise prescription (exercise mode or type, frequency, intensity, and duration) to produce the desired change.
2. The exercise prescription itself is faulty or inadequate.
3. The measures are not sensitive enough to the changes and perhaps need to be altered, replaced, or supplemented by other measures.

We believe that it is important to mention again that performing an exercise fitness test is a complicated task, and health counselors who have no medical or exercise physiology training should *never* attempt exercise testing on clinical clients without direct supervision by medical or exercise physiology specialists. Interested readers are encouraged to consult the publications of the American College of Sports Medicine (ACSM) on exercise testing and prescriptions (ACSM, 1978; 1980). Numerous special training courses on exercise testing, prescription, and program implementation are provided by ACSM around the country. Contact ACSM, P.O. Box 1440, Indianapolis, IN 46206, (317) 637-9200.

Attitudes and Beliefs about Exercise

Dishman, Sallis, and Orenstein (1985) suggest that those who believe in the value of exercise for *their* specific benefit have a greater likelihood of incorporating and maintaining exercise as part of their daily routine. Although the researchers are quick to note that education is not a salient factor in the individual's motivation to engage in exercise, they do include it as an element in the client's choice to participate in an exercise program.

Few people would disagree that Americans are underexercised. Often, excuses and faulty beliefs for neglecting exercise are at the root.

"It's no fun."
"It's for kids."
"I'm too busy."
"I'm too tired."
"I'm too fat."
"I look awful in running shorts."
"I can't afford it."
"I don't have anybody to play with."
"I tried it once and it didn't work."
"I don't know how."
"I'm afraid."

The health beliefs of exercise are a part of the individual's value system at the personal, interpersonal, and cultural levels. An interesting empirical finding is that a person's attitudes and beliefs about physical fitness are not a salient predictor of that person's adherence to an exercise program (Dishman, 1982;

Carter, Lee, & Greenockle, 1987). Although these attitudes are an effective indicator of initial involvement in an exercise program, they are not effective in identifying individuals who would adhere to a prescribed exercise regimen.

Interventions

Counseling

Although the evidence supports the many benefits of exercise, the bottom-line effectiveness of the exercise program depends on ensuring sufficient adherence to the regimen to produce the desired health benefits (Haynes, 1984). As previously discussed, research strongly suggests that the majority of people who begin a systematic exercise program, either on their own or in a structured program, will stop before any lasting benefits occur. This is probably the result of inappropriate, inadequate, or inefficient counseling, both in the all-important habit acquisition stage and during the maintenance stage or during the transition from a formal program to a self-managed program. It is likely that poor attention to the learning environment, personality characteristics, and behavioral techniques are responsible for these statistics.

As the counselor helps a client develop and implement an exercise program, consideration of the following variables is important: (1) be sure to program early enjoyability and reinforcement of the exercise habit; (2) move slowly and gradually shape the desired habit; (3) begin with low to moderate exercise intensity; (4) utilize social support whenever possible; and (5) ensure that the program and the facility are convenient.

> Exercise programmers often view adherence to the program as the natural outcome of initial health education and the motivation provided by improved performance and fitness. In our opinion, more often the opposite is true: fitness improvement and health education are the inevitable by-products of exercise programs that ensure long-term adherence. Reinforcement can come from being with others; from easy invigorating activity; or from praise by family and program members (Martin & Dubbert, 1987, p. 368).

General Principles of Training

According to Ribisl (1984), three important principles provide guidance in the design of exercise programs. They are overload, progression, and specificity.

For an adaptive response to occur, a system must be subjected to a load significantly greater than the load to which it is accustomed. This is the essence of the *overload* principle. At the initial stages of an exercise program, when a client is deconditioned from sedentary living, every little exercise is enough to create an overload. As the client's fitness level improves, greater amounts of work are necessary to create an overload and produce change.

The principle of *progression* states that an exercise program should be applied in a gradual, progressive manner in accordance with the level of fitness. This principle directly relates to overload. At the beginning of an exercise

program, the rate of progression should be relatively slow. The program should last for several weeks, especially for individuals who have been sedentary for a long period of time, because any change produces muscle soreness and injury to muscles that are unaccustomed to the stress and strain of vigorous exercise. To keep the client's attitude positive and enthusiasm high, effective counselors work hard to minimize the client's discomfort and soreness at the early stages of a training program. This is often a difficult challenge, as we live in an age of "drive-through" living in which we want everything done right away. It is important for the counselor to stop an individual from doing too much too soon and thus losing interest.·

The third principle, that of *specificity,* is based on the fact that the body adapts to an overload stimulus in a manner that is specific to the type of training (aerobic or anaerobic) as well as to the muscles involved in the training. Research by Fox (1980) reveals that there is little transfer of training effects, either from one type of training to another or from one muscle group to another. It appears that different types of exercise place different demands on the mechanisms for energy production. It is perhaps with this thought in mind that many exercise trainers are urging cross-training to develop whole-body fitness.

Developing the Exercise Prescription

In developing an exercise prescription, the counselor needs to tailor the exercise program to each client to increase client adherence to the program. The major components of an exercise prescription include the type or mode of exercise, its frequency, its intensity, and its duration.

Mode of Exercise

It is important to choose an exercise that will be appropriate and also appeal to the individual. The counselor can assess a client's previous exercise history, home and work schedules, and individual goals and preferences as part of the assessment process. We have found that it is very important to tailor the exercise to the client's personal goals, history, and life-style. Research by Thompson and Wankel (1980) supports the effectiveness of the tailoring process. In their research, clients who believed that their program had been specifically designed for them continued longer than those who were not given that same impression.

For an activity to be considered satisfactory aerobically, several criteria must be met. The exercise must involve vigorous activity of large muscle groups, be rhythmic in nature, and be performed aerobically. The activities that best meet these criteria are aerobic dancing, bicycling, cross-country skiing, racquet sports, rope skipping, swimming, walking, jogging, and running. Many other activities could be used to complement these activities, but most are probably not vigorous enough to produce an adequate aerobic benefit. These activities include backpacking, golfing, hiking, downhill skiing, and skin diving.

In some cases, the exercise mode is not a matter of choice. Clearly, some

exercises have superior efficiency, and some might be the only feasible alternative. For example, working in the Midwest, we have found that winter weather restricts many clients to inside exercise, and often we find that the only feasible alternative is stationary biking. When we are not able to tailor the exercise mode to the individual client, we work with the client to reframe this exercise and see its positive features.

Frequency of Exercise

Researchers consistently report that the ideal frequency of aerobic exercise for improving cardiovascular fitness is three times per week. This allows the client time to complete the exercise and then gives a reasonable period of time to recover and allow the body to rejuvenate. Less frequent exercise produces minimal gains in fitness, endurance, and other health benefits. A bigger problem, however, is that lower frequencies prevent the establishment of exercise as a habit. It is important for the counselor to help the client develop an exercise pattern that will be continued and adhered to for years. Unless a person is in competitive sports training, exercising three to four times per week seems optimal. When clients exercise more than four times per week, the likelihood of injury, fatigue, and nonadherence increases.

Most researchers believe that exercising briskly every other day and resting on the alternative days is the preferred schedule. This system is relatively easy to keep track of and easy to schedule and manage. There are exceptions to this suggestion. Some clients find it helpful to exercise on a daily basis, perhaps just after awakening, whereas others enjoy working out five days a week and resting on weekends. The important point is to understand each individual's life-style and develop a schedule of no less than three times per week. If individuals choose to exercise on a daily basis, it may be important to suggest lower intensities.

Another consideration in exercise frequency is the availability of programs. In large metropolitan areas, programs are available around the clock, whereas in urban and rural areas, programs may be limited. When tailoring an exercise program, counselors need to choose one that is realistic for an individual's schedule.

Intensity of Exercise

There are many suggestions for assessing the proper level of intensity for an exercise program. A general rule of thumb is for the client to exercise at a level that is around 70 percent higher than the client's resting heart rate. Exercising at this target heart rate will produce an aerobic, or cardiovascular, benefit. Researchers believe that lower intensities produce significantly fewer benefits but that exercising too intensely can be counterproductive; that is, the benefits are not any greater, and the increased intensity greatly increases the risk of injuries, which can lead to poor treatment adherence. A simple rule to follow with clients is that, if they find it difficult to talk while exercising, then it is likely that they are operating at too high a level of intensity.

To determine and monitor heart rate, the following is suggested. To obtain

a maximum heart rate, it is necessary to have a stress electrocardiogram. For those clients for whom this would be too costly and not warranted, a simple general calculation is to take the number 220 and subtract from it the client's age. The number obtained can be termed the *maximum heart rate.* In order to determine the *target heart rate,* subtract the individual's resting heart rate from the maximum rate. Determine 70 percent of that difference and add it back to the resting heart rate. The result represents the target heart rate. For example, the maximum heart rate of a 50 year old with a heart rate of 80 beats per minute is 170 (220 – 50 = 170). His or her target heart rate is 143 (170 – 80 = 90; 70% of 90 = 63; 63 + 80 = 143). Urge individuals to operate within 65 to 75 percent of their maximum heart rate. We suggest that individuals stop periodically and take their heart rate for ten seconds (and multiply by 6 to determine heart rate per minute). This should be done periodically throughout an exercise program until the individual feels comfortable just "feeling" what the proper exercise intensity level is. Individuals who have a difficult time taking their own heart rate can use any of the low-cost monitors that are available commercially.

Counselors can usually observe whether the intensity level is too great by noticing whether the client's face is bright red or whether there is profuse sweating or heavy breathing. If so, the exercise is probably being done too intensely. It is also important to caution all clients to be sure to drink plenty of fluids before, during, and after exercise to avoid dehydration. This is especially important during the summer months or in hot climates.

Duration of Exercise

The duration of exercise is closely related to mode, frequency, and intensity. The general rule of thumb is that exercise needs to be a minimum of 15 to 20 minutes in duration. However, it may be necessary to move gradually to that level. Programs such as Ken Cooper's (1968; 1977; 1982) aerobic point system for quantifying exercise levels effectively combines mode, frequency, intensity, and duration into a single scale. This allows the counselor and the client to tie all four components together effectively.

The duration of exercise will relate directly to how much time individuals have available. Many people in today's high-efficiency, fast society want to get the most out of an exercise program in the least amount of time. Cooper's program effectively shows which exercises produce the best results in the shortest period of time. On the basis of our personal experience, we believe, as would Cooper, that although 15 to 20 minutes is the minimum exercise duration, it is more likely that a duration of 30 to 45 minutes will produce the necessary aerobic effect.

In summary, selecting the proper mode, frequency, intensity, and duration can help tailor the exercise prescription and increase treatment adherence. Once an appropriate form of exercise has been chosen, the counselor needs to help the client think in a fashion that views exercise as an important part of daily living.

Developing Goals and Objectives

The importance of goal setting in exercise performance cannot be stressed enough. Common goals and objectives are to improve flexibility, muscular strength and endurance, cardiovascular endurance, and body composition and weight. However, other clients may start an exercise program with the intent of improving stress management, increasing social contacts, improving self-esteem, and so on. It is important to identify clearly the client's goals and, as we said earlier, to tailor the exercise prescription. Researchers believe that the more flexible, individually tailored, and achievable the goals are, the better the ensuing adherence. It is important to educate clients about reasonable goals and reasonable timetables for achieving results. Most clients expect immediate changes and benefits and are often quickly discouraged.

After helping the client establish overall goals of exercise, it is important to help set subgoals and establish just how the mental aspects of setting, achieving, or failing to achieve the goals might affect the client's sticking with the program. Often individuals who are allowed to create their own exercise goals continue patterns of failure that have plagued their entire exercise history. It is therefore important for counselors to help clients formulate subgoals. We have found that the more flexible these goals are, in terms of both specific sessions and hoped-for performance across time, the more effective they are in minimizing the occurrence of failures. For example, we would urge clients to state goals such as "I want to be able to run the Chicago Marathon in eight months" or "I want to be able to run three miles to my brother's house without stopping within one-and-a-half months." We encourage clients to concentrate more on adherence and regularity than on performance, because we feel that performance will be the by-product of adherence.

Cognitive Strategies during Exercise

Our experiences support the use of dissociative, or distraction-based, thoughts during exercise (Hendricks & Carlson, 1981). Research by Martin et al. (1984) found that individuals who were taught to dissociate their thoughts from the actual exercise or the bodily sensations connected with the exertion had significantly better class attendance, exercise adherence, and long-term maintenance of their regimen than did those who were taught to associate thinking of the exercise and how it felt and acted as their own coach.

Other studies (Martin & Dubbert, 1985) suggest that distraction during exercise enhances performance and increases exercise duration. During the initial stages of exercise, the feedback that the body provides is often negative, and individuals who pay attention to these signals are often quick to stop a program that appears so discouraging. Through the use of distracting cognitive strategies, this negative feedback can be minimized. Distraction activities might include exercising with others and talking, listening to a portable radio, reading or watching television while doing stationary exercise, participating in an ex-

ercise class, or exercising in a pleasant setting. It is important to mention that distraction activities such as these would *not* be appropriate for clients with serious physical problems who are taught and need to be trained to become very sensitive to their body signals.

Psychoeducational Strategies

Enduring patterns are sustained because they are cued and reinforced as aspects of the environment. This basic paradigm of antecedent behavior-consequence is a fundamental psychological principle. The basic strategy necessary in modifying behavior is to make changes in the environment that will both support the desired behaviors and weaken the competing behaviors. The process involved in identifying cues that will enhance the desired outcome while subsequently noting the cues that result in competing or less desirable behaviors is a complex task. In the lives of sedentary individuals, there are few effective cues for promoting exercise, as compared to the cues for the competing behaviors. Therefore, the counselor's job is to help the client build on and increase these cues. The more often a behavior occurs in a particular stimulus situation, the more powerful a cue the stimulus situation becomes. The counselor can help the client recognize the very process of conditioning that is occurring on a daily basis. Once the client is cognizant of this, he or she can be more open to the psychoeducational process.

The initial step in the process is to have clients spend a discrete period of time engaged in self-monitoring. After clients have had sufficient time to observe and record their exercise behaviors, the antecedent variables, and any cueing that they may have been aware of, they can work with the counselor to arrange an environment that is conducive to promoting exercise (Dishman, 1988). As with any self-monitoring activity the performance of the desired behavior almost predictably increases.

The time, place, and people involved in an exercise program will come to represent the cues for those who adhere to the program. Yet, structured exercise programs have a built-in, unfortunate drawback, and that is that, once the structured program ends, so do the cues it provides. One way to deal with this problem is to provide a variety of cues within the environment. The counselor should attempt to generalize the stimulus control of exercise to other settings before the program is concluded. To expect people to continue to exercise following the sudden withdrawal of their cues is naive.

Another important factor to attend to is the decreasing of cues for competing behaviors (Martin & Dubbert, 1984). The counselor can promote this process by helping the client identify concretely the specific time and location that he or she will be relatively isolated from competing cues and can engage in exercise. Dishman (1988) suggests that early morning seems to be a good time for most people, especially for the busy Type A individuals who are increasingly being seen for cardiac rehabilitation. It is also useful to help the client set up an elaborate set of environmental cues to decrease competing cues—for example, equipping one's office with exercise photos and carrying a gym bag complete with exercise clothes for any occasion.

In general, punishment without simultaneous reward for the desired behavior is ineffective in eliminating a high-frequency undesired behavior. Therefore, the elimination of the natural discomforts that accompany increased physical activity is essential. Intervention at the level of the behavior itself, in the form of an individualized exercise prescription and educative process, may help lessen the natural discomforts that are associated with increased physical activity. Cognitive restructuring that eliminates negative self-talk (such as: "I hate running," "I'm so tired," and "Why does this have to hurt so much?") and then teaches some well-needed skills in temporary dissociation appear to be the most effective interventions (Dishman, 1988).

Reinforcement and encouragement are another important aspect of the psychoeducational process. Again, it is important to encourage the client not to rely on the counselor as the primary agent of change. For example, clients are often encouraged to sign written contracts that serve primarily as reinforcers for exercise adherence. An often overlooked disadvantage of written contracts is that they are dependent on external forms of reinforcement; when the client is without an external agent of reinforcement, she or he will almost certainly relapse. A further complication of the contract system is that clients may come to view the counselor as responsible for their success. Clients may find themselves unable to gain a sense of self-efficacy that will allow them to succeed independently of the counselor.

Preventive and therapeutic exercise programs are increasingly found in the community at large, in the school, and in the workplace (Iverson, Fielding, Crow, & Christenson, 1985). Very few exercise programs are available in medical-care settings such as hospitals or with outpatient clients. Physicians prescribe exercise programs to fewer than 10 percent of the patients they see, and a number of studies suggest that part of the reason is that physicians do not believe that they can alter the behavior of their patients. Interestingly, patients want their physicians to be concerned about their health habits, and it seems quite likely that the influence that physicians have on their patients' behavior is substantially greater than the physicians themselves believe.

Most people who are trying to locate physical activity programs for maximum benefit conclude that the single most important setting for such programs is the school. Well-run physical education programs for school-age children can set the stage for a lifetime of interest and involvement in exercise. Yet, in spite of the fact that most states require the teaching of physical education at some point in the school curriculum, only about one-third of the young people between the ages of 10 and 17 participate in daily physical education programs in school (Iverson et al., 1985).

The newest setting for the development of physical activity programs is the workplace. Nearly three-quarters of adults between the age of 18 and 65 are now employed, and workplace physical-activity programs have been shown to provide health and economic benefits to employees and both economic and noneconomic benefits to employers (Iverson et al., 1985).

An additional special community resource is the YMCA. This organization has been involved with the development and implementation of exercise programs across the United States for years and many of its programs have been

recently updated. Further information can be obtained by calling (708) 823-2973 or writing to the YMCA of the U.S.A., Program Resources, 6400 Shafer Court, Rosemount, IL 60018.

Case Example

Bill is a 31-year-old married white male who sought out counseling for depression. The precipitating event was a physical exam in which his physician felt that Bill was at considerable risk for cardiovascular problems. Bill was, apparently, confronted with his mortality for the first time in his life. Bill reported that he was a good high school athlete and that he had participated in three different sports events. Since graduating from high school, he has participated in physical activities only on an irregular basis. He has attended a state college and earned a business degree. He has been relatively successful in business and was receiving a routine executive fitness exam when he learned of his high risk for cardiovascular problems. In addition to describing his high-stress job and lack of exercise, Bill reported tension in his marriage of seven years and high stress with his three preschool-age children. Although Bill did say that he loved his wife, he also indicated that he didn't like her all the time. There is a history of cardiovascular problems in Bill's family of origin. Bill's father had suffered a near-fatal heart attack at age 52 and had died of cardiovascular complications at age 56.

The biopsychosocial treatment formulation addressed the many problem areas that Bill faced. The counselor believed that Bill, as had Bill's father, had taken his physical health for granted and had focused heavily on being a good provider. Although his health habits were not necessarily bad, they were not very good either, and it was likely that he did have some inherited cardiovascular weakness. It was also likely that, given the high stress caused by Bill's current living situation—three young children, a high-pressure job, and some marital conflict—he might be reluctant or incapable of taking on any new challenges such as an exercise program.

With the above information in mind, the counselor began to talk with Bill about the kind of exercise program that he could realistically become involved in. Bill indicated that two of his close friends had been skipping business lunches and going to the local YMCA, riding the stationary bicycles and using the rowing machines. He thought that this was something that he too would be able to do on roughly four out of every five working days. He indicated that he was not too interested in either rowing or biking but did feel that the Y was convenient and that having his close friends along would make the whole experience more enjoyable. The counselor suggested that Bill talk specifically with the director of the Y and ask him or her to contact his physician regarding setting up a specific exercise program. Bill and his counselor eventually decided that he would begin slowly, riding the bike for seven minutes and doing some walking, and then gradually build up his workout to be in the 35- to 40-minute range at the end of four months.

The counselor helped Bill find out what might be a good reward if he was

successful in his exercise program. Bill indicated that he was planning to go to the Caribbean on business and that he was thinking of taking his wife along. He thought that just feeling good while outdoors and being comfortable in summer clothes might be worthwhile. Bill agreed to meet with the counselor on a weekly basis to deal with other presenting issues but indicated that five minutes of each session would be devoted to reporting on and continuing to tailor the exercise prescription. The ongoing contact would also help eliminate and fend off problems of relapse.

Adherence to Exercise Programs

Regardless of the setting in which physical activity and exercise programs take place, researchers consistently express a major concern with the low rate of adherence to such programs (Epstein & Wing, 1980; Haskell, 1985; Mirotznik, Speedling, Stein, & Bronz, 1985). Three sets of factors have been studied in terms of their roles in predicting adherence: personal factors, social-environmental factors, and characteristics of the exercise program itself. Unfortunately, the most obvious personal factor—attitude toward exercise—appears to be unrelated to whether a person adheres to an exercise program. That is, most people who lead sedentary lives have extremely favorable attitudes toward exercise (Dishman & Gettman, 1980).

Of the personal factors, perhaps the most accurate predictor of nonadherence is low motivation. A second important personal factor is the extent to which the person is achieving his or her exercise objectives. Low motivation and the failure to appear to be making progress toward one's goals may be a near-fatal combination. In the behavioral domain, predictors of dropping out of exercise programs include smoking, having inactive leisure-time pursuits, and exhibiting Type A behavior (Martin & Dubbert, 1982). Being overweight is a biological factor that is associated with a high dropout rate. Combining the measures of body weight, motivation, and smoking behavior will result in 80 percent accuracy in predicting who will adhere to an exercise program and who will drop out.

The major social-environmental factors that appear to predict adherence to an exercise program include support by family members, geographic stability, absence of family problems, and exercise done in a group setting, as opposed to exercise done alone.

Finally, with regard to the characteristics of the exercise program, adherence is highest when the program is conveniently located and moderate in intensity—not too easy and not too hard.

In their general conclusions regarding the current status of exercise programs, Martin and Dubbert (1982) indicate that:

1. Aerobic exercise (Cooper, 1968) appears to be beneficial in the treatment and prevention of a variety of health disorders.
2. Problems of low adherence rates are so severe that, even though the evidence is clear that exercise is helpful, the overall effectiveness of exercise programs is in doubt.

3. Comparison among studies is difficult because of the failure to establish standardized ways of measuring both the exercise program and adherence to it.
4. There is some evidence that behavioral strategies, such as self-control procedures, can increase adherence, but the effects appear to be temporary.
5. Many of the studies of the effectiveness of exercise programs are methodologically unsound in that, without appropriately selected control groups, it is not possible to identify the specific effects of a particular exercise versus the effects of participating in a program of any kind (Bloom, 1990).

Adherence-Promoting Program Structure

Martin and Dubbert (1987) explain that, if clients are to establish the exercise habit effectively, their specific concerns about the program and the facility need to be addressed. Several considerations and recommendations are listed as follows:

1. the overall convenience of the program facility and regimen
2. the use of group exercise format
3. the supervision of participants by counselors
4. an emphasis on shaping individual responsibility for the exercise program
5. the liberal use of behavioral technologies to prompt and reinforce the exercise habit
6. the utilization of early generalization training
7. the use of continued contact and testing for those who have graduated from the program

Even in the best prescribed programs, it is important that individual clients be prepared to take responsibility for self-motivated home- or work-based exercise programs. As part of this preparation, clients need to be "inoculated" against relapses or slips (Marlatt & Gordon, 1985). Studies suggest that many breaks in the exercise routine are due to injury or sickness, much of which is, in turn, the result of exercising too intensely. Therefore, Martin and Dubbert (1987) believe that a number of these relapses might be prevented through a more careful shaping and monitoring of the exercise program design. The remainder of the slips or relapses are generally related to (1) work and home changes (such as a job transfer and marital conflicts) or (2) motivational problems and loss of interest in the exercise.

If slips or relapses occur, it is helpful to use the following strategies (Martin & Dubbert, 1987).

1. Participants should admit and take responsibility for the exercise slip, which includes letting go of guilt, blame, and so on. They are encouraged to call a friend and talk about the slip in objective (not self-loathing) terms: "it happened; it was no one's fault; now what do I do about it?"
2. Participants should plan to exercise the following day or as soon as possible. This includes planning when, where, what, for how long, and with whom. Participants are encouraged to write these plans down and/or share them with another.

3. Participants could arrange to exercise with someone else. Exercising with someone at an equal fitness level or who will agree to exercise at the same intensity enhances reinforcement and distraction. The first day after the slip, the individual should not attempt the highest level of intensity, frequency, or duration of exercise previously achieved, especially after an extended layoff. This is courting trouble, burnout, and injury. The first several weeks of exercising should be especially easy and enjoyable to solidly reshape the exercise habit.

4. Participants should prepare completely for exercise on the planned return day, both cognitively and physically. They should get a good night's rest, eat well, go over each step of the return event mentally, lay out proper clothing, clear away competing events, show up early, warm up properly, and give it their best.

5. Participants should be reinforced for showing up. No matter how little or how much they accomplish in the early return to exercise sessions, participants should praise themselves and encourage others to praise them for their positive steps. Participants could plan some reinforcing event following each session, such as going to the movies or to a favorite dinner spot or taking a nice, hot bath.

Our concern is not whether our clients will slip; we expect a period of time in which they will stop exercising. We are more concerned with what they can do when this occurs. We have often found it helpful to rehearse with clients, before the termination of counseling, how relapses will be dealt with.

Dishman (1988) notes that the ongoing focus of much of the research in the field of relapse prevention has been the attempt to construct a profile of "the client most likely to . . ." This not only is a fruitless exercise but also demonstrates a total disregard for the uniqueness and individuality of each client. This attempt to isolate the profile of the client most likely to experience relapse problems has done nothing to advance the concept of cooperation in the treatment process and has done much to further the notion of the counselor as the only active agent in the treatment process (Sperry, 1985). This problem was alluded to when the concept of relapse prevention strategies was explored earlier in this chapter (Dishman, 1988). Previous suggestions as to the preferred approach to relapse prevention have viewed the client as the main operative in the process, with the counselor's participation being limited to that of an interested—albeit ineffectual—observer. Current wisdom (Dishman, 1988; Belise, Roskies, & Levesque, 1987) emphasizes the mutual participation of counselor and client in treatment. Sperry (1985) quotes Rudolf Dreikurs: "When the goals and interests of the patient and therapist clash, no satisfactory relationship can be established. . . . What appears a 'resistance' constitutes a discrepancy between the goals of the therapist and those of the patient."

One frequent oversight in the process of relapse prevention is the failure to identify conditions that militate against adherence to treatment (Dishman, 1988; Sonstroem, 1988). Fatigue, sore muscles, and time spent away from the television can be powerful aversive factors in treatment adherence. Without the proper identification of these factors, no interventions or inoculation measures

can be instituted. Questions such as "What will you miss by exercising?" or "What will be the worst part about starting to exercise?" should help pinpoint these troublesome areas.

Very little research exists to provide specific information on the *one* best adherence program. Several characteristics of successful exercise programs have already been mentioned. Additional characteristics that receive considerable attention in the literature are locus of control, perceived self-efficacy, and the exercise setting.

Locus of control.   Not surprisingly, Carter, Lee, and Greenockle (1987) found that the expected adherence of clients who are engaged in the exercise program is consistent with their understanding of how able they are to control the outcome of their efforts. Subjects in the study who saw themselves as able to change, particularly with regard to exercise-related behaviors, had the highest actual performance rate. Other studies note that the individuals who are best able to internalize their own reinforcements or are able to better motivate themselves experience a higher internal locus of control than those who are primarily other-oriented in their reinforcement process (Dishman, 1982; 1988).

Perceived self-efficacy.   Perceived self-efficacy is the internalization of the concept that one can succeed at a given task with a given set of circumstances. Research supports self-efficacy as an essential component in the process of treatment adherence and relapse prevention (Dishman, 1988; Sonstroem, 1988). The self-evaluative process is a part of the client's set of expectations for treatment, and it is an area that deserves considerable explanation at the beginning of treatment. Although the client may have a firm sense of his or her ability to be efficacious in an exercise program, this does not mean that the counselor and the client cannot make the appropriate interventions that would affect positively the continuation of this motivation early in the program. Dishman (1988) suggests that the client learn some cognitive restructuring techniques. These attempts at altering the client's self-perception should be made with the client's knowledge and, perhaps more importantly, cooperation. Guided imagery is an excellent way to intervene on a cognitive level. The counselor can also carefully arrange exercise assignments that are easily attainable for the client, thereby enhancing his or her sense of self-efficacy.

Exercise setting.   Many researchers in the field have identified the exercise setting as one of the problematic areas in relapse prevention and exercise adherence. It should be noted, though, that while it certainly is an important component, it is not the only one affecting adherence. Many writers suggest that those who tailor exercise programs need to pay close attention to varying the setting in which the exercise is performed in order to alleviate boredom. Ardell (1986) suggests that the counselor utilize a variety of exercises and be careful not to rely on just one or two modalities of exercise. Many writers advocate cross-training, which involves using several exercise modalities as part of an exercise program (for instance, bike one day, run another, swim on a third day, and so on).

Another concern with the setting is that it be readily accessible and an almost obvious choice for the client (Dishman, 1982). Whereas some people prefer the convenience of their home, others would much rather have another location. Counselors must be very sensitive to the client's individual needs and develop a location for exercise that is convenient for the client. A program based solely on one's physical ailments and exercise needs has high probability of failure.

Summary

Counselors can play an important role in helping clients develop the behavioral and motivational aspects necessary to initiate and maintain an exercise program. Although most people acknowledge the importance of exercise, few adhere to a regular program. This is the greatest challenge for the counselor. By tailoring exercise prescriptions with regard to mode, frequency, intensity, and duration, counselors can increase the likelihood of habit formation.

References

AMERICAN COLLEGE OF SPORTS MEDICINE (ACSM). (1978). Position statement on the recommended quantity and quality of exercise for developing and maintaining fitness in healthy adults. *Medicine and Science in Sports and Exercise, 10,* 7–10.

AMERICAN COLLEGE OF SPORTS MEDICINE (ACSM). (1980). *Guidelines for graded exercise testing and exercise prescription.* Philadelphia: Lea and Febiger.

ARDELL, D. B. (1986). *High level wellness.* Berkeley: Ten Speed Press.

ASMUSSEN, E. (1981). Similarities and dissimilarities between static and dynamic exercise. *Circulation Research, 48*(II), 1–3.

BANDURA, A. (1977). Self-efficacy: Toward a unifying theory of behavioral change. *Psychological Review, 84*(2), 191–215.

BELISE, M., Roskies, E., & Levesque, J. M. (1987). Improving adherence to physical activity. *Health Psychology, 6*(2), 159–172.

BLOOM, B. L. (1990). *Health psychology: A psychosocial perspective.* Engelwood Cliffs, NJ: Prentice-Hall.

CARLSON, J., & Ardell, D. B. (1981). Physical fitness as a pathway to wellness and effective counseling. *Counseling and Human Development,* March, 1–12.

CARTER, J., Lee, A., & Greenockle, K. (1987). Locus of control, fitness values, success expectations, and performance in fitness class. *Perceptual and Motor Skills, 65,* 777–778.

COOPER, K. H. (1968). *Aerobics.* New York: Bantam Books.

COOPER, K. H. (1977). *The aerobics way.* New York: Bantam Books.

COOPER, K. H. (1982). *The aerobics program for total well being.* New York: Bantam Books.

DISHMAN, R. (1982). Compliance-adherence in health-related exercise. *Health Psychology, 1*(3), 237–267.

DISHMAN, R. (1988). *Exercise adherence: Its impact on public health.* Champaign: Human Kinetics Publishers.

DISHMAN, R. K., & Gettman, L. R. (1980). Psychobiologic influences on exercise adherence. *Journal of Sports Psychology, 2,* 295–310.

DISHMAN, R., Sallis, J., & Orenstein, D. (1985). The determinants of physical activity and exercise. *Public Health Reports, 100*(2), 158–171.

EPSTEIN, L. H., & Wing, R. R. (1980). Behavioral approaches to exercise habits and athletic performance. In J. M. Ferguson & C. B. Taylor (Eds.), *The comprehensive handbook of behavioral*

medicine: Volume 1—Systems interventions (pp. 125–137). New York: S. P. Medical and Scientific Books.

FOX, E. L. (1980). Physiological effects of training. In G. A. Stull & T. K. Cureton (Eds.), *Encyclopedia of physical education, fitness, and sports.* Salt Lake City: Brighton.

HASKELL, W. L. (1985). Exercise programs for health promotion. In J. C. Rosen & L. J. Solomon (Eds.), *Prevention in health psychology* (pp. 111–129). Hanover, NH: University Press of New England.

HAYNES, R. B. (1984). Compliance with health advice: An overview with special reference to exercise programs. *Journal of Cardiac Rehabilitation, 4,* 120–123.

HENDRICKS, G., & Carlson, J. (1981). *The centered athlete.* Engelwood Cliffs, NJ: Prentice-Hall.

HEYWARD, V. (1984). *Designs for fitness.* Minneapolis: Burgess Publishing.

IVERSON, D. C., Fielding, J. E., Crow, R. S., & Christenson, G. M. (1985). The promotion of physical activity in the United States population: The status of programs in medical, worksite, community, and school settings. *Public Health Reports, 100,* 212–224.

MARLATT, G. A., & Gordon, J. R. (1985). *Relapse prevention: Maintenance strategies in the treatment of addictive behaviors.* New York: Guilford Press.

MARTIN, J. E., & Dubbert, P. M. (1982). Exercise applications and promotion in behavioral medicine: Current status and future directions. *Journal of Consulting and Clinical Psychology, 50,* 1004–1017.

MARTIN, J. E., & Dubbert, P. M. (1984). Behavioral management strategies for improving health and fitness. *Journal of Cardiac Rehabilitation. 4*(5), 200–208.

MARTIN, J. E., & Dubbert, P. M. (1985). Adherence to exercise. In R. L. Terjung (Ed.), *Exercise and sports sciences review* (Vol. 13, pp. 137–167). New York: McMillan.

MARTIN, J. E., & Dubbert, P. M. (1987). Exercise promotion. In J. A. Blumenthal & D. C. McKee (Eds.), *Applications in behavioral medicine and health psychology: A clinician's source book* (pp. 361–398). Sarasota, FL: Professional Resource Exchange.

MARTIN, J. E., Dubbert, P. M., Catell, A. O., Thompson, J. K., Raczynski, J. R., Lake, M., Smith, P. O., Webster, J. S., Sikora, T., & Cohen, R. E. (1984). Behavioral control of exercise in sedentary adults. Studies 1–6. *Journal of Consulting and Clinical Psychology, 52,* 795–811.

McARDLE, W. D., Katch, F. I., and Katch, V. L. (1981). *Exercise physiology.* Philadelphia: Lea and Febiger.

MIROTZNIK, J., Speedling, E., Stein, R., and Bronz, C. (1985). Cardiovascular fitness programs: Factors associated with the participation and adherence. *Public Health Reports, 100,* 13–18.

MONTOYE, H. J. (1978). *An introduction to measurement in physical education.* Boston: Allyn & Bacon.

OLDRIDGE, N. B. (1984). Adherence to adult exercise fitness programs. In J. D. Matarazzo, S. M. Weiss, J. A. Herd, N. E. Miller, & S. M. Weiss (Eds.), *Behavioral health: A handbook of health enhancement and disease prevention* (pp. 467–487). New York: Wiley.

RIBISL, P. M. (1984). Developing an exercise prescription for health. In J. D. Matarazzo, et al. (Eds.), *Behavioral health: A handbook of health enhancement and disease prevention* (pp. 448–466). New York: Wiley.

SIME, W. E. (1984). Psychological benefits of exercise training in the healthy individual. In J. D. Matarazzo, et al. (Eds.), *Behavioral health: A handbook of health enhancement and disease prevention* (pp. 488–508). New York: Wiley.

SONSTROEM, R. J. (1988). Psychological models. In R. Dishman (Ed.), *Exercise adherence: Its impact on public health.* Champaign, IL: Human Kinetics Publishers.

SPERRY, L. (1985). Treatment noncompliance and cooperation: Implications for psychotherapeutic, medical, and lifestyle change approaches. *Individual Psychology, 41*(2), 228–236.

TAYLOR, C. B., Sallis, J. F., & Needle, R. (1985). The relation of physical activity and exercise to mental health. *Public Health Reports, 100,* 195–202.

THOMPSON, C. E., & Wankel, L. M. (1980). The effects of perceived activity choice upon frequency of exercise behavior. *Journal of Applied Social Psychology, 10,* 436–443.

7

Sleep

Tis sleep that knits up the ravell'd sleave of care . . . balm of hurt minds, great nature's second course, chief nourisher in life's feast.

Shakespeare

For many, good health has become a preoccupation and even an obsession. Today, people count calories, jog, eat healthy food, work out with weights, and take their own pulse and blood pressure readings. Yet, the quest for fitness by day can be undermined by poor sleep at night. Sleep loss can shatter an individual's timing, resilience, zest for life, and sense of well-being. Good sleep, then, appears to be a basic requirement for feeling good. But, according to an Institute of Medicine report (1979), disturbed sleep is one of the most common health complaints noted in surveys of general population. Whereas short-term or transient insomnia is virtually a universal human experience, chronic and severe insomnia affect about 20 percent of American adults (Drugs and insomnia, 1984). When compared with the prevalence of major psychiatric disorders—depression, anxiety, schizophrenia, and alcohol and substance dependence—the prevalence of chronic insomnia and other sleep disorders is greater. Not surprisingly, research indicates that sleep disorders are relatively common among individuals who manifest psychiatric disorders (Wehr & Goodwin, 1983; Roffwarg, 1979).

Although individuals with sleep disorders typically seek treatment from physicians, health counselors and other mental-health clinicians can play an important role in the treatment of these problems. It is unlikely that many mental-health counselors will work in sleep clinics or specialize in the treatment of sleep disorders. But it is very likely that counselors will encounter disordered sleep—particularly insomnia—among the concerns of clients or patients who seek counseling for other reasons. Thus, this chapter focuses on background information and treatment strategies for insomnia that are applicable, in both individual and group settings, to clients who present with various health or mental-health concerns.

Characteristics of Sleep

Despite the importance of sleep in our lives, researchers have not been able to answer the basic question, Why do we sleep? The function of sleep has been the basis for much speculation and research. Webb (1979) has reviewed five of the most common theories. The *restorative* theory regards sleep as a time of rest, recovery, or restoration. The *protective* theories of sleep suggest that sleep protects the body from tissue damage caused by exhaustion. The *energy conservation* hypothesis suggests that the purpose of sleep is to conserve metabolic energy. The *ethologic* theory holds that sleep is a controlled system that enhances survival. And the *instinctive* theory postulates that sleep is an instinct, like migration, courtship dances, or imprinting.

Many of these theories are compatible, and it seems likely that sleep serves many functions. It may well be that a certain minimal amount of sleep is required to restore some bodily processes and that additional sleep may vary according to ethological requirements or specific needs to conserve energy (Hauri, 1982).

Stages of Sleep

Sleep consists of types and stages that are traditionally measured and defined by an electroencephalogram (EEG). There are two basic types of sleep, rapid eye movement (REM) and nonrapid eye movement (NREM), as well as a transition phase between sleep and wakefulness. NREM sleep begins when a person falls asleep and becomes disengaged or decreasingly conscious of the outside world. This moment of disengagement is sudden and precise and signals the onset of sleep. Following the onset of sleep, the NREM stage involves a descent into periods of decreasing brain activity that are categorized into four stages (Kales & Kales, 1984).

In stage one, EEG activity slows from alpha waves, which are the dominant resting-waking pattern, to beta and pheta waves (one to six cycles per second). Activity slows further with the onset of stage-two sleep, which occurs within several minutes after falling asleep. A person awakened from stage-one sleep usually reports a feeling of having been awake all along.

Stage-two sleep is the longest of the sleep stages and occupies 50 percent to 70 percent of adults' sleep. EEG activity at this stage consists largely of beta waves and two electrical phenomena called spindles and K-complexes, which are thought to be a response to both external and internal stimuli. People awakened from this stage usually report having had short, fragmented, and mundane thoughts.

Stage-three sleep is characterized by the presence of slow, high-amplitude delta waves (one to four cycles per second). Delta sleep is the deepest type of sleep and is commonly believed to be the most restorative. It occurs primarily in the early part of the night and occupies about 20 to 50 percent of adults' sleep.

Stage-four sleep is considered to have the lowest level of physiological, neurological, and psychological activity. The threshold for arousal by external stimuli is higher at stage four than at any other time, and sleep deprivation studies suggest that this stage may be the most necessary element of sleep. After several nights of total sleep deprivation, the length of stage-four sleep increases dramatically on the first recovery night. So, a person permitted only four or five hours of sleep over several nights will soon exhibit a "rebound" effect, meaning that when allowed to sleep undisturbed, the person will compensate by having about 60 percent more REM sleep than he or she normally would.

REM sleep is characterized by rapid eye movement, which usually occurs in bursts. Although muscle tone is lowest during REM sleep, small twitches may be noted in many muscle groups. Heart rate and respiratory rates are higher and more variable during REM than during NREM sleep. REM sleep is associated with dreaming, and 80 percent of those awakened from REM sleep report having had vivid dreams.

A single night of sleep consists of four to six cycles of NREM/REM sleep. The first sleep cycle is as follows: stage one, stage two, stage three, stage four, stage three, stage two, and REM. On going to bed, the normal sleeper enters stage one and then passes into stage two. After ten to thirty minutes in stage two, the sleeper gradually enters delta sleep in stages three and four. Within 90

minutes, the sleeper cycles to stage two and then enters a REM period that lasts only a few moments. This first REM period is the least intense REM stage, in terms of both physiological manifestations and dream intensity. The remaining sleep cycles are the same, but they follow a slightly different course: REM, stage one, stage two, stage three, stage four, stage three, and stage two. Each sleep cycle lasts approximately 90 minutes and, as the night progresses, stages three and four decrease, but each REM episode lasts longer. REM sleep becomes more intense both physiologically and psychologically toward morning, whereas delta sleep is rarely seen in these later sleep cycles (Hauri, 1989). Five or more spontaneous awakenings· are spread throughout these sleep cycles. In good sleepers, these awakenings typically last for a few seconds to a few minutes each. Although the sleeper is responsive to environmental stimuli during these periods of arousal—for instance, removing a blanket if it is too warm in the room—the brief awakenings are seldom recalled in the morning. Figure 7-1 visually depicts the sleep cycles in a normal adult.

Sleep Needs across the Life Span

The physiology of sleep changes noticeably across the developmental span. Total sleep time increases as the individual matures and then gradually decreases. A child sleeps about 18 hours a day when newborn, 10 to 12 hours a day by age 4, 9 to 10 hours at age ten, and about 7½ to 8 hours by adolescence. From adolescence on, there is a very gradual decline in the amount of sleep needed, to 6½ hours in the elderly adult (Hauri, 1982). Although time spent asleep decreases over the adult years, time spent in bed increases after about age 40, so that the older adult spends more time in bed but gets less sleep.

The configuration of sleep of the older adult is unlike that of the adolescent or young adult. Typically, the elderly experience decreases in periods of deep, or delta stage, sleep and experience increases in light, or stage one and two, sleep. At age 70, the delta stage makes up less than 10 percent of sleep, as

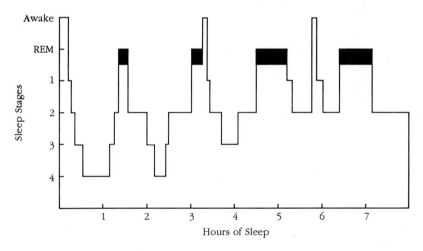

Figure 7-1. Sleep cycles in a normal adult

compared with 15 to 25 percent during adolescence and young adulthood. As a result of this increased percentage of light sleep, the elderly find themselves awakening more often during the night (Walsh, 1983).

As the type and amount of sleep change with age, the incidence of sleep dysfunction increases. Typical sleep dysfunction in young children includes nightmares, enuresis (bed-wetting), and bedtime fears. Because adolescents often underestimate their sleep needs and become sleep deprived, they often have difficulty getting up in the morning. For young and middle-age adults, transient and chronic insomnia are very common. Among the elderly, there is a sharp increase in the incidence of sleep apnea (cessation of breathing), nocturnal myoclonus (muscle spasms), and chronic insomnia. With reference to insomnia, the elderly suffer more from frequent and longer midcycle awakenings or early morning awakenings, whereas insomnia in younger adults is characterized by initial insomnia, meaning difficulty falling asleep. All of these changes seem to occur, at an earlier age in females than in males (Dement, 1983).

How much sleep does the average individual need to be alert and energetic throughout the day? The consensus in Western culture is that eight hours is the optimum amount of sleep. However, many individuals require smaller or larger amounts of sleep but worry needlessly because their sleep pattern does not match the norm of eight hours. Normal sleep across individuals ranges from 3 to 10 hours per night. Each individual, whether child or adult, has a personal ideal amount of sleep. The best measure of sufficient sleep is adequate daytime functioning; an individual who remains alert and energetic during wakefulness is probably getting sufficient sleep (Hauri, 1982).

Circadian Rhythms

There are many biological "clocks" in our brain that must be regularly synchronized for us to remain in a state of health. *Circadian rhythms* are biological cycles that require about 24 hours to complete, and of the body's various circadian rhythms, the sleep/wake cycle is one of the most important. When normal individuals live with no time cues, they usually show a sleep/wake rhythm that lasts 25 hours. Most individuals who work in the daytime have a circadian system with a diurnal orientation, which means that they sleep at night and are awake during the day. Individuals who work at night must acclimate to a nocturnal orientation, which means being awake at night and asleep during the day. Over time, this circadian system can accommodate a change from a diurnal to a nocturnal orientation. But the inborn clock that controls this circadian system does not reset itself immediately after abrupt changes in the sleep/wake cycle. Until it does, the individual may experience sleep deprivation, mood changes, difficulty with concentration, and poor work performance. In short, the circadian system has a profound influence on sleep/wake cycles.

Entrainment is the mechanism that keeps the circadian system on a 24-hour diurnal orientation. Entrainment relies on *zeitgebers*—a German word for *time giver*—to allow the circadian system to become oriented accurately. Zeitgebers may be physical phenomena, such as the alternation of daylight and

darkness, or social practices involving cultural patterns and knowledge of clock time. Zeitgebers must be experienced by the individual for entrainment to follow. Thus, an individual who is socially isolated, has an irregular routine, and has little exposure to daylight could not be entrained to a 24-hour cycle (Kales & Kales, 1982).

Sleep Disorders and Irregular Schedules

The endogenous, self-sustaining nature of the circadian system and the need for an entrainment mechanism to keep it cycling on time suggest how sleep disorders can arise from irregular schedules. When major changes in the sleep/wake cycle occur, significant changes in the circadian system can be expected. Accordingly, the individual's biological clock will no longer be running "on time." The individual's sleep, daytime alertness, and well-being become impaired, and that impairment is often chronic. Life-style changes, jet lag, shift work, and depression are all associated with circadian dysfunction.

Changes in Life-Style
If an individual's life-style is such that the normal and necessary physical and social zeitgebers are disregarded and replaced with a cavalier attitude toward the timing of sleep, insomnia is very likely to occur. On the other hand, a regimen of both indoor and outdoor activity that allows an adequate exposure to the necessary zeitgebers and ensures a regular daily pattern of sleep is all that is necessary to realign the circadian system.

Jet Lag
Because of the increase in air travel across time zones, jet lag is becoming a major source of circadian disregulation (Hales, 1981). A distinction must be made between the effects that result from the particular environmental conditions of air travel and the effects that result from the need to realign the circadian system, because it is the latter that has the most direct impact on the individual's sleep and that lasts the longest. Jet lag is not limited to sleep deprivation; it is also a problem of daytime functioning, which is affected by two other processes.

The first process concerns inappropriate phasing and the physiological and psychological functions associated with alertness, well-being, and performance efficiency exhibiting endogenous, self-sustaining circadian rhythms. These rhythms are timed in such a way that the down phase of the sleep/wake cycle normally coincides with the timing of sleep. But, after a flight to a new time zone, the down phase may coincide with a time that is normally meant for daytime activities. Therefore, performance and mood can be impaired by the individual's shift into the down phase of the cycle.

The second process that affects daytime functioning is called *dissociation,* in which there is rhythmic disharmony in the circadian rhythms. A good analogy is that of a symphony orchestra that is not playing in concert. Circadian dissociation is characterized by feelings of tiredness and malaise, gastrointestinal

dysfunction, and irritability. All of these symptoms are likely to result in impaired mood and performance (Wever, 1979).

For most travelers, jet lag is an acute problem that lasts only a few days. The sleep pattern can be improved by speeding up the process of circadian realignment. Regardless of the time zone they're in, travelers have the advantage of physical and social *zeitgebers* working on their behalf. Thus, by rigidly avoiding daytime napping and maximizing exposure to physical and social zeitgebers, travelers can greatly reduce the duration of circadian misalignment and its adverse effects. But resolving the sleep problem eliminates only one of the three components of jet lag. Inappropriate phasing and circadian dissociation can be improved only by speeding up the process of circadian realignment or, in the case of inappropriate phasing, by careful scheduling of activities.

Shift Work

When compared to jet lag, the sleep problems of workers on rotating or night shifts are far more complex (Monk & Folkard, 1983). For people engaged in shift work, sleep deprivation is chronic, and physical and social zeitgebers are impervious to nocturnal circadian realignment. At this point, it is not clear whether a perfect realignment can ever be accomplished. Some studies on the circadian rhythm in shift-workers show that complete circadian realignment never occurs (Nauth & Rutenfranz, 1976). The primary impact of the circadian system on sleep results from the system's inability to adjust instantly to the change from a diurnal to a nocturnal routine. However, circadian factors are not the only determinants of the shift-worker's sleep problems. The worker's ability to cope with the rotating or permanent night-shift schedule is influenced by three interrelated factors: circadian realignment, sleep hygiene (the behaviors and rituals involved in falling and staying asleep), and domestic and social factors.

As with jet lag, during this adjustment period, there are three mechanisms by which mood, well-being, and performance efficiency can be greatly affected. First, sleep becomes disrupted, which results in a stage of partial sleep deprivation. Second, nighttime wakefulness overlaps with the down phases of various psychological functions that are normally associated with sleep in the day-oriented individual. Third, the various individual components of the circadian system become disordered, so that the normal harmony of appropriate phase relationships is significantly changed.

If the shift-worker resides in a well-adjusted household, his or especially her—sleep is likely to be interrupted by the demands of child care, shopping, and household management. Unfortunately, domestic disharmony is frequently blamed on the shift-worker's need for sleep at a time when households are usually rather noisy. The shift-worker is also socially isolated from day-working friends, which compounds shift-work intolerance. On the other hand, in "company towns" where shift work is the rule rather than the exception and social and community events are scheduled accordingly, shift work seems to be better tolerated (Monk, 1986).

If the effects of shift work and circadian disregulation were felt only by shift-workers and their families, the general public might be disinterested. But

the fact of the matter is that shift work and circadian disregulation have profound implications for the environment and the world's population. The recent tragedies at Bhopal, Chernobyl, Three Mile Island, and the *Valdez*–Alaskan oil spill are examples of the hazards of shift work. All of these disasters occurred around 4:00 A.M. and have been attributed to errors in judgment by shift-workers.

Treatment for sleep deprivation in the shift-worker is not only complex but also difficult. Treatment is difficult because of chronic sleep loss and the inability of natural daytime zeitgebers to realign the circadian system to a nocturnal orientation. Other factors, such as daytime, domestic, and social functions, can encroach on the shift-worker's sleep time and further compound the problem. In addition, shift-workers find it difficult to remain on a night-shift schedule on their days off. Research shows that most revert to a day-oriented routine and fail to maintain their nocturnal circadian orientation (Nauth & Rutenfranz, 1976).

Shift-workers must be encouraged to adhere to a regular sleep schedule and receive sufficient support and cooperation from those with whom they live to honor the sleep schedule. Finally, supervisors and those involved with scheduling workers' shifts must become more knowledgeable of the effects of shift work on circadian rhythms. Those who work in law enforcement and in the nursing and medical fields become prime candidates for chronic sleep disturbances when they are asked to work on rapidly rotating shifts. Monk (1986) reviews a number of healthy and realistic ways of scheduling shift work that avoid the circadian disregulation.

Depression

In addition to irregular life-styles, jet lag, and shift work, certain illnesses are greatly influenced by the circadian system. In particular, depression is strongly linked to circadian system dysfunction (Wehr & Goodwin, 1983). Although there is not a one-to-one correspondence between circadian disregulation and depression, it is clear that inappropriate circadian functioning is a primary symptom of depression and may also be a contributing factor. Circadian-related symptoms of depression include early morning awakening, diurnal mood swings, and insomnia or hypersomnia. Clearly, the sleep patterns of depressed patients are significantly changed. For many of them, sleep latency (the amount of time required to move from wakefulness to the onset of REM sleep) is reduced. Depressed patients must be educated in the importance of sleep hygiene in the reversal of their depressive symptoms. The use of tricyclic antidepressant medication has been shown to be useful in regulating circadian rhythms and sleep patterns.

In short, sleep deprivation involves a major disruption in the sleep/wake cycle and is a common problem of travelers and shift-workers. In some cases, it is a symptom of an underlying illness—depression. The difficulties in adjusting to the altered sleep/wake schedule are closely related to an endogenous circadian system that can be very resistive to change. Proper exposure to physical and social *zeitgebers* encourages circadian realignment to normalcy.

Biopsychosocial Factors in Sleep

Numerous factors have been found to relate to sleep difficulties. If we take a biopsychosocial perspective, it is possible to consider these factors in an orderly and comprehensive fashion. We begin with biological factors.

Biological Factors

Medical conditions that cause pain, breathing difficulties, or other discomfort can disrupt sleep. These conditions include asthma, ulcers, arthritis, angina, migraines, and cluster headaches. Some medications used to treat these problems may also adversely affect sleep. For instance, prescription medication for the treatment of asthma often contains adrenaline, which causes arousal and interferes with sleep. Other medications that interfere with sleep include the thyroid medications synthroid and cytomel; cancer chemotherapy agents; oral contraceptives; anticonvulsant agents, such as Dilantin; and Inderal, a beta blocker commonly used for hypertension and other cardiovascular conditions. These medications interfere with sleep onset and often cause frequent sleep interruptions. In addition, sleep problems can develop from withdrawal of some medications such as Valium, Librium, Tranzene, and other minor tranquilizers; sedating tricyclic antidepressants such as Elavil and Sineqaun; street drugs such as marijuana, cocaine, and heroin; and, occasionally, medications that contain aspirin. Some of these medications also suppress REM sleep, which leads to intense, vivid dreaming during withdrawal of the medication. Some drugs used to treat insomnia can actually worsen other medical disorders. Finally, some sleeping medications suppress the brain's respiratory centers, compounding the breathing difficulties of asthmatics (Roffwarg, 1979).

Another cause of sleeping difficulty is the regular use of central nervous system stimulants. The most common of these is caffeine, whether in the form of coffee, tea, or soft drinks. In amounts equivalent to four cups of coffee taken before bed, caffeine increases awakenings from sleep. Cigarette smoking has also been associated with sleep difficulties. For instance, when the sleep difficulties of smokers and nonsmokers who were matched in terms of personality pattern and drug consumption were compared, the smokers spent an average of 15 minutes longer falling asleep and nearly 20 minutes longer being awake during the night than did nonsmokers. Presumably, these differences were caused by the stimulative effects of nicotine. Finally, it has been noted that smoking cessation leads to improved sleep patterns (Soldatos, Kales, Scharf, et al., 1980).

Although the occasional use of alcohol may aid sleep in some individuals, excessive alcohol intake has been noted to severely interfere with normal sleep patterns. Those who regularly use alcohol complain that, although they may fall asleep quickly, they experience frequent episodes of awakening during the night and difficulty falling back to sleep. They often sleep no more than two to four hours a night. EEG sleep recordings of these individuals show fragmented REM sleep and reduced total REM. In addition, deep NREM sleep has been shown to be diminished during withdrawal from alcohol.

Medications aimed at relieving insomnia have also been shown to disrupt sleep. This rebound phenomenon is called *drug dependency insomnia* (Bootzin & Nicassio, 1978). Typically, sleep medication is effective for the first few nights but becomes less effective after about 14 days of continuous use. In fact, larger and larger doses of medication are required to achieve sleep, which means that drug tolerance has developed. When the medication is abruptly withdrawn, the result is "rebound insomnia," which is the reappearance of disturbed sleep but now with frightening nightmares. These disturbing experiences reinforce the individual's sense of need for the medication. Not surprisingly, the individual continues to take the medication despite obtaining only light, disturbed sleep.

Finally, external factors can affect biological and physical processes and subsequently alter the quality of sleep. Bedroom ventilation, humidity, temperature, and similar conditions and interfering noises can all alter the quality of sleep. The comfort of one's bed, especially the softness or hardness of pillows and mattress, can affect sleep. For some sleep problems, a simple environmental modification of one of these factors may be sufficient to reestablish a restful pattern of sleep.

Psychological Factors

Most sleep problems involve an interaction between physiological and psychological factors. When an individual undergoes serious and prolonged stress, such as with the loss of a job or the ending of a relationship, the brain's arousal system responds with increased activity, which results in changes in sleep patterns. If the stress continues for several weeks, other factors usually interfere to cause temporary insomnia. Frequently, a dysfunctional habit of "trying too hard to fall asleep" develops. The more individuals are sleep deprived, the harder they try to sleep, which further increases arousal and results in less sleep. Such individuals usually fall asleep easily when not trying to sleep, but become alert whenever they make a conscious decision to fall asleep. Maladaptive conditioning often results when an individual lies in bed unable to sleep. When this occurs, the bedroom environment becomes associated with frustration and arousal rather than with relaxation and sleep. Similarly, the individual's usual bedtime rituals, such as brushing teeth and setting the alarm clock, become stimuli that anticipate frustration and tension rather than relaxation. Often, individuals who suffer from such conditioned insomnia sleep better away from their usual sleep environment, such as in the living room or in a hotel. In addition, when individuals sleep poorly because of stress, they often fall asleep in the early morning hours and then oversleep or need daytime naps to "catch up." Not surprisingly, these behaviors lead to circadian disregulation.

As long as sleep is basically adequate, an occasional poor night's sleep is usually tolerated. However, for individuals who believe that they suffer from insomnia, a poor night's sleep only serves to reconfirm this belief, and the fear of insomnia becomes a self-fulfilling prophecy (Kales & Kales, 1982).

These behavioral factors contribute to almost all chronic insomnia. Whether the insomnia results from psychological upheaval, environmental stress, a medical condition, or medication, behavioral factors reinforce the

pattern of insomnia. Therefore, behavioral factors need to be considered and treated even if the original cause of the insomnia was not behavioral in nature. It should not be surprising, then, that the treatment of chronic insomnia requires behavioral interventions in addition to treatment of the primary cause of the insomnia.

Social Factors

There has been relatively little written about social factors involved in sleep disorders, with the exception of some research that has been reported on marital functioning and the effects of shift work on marital and family life.

Marital problems have been shown to be commonly associated with insomnia, and various explanations for this association have been given. One explanation is that poor sleepers are frequently unable to express their feelings and consequently have unsatisfactory interpersonal relationships (Kales, Soldatos, & Kales, 1981). Another explanation is that the partner who anticipates problems with sexual performance may consciously or unconsciously delay going to bed in order to avoid sexual intimacy, which then leads to a sleep disorder. Furthermore, couples with poor sexual relations tend to suffer from continuous deprivation of affection and closeness, which leads to tension and feelings of being neglected that in turn result in insomnia (Kales & Kales, 1982). A third explanation involves social support factors. Berkowitz and Perkins (1985) found that interpersonal role conflicts, lack of support from their husband, and decreased marital satisfaction were associated with increased reports of insomnia and other psychosomatic symptoms in wives.

Another explanation for marital disharmony involves the degree to which the spouses are out of phase with each other's circadian rhythms. There is extensive research comparing "larks," or morning individuals, with "owls," or late-night individuals (Folkard, 1983; Monk & Folkard, 1983). Larks tend to live by the maxim "Early to bed and early to rise," whereas owls tend to retire late and arise late.

Needless to say, out-of-phase couples tend to have fewer serious conversations, fewer shared activities—including time together in bed—more marital conflict, and less frequent sex (Larson, Crane, & Smith, 1991). Not surprisingly, shift-workers are often "owls." They tend to sleep less than seven hours per night and have many health complaints. Monk and Folkard (1983) have shown that shift work not only exacerbates existing health and relational problems but also creates new problems and sets the stage for conflicts not likely to be faced by couples who are in phase. One of the most common problems is that the shift-worker's need for peace and quiet conflicts with the spouse's and family's normal morning activities, which are usually noisy and chaotic. In addition, the female shift-worker is often expected to attend to housekeeping responsibilities in addition to her job, which adds to her sleep debt.

Sleep apnea is a more serious disorder, characterized by breathing cessation that occurs more than five times per hour during sleep and can last for more than ten seconds. People with sleep apnea tend to snore loudly, which disturbs the sleep of their bed partners. Although marriage generally buffers

the impact of external stressors for spouses, this is seldom the case for individuals with sleep apnea. People with sleep disorders like sleep apnea often experience significant marital dissatisfaction. Sleep apneic spouses are found to be significantly more depressed, exhausted, and socially isolated than are their divorced counterparts. Also, both marital spouses show poor adjustment in their marital, social, and leisure activities, and the sleep apneic spouse also shows poor adjustment in parental growth (Cartwright & Knight, 1987).

Another social factor involves the compatibility or incompatibility of a couple's sleep styles. Studies have shown that wives don't sleep as well as their husbands do. Typically, deep NREM sleep is often briefer for wives than for husbands. This is probably because men tend to snore more than women and are more prone to movement disorders in their sleep—called sleep myoclonus. Or, perhaps because of his sheer weight, each time the husband rolls over, his movement jars his wife to the point of waking her. The exception to this set of observations is the post-intercourse couple, who sleep in tandem, with their body positions and sleep cycles tightly synchronized throughout REM and NREM sleep. Presumably, lovemaking maintains the couple's emotional as well as physical closeness (Hales, 1981).

The way that couples sleep together may change dramatically over time, and sleep positions that couples choose at the start of the night may reflect their relationship during the day. According to Dunkell (1978), new couples may sleep nestled together, with one spouse tucked into the contours of the other spouse's body. This coziness provides each spouse with reassurance by offering maximum physical intimacy. After five years or so, the spouses begin to drift apart, and there is a widening gulf between their bodies when they cuddle. This physical retreat does not necessarily represent an emotional separation, but it may indicate a mutual security that the couple has achieved.

Finally, many believe that sex is an effective sleep inducer. Research shows, however, that the male is more likely to fall asleep and have unchanged sleep stages after intercourse than is the female, who is likely to drift into sleep but experience less deep NREM sleep and spend more of the night in REM sleep. This difference between men and women may be partly a matter of sexual satisfaction. After climaxing, a man may feel so relaxed that he falls asleep quickly and easily; if the woman has not climaxed, she may feel physically restless and frustrated. The sleep clinic at Baylor University has reported a high correlation between sexual and sleep problems in females. Sixty to seventy percent of females who complained of insomnia also reported sexual frustration. Hales (1981) suggests that sexual frustration and dysfunction may be the cause of disturbed sleep.

Assessment

Before we proceed, it is important to define and classify insomnia. Usually, three categories are acknowledged by sleep experts. They are transient insomnia, short-term insomnia, and chronic insomnia. Transient insomnia is sleep loss that

lasts one to three days and is triggered by excitement, nervousness, or travel. Christmas Eve, jet lag, the night before a key meeting, or the prospects of having surgery may trigger transient insomnia. By definition, transient insomnia is insomnia that clears spontaneously. Short-term insomnia, on the other hand, disturbs sleep for up to three weeks and is common during times of personal stress or serious medical illness. It is often resolved when the stress is elevated or the medical illness is treated. However, chronic insomnia may persist for years. In the face of chronic stressors, some individuals develop insomnia, whereas others develop peptic ulcers or tension headaches (Hauri, 1989). On the other hand, many insomniacs are not overly stressed but develop sleep problems as a result of "learned" or conditioned insomnia.

An Assessment Strategy

As noted earlier, individuals with sleep problems usually present themselves to physicians for assessment and treatment. Over the past ten years, sleep disorders clinics staffed primarily by physicians have helped thousands of individuals with serious and relatively rare sleep conditions return to a more normal pattern of life. There are times when referral to a sleep disorders clinic is essential, particularly when excessive daytime sleepiness is reported or when there are indications of sleep apnea. Generally speaking, health counselors and therapists should be able to recognize and treat most cases of insomnia.

Speilman (1986) suggests a conceptual strategy for the assessment of insomnia. He suggests that case material be categorized into a schema of predisposing conditions, precipitating circumstances, and perpetuating factors. We will briefly review this assessment scheme.

Predisposing conditions are those that precede the onset of the sleep disturbance and set the stage for recurrence by lowering the thresholds for triggering insomnia. Although the intensity of the predisposing condition is not sufficient to produce the insomnia, it establishes a vulnerability or serves as a contributing factor in the development of the insomnia. *Precipitating circumstances* are the triggering events of the symptoms of insomnia. Precipitating circumstances are traditionally at the center of the assessment process, because these triggering factors are often the best clue to pathophysiology and subsequent treatment. However, in chronic insomnia, the current sleep problem may function autonomously from its origins. *Perpetuating factors* are those features that sustain or support the insomnia. Therefore, Speilman believes that influences that currently maintain the sleep disturbance are the necessary and sufficient factors that must be countered for effective treatment.

For example, an insomnia triggered by the anticipation and worry involved in buying a new house may persist for a number of months after the excitement and turmoil have subsided. If these precipitating influences are no longer present and an irregular sleep/wake schedule can be assessed as the factor responsible for the persistence of the insomnia, effective treatment for the current problem can disregard the initial reason for the development of the sleep problem. By the same token, if the house purchase has turned out to be a disaster and the ruminative worrying continues, then features of the precipitat-

ing condition have become perpetuating factors, and treatment needs to focus on these problems. Speilman (1986) lists several factors that may perpetuate insomnia: excessive time in bed, irregular timing of retiring and arising, unpredictability of sleep, worry over daytime deficits, maladaptive conditioning, increased caffeine consumption, hypnotic and alcohol ingestion, and multiple episodes of sleep (such as naps or fragmented sleep).

Biological Assessment

The biological assessment of insomnia should include a health history, drug history, family history, and possibly a referral for a medical evaluation. The assessment of insomnia begins with a review of the client's health history. It is common practice for medical and health practitioners and clinics to have clients complete a standardized health history form. This form can be a useful screening device for the health counselor to use to collect additional information from the client.

The pain and discomfort associated with a number of medical conditions, such as arthritis, asthma, angina, cancer, and various types of headaches, often contribute to insomnia. Pain experienced during the day may be intensified at bedtime because environmental stimuli are diminished and the client's attention becomes more internally focused. Individuals with cancer, in addition to being in pain, are often overwhelmed with fear and anxiety over the ultimate consequences of their illness. Similarly, people with angina or cardiac arrythmia often fear going to sleep, afraid of a possible attack during the night, which makes them feel even more vulnerable and helpless.

As described earlier, sleep can be disturbed by a number of medications, including sleep medications that are misused. A sleep evaluation should therefore include a thorough drug history. Stimulant drugs, steroids, energizing antidepressants like Prozac, and beta blockers like Inderal are more likely to cause sleep problems when they are taken close to bedtime, even if taken in therapeutic doses. Caffeine-containing substances taken close to bedtime can also cause difficulty falling asleep, whereas alcohol ingestion can result in an inability to stay asleep. Rebound insomnia may follow the withdrawal of even a sedative hypnotic (such as Valium or Halcion) for more than a few nights. The abrupt withdrawal of high doses of other sleeping medications may cause both insomnia and nightmares. Finally, the improper doses or scheduling of certain sleep medications or sedating antidepressants can cause excessive daytime sleepiness. Since these can be mistaken for the excessive sleep of hypersomnia or narcolepsy, the health counselor needs to inquire not only about the type of drug but also about the dosage and the scheduling of the drug. It is here that the *Physicians' Desk Reference* or a call to a pharmacist or physician may be useful and necessary.

A family history of sleep disorders should be taken from anyone in whom insomnia is suspected, since it can aid in the diagnosis of the client's problem and could uncover treatable sleep problems in other family members. Families of both narcoleptic and hypersomniac patients have been found to have a higher incidence of sleep disorders as compared to the general population. Similarly,

individuals who experience sleep apnea, nightmares, and somnambulism (sleepwalking) often have positive family histories (Kales & Kales, 1984).

To help individuals assess their sleep, health counselors should obtain a 24-hour sleep/wake history and not just learn about the 8-hour sleep period. For instance, elderly patients often complain of severe listlessness at night, but they take several naps during the day. Insomniacs frequently have a history of irregular habits, including erratic bedtime schedules. They also report low or inconsistent levels of physical activity during the day. In addition, the 24-hour sleep/wake history may reveal that excessive physical exercise or stimulating mental activity close to bedtime is causing initial insomnia (difficulty falling asleep).

Sleep Disorders Clinics

We have previously noted that excessive daytime sleepiness, excessive snoring (which may indicate sleep apnea), myoclonus, and narcolepsy are common indications for referral to a sleep clinic. To this we might add impotence, which can have either psychological or physiological origins. Occasionally, clients with psychological impotence may be convinced of the nonorganic nature of their disorder only when confronted with laboratory evidence of nighttime erections (which rule out the possibility of an organic cause for impotence).

The mainstay of sleep centers is the polysomnogram (PSG). PSGs monitor brain waves, heart rhythm, respiration, temperature, and body movement throughout the night (Walsh, 1983). Typically, clients report to the sleep clinic late in the evening, change into their bed clothes, and have several electrodes applied to their face and body. The electrodes are arranged in pairs and are placed on the chin to record muscle tone, on the corners of the eyes to measure eye movement, on the top of the scalp to detect brain waves, and on the upper-right and lower-left areas of the chest to measure heartbeats. Temperature-sensitive devices are taped under the nostrils and mouth to record the rate and volume of inhaled air, and electrodes on each leg record leg movement before and after sleep. Finally, a beltlike gadget around the lower chest monitors the movement of the diaphragm. If sleep apnea is suspected, a small microphone is placed underneath the nose to record breathing. The PSG records continuously throughout the night, and electrical impulses appear as wavy lines on a continuous sheet of paper fed into the PSG machine. The data from the PSG is processed by computer, which calculates sleep latency, time in each sleep stage, number of awakenings, number of breathing stoppages, changes in heart rate, and final awakening. These data, plus the patient's sleep history and other available information, are then assessed by sleep specialists. The diagnostic workup and consultation at the sleep clinic may range in price from $800 to $1200.

Psychological Assessment

Psychological assessment of insomnia usually includes information gathered from sleep diaries, rating scales, behavioral observations, psychological inventories, and interview data.

Sleep diaries.   Having clients keep a sleep diary for a one- or two-week period of time can help the counselor assess clients' 24-hour sleep/wake patterns. The sleep diary or logs are filled out each morning. Clients typically self-monitor such behavior as the time they went to bed, the time they fell asleep, the number of times they awakened during the night, the number of minutes needed to resume sleep, the number of nightmares, the time they awakened in the morning, and the time at which they actually got up in the morning (Lawrence, 1982). The health counselor may also want clients to monitor their physical activity throughout the day and record any naps that are taken. For cases of insomnia, the client's sleep diary may be particularly useful in detecting sleep difficulties related to disordered schedules and routines. When excessive sleep is the problem, the diary documents not only the symptomology of the condition but also the number of naps taken and the client's general activity patterns. The health counselor will have to determine whether clients with obsessive/compulsive or hyperchondriacal traits should be asked to keep a sleep diary, as it could reinforce the tendency to focus and ruminate on sleep difficulties.

A spouse or roommate may be asked to verify the accuracy of the client's sleep diary. The counselor may provide them with a separate diary on which to record sleep data.

Rating scales.   A variety of rating scales have been developed to measure various sleep difficulties. These scales are primarily useful in evaluating the subjective feelings of patients when more objective measures are not possible. Scales typically measure the degree of restedness in the morning, general satisfaction with the night's sleep, difficulty in getting to sleep, and pleasantness of dreams. Four- to nine-point scales generally are used. Two rating scales will be highlighted here. One is the Sleep Behavior Self-Rating Scale by Kazarian, Howe, and Csapo (1979). This instrument is useful in assessing various sleep-compatible behaviors associated with an individual's bedroom or bed. This scale appears to be a valid indicator of sleep latency that is relatively independent of anxiety or depression. A second scale is the Sleep Hygiene Awareness and Practice Scale developed by Lacks (1987). This scale includes several items on an individual's knowledge of sleep hygiene, knowledge about caffeine and its effect on sleep, and factors related to the client's practice of sleep hygiene.

Behavioral observations.   Aside from having irregular and inconsistent bedtimes, the insomniac may engage in daytime napping, which further disturbs circadian rhythms. Other poor sleep habits may include using the bed for purposes other than sleep, such as reading, watching TV, eating, conversing, or worrying about the next day's events. As a result, the bed becomes a cue for a variety of activities other than sleep. Although it is useful to elicit information of this nature from the client, it is also helpful to have corroborating data from another party, such as a spouse, family member, or roommate. Health counselors suggest that this individual, typically a spouse, be interviewed independent of the client for purposes of collecting corroborating information. Perhaps the most objective behavioral observation occurs in sleep clinics, where a contin-

uous videotape recording is made of the individual concurrent with the PSG monitoring (Lawrence, 1982).

Psychological inventories.   The experience of disrupted sleep is often associated with anxiety, mood changes, ruminations, and psychopathology—particularly depression. To aid in the assessment of insomnia, the health counselor may consider the use of psychological inventories. The most frequently used inventory for the description of personality and the diagnosis of psychopathology is the Minnesota Multiphasic Personality Inventory (MMPI). If depression is suspected, the Beck Depression Inventory (Beck, 1967) can be very useful. It is important to remember that insomnia may develop either independently or as a result of depression. Thus, it is important to determine whether the course of the sleep problem parallels the course of the mood disturbance, or whether the sleep problem predated the depression. Subsequently, health counselors should be aware that many depression inventories include sleep disturbance items that may artificially increase the depression scores of individuals who suffer from insomnia.

Interview data.   The interview plays a significant role in the assessment of sleep disorders, particularly of insomnia. In addition to collating and clarifying data from health-history forms, sleep diaries, rating scales, and personality inventories, the interviews can supply important additional information. Determining whether a sleep difficulty is associated with psychological problems is critical. Insomnia is common in many psychiatric conditions, including anxiety disorders, depressive disorders, mania, acute schizophrenia, and organic brain syndrome. Roffwarg (1979) has found a number of correlations between psychiatric diagnoses and sleep difficulties. For instance, neurotic patients typically experience initial and midcycle insomnia—that is, difficulty falling asleep and awakening frequently at night. Excessive bedtime rituals, common in obsessive/compulsive personalities, also tend to interfere with sleep. On the other hand, depressed patients often complain of early morning awakening, and bipolar depressives frequently sleep excessively but awaken unrefreshed. Manic patients frequently show a very long sleep latency but, once asleep, awaken refreshed after only two to four hours of sleep. Roffwarg also notes that severely depressed and anxious patients often take psychotropic medications, which may further complicate their sleep difficulties. It is assumed that the counselor has the clinical skills and knowledge base necessary to conduct such a diagnostic interview or will refer the patient to another professional who can make this determination.

A variety of cognitive factors are implicated in sleep disorders. Chronic insomniacs typically blame their insomnia on cognitive arousal rather than on somatic factors. Some of these insomnia-producing dysfunctional beliefs or misconceptions are: "Everyone needs eight hours of sleep"; "We have to think, worry, analyze, and plan while lying in bed"; "We can't function well after a poor night's sleep"; "We should keep the same sleep schedule as others in our family"; "All sleep difficulties are stress-related"; and "Occasional insomnia indicates chronic insomnia" (Lichstein & Rosenthal, 1980). Assessment of specif-

ic cognitive factors related to sleep difficulties suggest that cognitively oriented interventions, such as cognitive restructuring, paradoxical intention, and thought stopping, can be particularly useful with insomnia.

Assessment of Social Factors

As mentioned in the section on behavioral observation, other important information that the client might not be able to provide can sometimes be obtained from a corroborator, such as a spouse or roommate. For example, when a client complains of sleeping too much during the day, the corroborator can be questioned about the possibility of sleep apnea. If the corroborator indicates that the client snores heavily and that periodic snorting sounds occur in intervals of more than ten seconds, sleep apnea can be suspected. Similarly, regarding complaints of insomnia, the corroborator could provide useful information about the quantity and quality of the client's sleep.

Earlier we discussed the impact of marital functioning on sleep and indicated that it is essential that the spouse of the insomniac be interviewed. It was suggested that the spouse be interviewed separately regarding the marital relationship, family stresses, work demands and stresses, the regularity or irregularity of daily schedules, the use of prescription medication and other substances that could interfere with sleep, as well as sleep and sexual styles and patterns. In a conjoint interview, a counselor should be able to ascertain the degree to which the couple's energy levels are in phase or out of phase and the extent to which each is a "lark" or an "owl."

Treatment Strategies

Biological Interventions

Three types of medication are generally used to induce sleep. Nonprescription or over-the-counter "sleep aids" can cause drowsiness but do not directly induce sleep. These medications sometimes allow the individual who tries too hard to fall asleep to actually relax and then fall asleep. Prescription medications, often referred to as hypnotics, are a second type of sleep medication. Even though five million or more individuals a year receive prescriptions for hypnotics, their use appears to be declining. Medications like Valium, Librium, and Tranzene, which were originally marketed to relax muscles and relieve anxiety, have replaced barbiturates as the most frequently prescribed hypnotic. Barbiturates are the third type of sleep medication. Because of their high potential for abuse and overdose, they are seldom prescribed today.

Occasional use of hypnotics is considered quite acceptable, whereas chronic use of hypnotics to treat insomnia should be avoided. We have already noted that the efficacy of hypnotics decrease over time, that most hypnotics distort natural sleep, and that hypnotics often result in "rebound insomnia" when the medication is withdrawn or wears off. In addition, it should be noted that hypnotics can impair waketime performance of activities, such as driving, and mental concentration. In fact, there are a number of reported cases of transient amnesia associated with the use of medications like Halcion and

Valium. There is also concern that hypnotics also mask the insomniac's medical, behavioral, and psychological problems, which can delay appropriate treatment. Finally, sleep medications carry the risk of medical complications including overdose, adverse reactions with other medications, and withdrawal symptoms (Kales & Kales, 1984).

It is currently considered acceptable medical practice to prescribe hypnotics to help the patient get through an acute crisis as long as the patient is also followed and supported through the withdrawal period. A nightly prescription of hypnotics over months or years is rarely indicated, although there are a few patients who seem to benefit from long-term low doses of a hypnotic. On the other hand, occasional use of hypnotics, such as once or twice a week, sometimes helps to reduce the insomniac's fear that he or she may never sleep again and allow him or her some needed rest. The benzodiazepine medications, such as Halcion and Dalmane, are now generally preferred over other medications because of their relative safety and lack of interaction with other drugs. However, benzodiazepines should not be taken with alcohol, which could result in lethal overdose. Barbiturates, such as Seconal and Phenobarbital, may be prescribed for those patients for whom benzodiazepines are ineffective.

Psychological Interventions

The psychological approaches and interventions found useful in the treatment of insomnia include relaxation training, stimulus control, cognitive-behavioral strategies, sleep restriction, homework, and psychotherapy. Each of these will now briefly be described.

Relaxation training.   Teaching patients to relax is probably the most common behavioral treatment for insomnia. The rationale for relaxation training is based on the theory that all insomniacs are muscularly tense or physiologically aroused at the time of sleep onset. Accordingly, relaxation training is focused on reducing the level of arousal and tension. The type of relaxation training chosen is relatively unimportant. Progressive muscular relaxation, controlled breathing, hypnosis, and EMG (electromyography) biofeedback have all been proven effective. It seems that these relaxation techniques are effective mainly because they focus the insomniac's attention away from tension-inducing thoughts and onto a repetitive, nonthreatening stimulus.

The health counselor is cautioned that relaxation training is considerably more of a challenge for the insomniac than for other anxious clients. Simply giving the insomniac a relaxation tape or conducting a single practice session is rarely sufficient. Hauri (1989) notes two reasons for this difficulty. First, insomniacs seem to be much slower in learning relaxation techniques than are patients with other physiological disorders, and they need to apply these skills around desired sleep onset, at a time when voluntary control is waning.

Cognitive-behavioral strategies.   For many insomniacs, anxious concerns and ruminative thoughts are the most distressing signals that sleep will not come easily. Their worry may reflect realistic reactions to external events, such as real or imagined interpersonal, financial, or health problems. Not sur-

prisingly, some insomniacs report that their worries focus primarily on whether or not they will be able to fall asleep. Whatever the source of anxiety, a vicious cycle occurs; concern over not sleeping leads to a disruptive night's sleep, which in turn reinforces the conviction that insomnia persists. Cognitive-behavioral strategies can be helpful in allaying these concerns and ensuring the onset of sleep (Lacks, 1987). For instance, if the insomniac is overwhelmed with tension-inducing thoughts, a distraction procedure might be used. Clients might be advised to read or watch TV in bed until sleep overcomes them. Similarly, the insomniac typically looks at the clock every five to ten minutes and then becomes upset about the fact that sleep is not forthcoming; simply removing the clock may be more important than extensive training and relaxation. On the other hand, if specific anxious thoughts keep the insomniac awake, these thoughts need to be dealt with individually. For example, one might prescribe a 20-minute, presleep worry time, during which the client sits down—undistracted—writes down all random thoughts, and then deals with and thinks about each troubling thought. In contrast to good sleepers who think nonthreatening thoughts when they awake in the middle of the night, poor sleepers immediately become angry and upset that they are awake. These arousing thoughts then turn a five-second arousal into a two-hour catastrophe. In this situation, cognitive reframing techniques are quite effective. However, other cognitive methods such as thought stopping may be contraindicated when the patient is at the threshold of sleep.

In those clients for whom the maladaptive, conditioned association between bedroom stimuli and arousal is the major problem, *stimulus control* may be effective. This association is typically diagnosed in patients who sleep well away from their own bedrooms but poorly in their usual environment. When this is the case, the counselor educates clients about the mechanisms that keep them awake. Stimulus-control instructions (Bootzin & Nicassio, 1978) have been developed to ensure that bedtime becomes associated with rapid sleep onset. These instructions are listed below.

1. Go to bed only when sleepy.
2. Use the bed for no other purpose than sex and sleep. Do not read, eat, watch TV, knit, or talk with bed partner.
3. If you are not asleep within ten minutes of getting into bed, get up and leave the bedroom. Stay in another room until you feel sleepy; then go back to bed.
4. Set the alarm and get up at the same time every morning.
5. Do not nap during the day.
6. Fill out a sleep log each morning.

Sleep restriction. It is common for insomniacs to believe that extending bedtime will help compensate for long sleep latencies for disrupted sleep, believing that they have an opportunity to "catch up" on lost sleep. Although extra time in bed may yield more sleep, it adds potentially deleterious effects. An assumption of sleep-restriction therapy is that extra bed time often leads to increased wakefulness and results in fragmented sleep and variability in the timing of sleep and wakefulness. Sleep restriction aims to consolidate sleep and constrain its occurrence to a specific time by restricting time spent in bed.

Clients are first asked to fill out a one- or two-week sleep log describing each night. Then they are instructed to stay in bed only for as long as they are actually sleeping. For instance, suppose an insomniac reports that he sleeps only two-and-one-half hours per night and gets up around 6:30 A.M. During the first week of treatment, this client would be asked to remain out of bed and awake until 4:00 A.M. He or she would then still have to rise at 6:30 A.M. and would not be allowed to take any naps.

Each morning clients on a sleep-restriction regimen report their sleep to their counselor (or to the counselor's answering machine). When they report at least 90 percent sleep efficiency—that is, when they spend at least 90 percent of their restricted time in bed actually sleeping—their bed time is lengthened in 15 minute intervals until they sleep normal amounts again (Hauri, 1990).

Homework.   Monitoring and charting sleep-related behaviors is necessary not only to develop a sense of self-control but also to develop new and better sleep habits. As in other life-style-change and health-promotion programs, homework tasks are a cornerstone of the treatment of insomnia and other sleep disorders. Clients must learn that they may need to spend up to an hour a day monitoring and practicing behaviors if they are to be successful in overcoming their insomnia. Similarly, the health counselor must establish and reinforce the expectation that homework and other between-session tasks are vital to the change of processes (Bootzin & Nicassio, 1978).

Psychotherapy.   Because psychopathology reflects unresolved emotional conflict that can underlie chronic insomnia, psychotherapy can play an important role in its treatment. The general goals of psychotherapy for insomniacs include: (1) the improvement of the patient's ability to express emotions appropriately; (2) the development of insight regarding the patient's personal vulnerability; (3) the improvement in the quality of the patient's interpersonal relationships; and (4) the restructuring of the patient's life-style so that it no longer revolves around the symptom of insomnia.

There are a number of common psychotherapeutic issues involved in the treatment of insomnia: (1) denial of problem areas other than insomnia; (2) strong resistance to the exploration of these other problem areas; (3) need for control, which is often expressed in demands for sleeping medications, failure to stay on medication withdrawal regimens, or lack of compliance with homework assignments; (4) excessive dependence upon the counselor and reluctance to become an active participant in the therapy process; and (5) withholding of direct expression of negative feelings (Kales & Kales, 1984).

Social Interventions

In earlier sections, we noted the impact that the marital relationship has on the disorders of sleep like insomnia and suggested that insomnia and other sleep disorders impact on marital relationships. Therefore, it is essential that the spouse or other significant individual be involved in the treatment process. It was suggested that the health counselor first interview the spouse individually and then conjointly with the patient about the nature of the insomnia and its

impact on the relationship. In some cases, it may be necessary to address the relationship issues with the couple. At other times, a referral for marital therapy is made when marital discord is an important factor in the insomnia. Kales and Kales (1984) indicate that the insomniac often develops unexpressed hostile feelings toward the spouse.

Traditionally, the treatment of insomnia has taken place within an individual format. Lacks (1987) argues that the group format is superior to the individual treatment of insomnia. She compared insomniacs treated with the same therapy protocol in individual formats and in group formats and concluded that, on measured treatment outcomes, individually treated patients fared the same as patients who were treated in groups. Yet she believes that the group participants appeared to profit more from treatment than those in an individual format because of group cohesion and mutual problem solving and support.

Lacks (1987) describes a four-session treatment protocol involving five to seven patients in which a single therapist facilitates the group. Lacks notes that the more homogeneous the group, with respect to background and type of sleep problem, the better the result. The program combines psychoeducation, self-monitoring, stimulus control, and cognitive methods. Clients are expected to have been weaned off of any sleeping medications and to be drug-free before beginning the program.

The first session lasts approximately 90 minutes, and subsequent sessions require about 60 minutes. The first session is the most important, in that the behavioral treatment of insomnia is explained and the concept of stimulus control is highlighted. The group members are instructed in the rules of sleep hygiene and the expectation that they will monitor their sleep patterns by means of a sleep diary and complete other homework assignments during the course of the group. The next three sessions focus on collaborative troubleshooting of problems that group members have encountered in adhering to the treatment during the previous week. Although new material is introduced into each of these three sessions, problem solving and troubleshooting are the mainstay of the sessions.

Typically, the second session is the most difficult. Many clients feel frustrated and discouraged, particularly if their symptoms and distress have worsened during the previous week. Issues of treatment adherence or noncompliance, especially with self-monitoring, need to be addressed. An important part of the second session is to help group members establish a set of prebed routines. It is during this session that the stimulus-control theory of insomnia becomes personalized in the sleep lives of each individual group member. As in the other sessions, the expected minimum homework involves the daily sleep diary, which logs the number of hours of sleep and the number of times that the client is out of bed each night, as well as the responses to these items:

- How sleepy were you when you first went to bed last night (on a 1 to 5 scale from "not too sleepy" to "very sleepy")?
- What time did you get up this morning?
- Briefly list your activities in getting ready for bed.

- Briefly list your activities from dinner to bedtime.
- List any activities you carried out in bed yesterday.
- What were you thinking about in bed last night?

Session three begins with the review of the sleep diaries and the troubleshooting of any problems clients encountered. The new material for the session involves discriminating behaviors associated with good and poor sleep. Clients discuss ways to make behaviors associated with good sleep a part of their daily routine.

In session four, the problem solving/troubleshooting format continues. In addition, the clients are prepared for the maintenance and follow-up phase of the treatment. They have to continue to fill out their diaries during this last week and then begin to phase out the use of this self-monitoring as the new routines become automatic parts of their behavior. The group counselor then approaches the subject of relapse. The clients are told that, from time to time, everyone has a night or a brief period of sleep difficulty, especially during periods of increased stress. And if the clients use the techniques they have learned during the session and can avoid the tendency to develop performance anxiety, they are very likely to avert any more serious or persistent sleep disturbance. Finally, they are to expect a follow-up call in six weeks to give the counselor feedback about their continued progress.

Lacks notes that four weeks is the average length of time for improvements in sleep to become apparent, even though some individuals take less and some take more time. In short, this treatment protocol combines stimulus-control techniques with cognitive methods and psychoeducation. It has been found to be effective in both individual and group formats.

Relapse Prevention

Relapse does not appear to be as problematic in the treatment of insomnia as it does in exercise programs, weight control, smoking cessation, or pain control. Thus, there is relatively little written in the treatment manuals on this subject. Lacks (1987) indicates that the group process has a distinct impact on treatment adherence. When seen individually, clients who are noncompliant in self-monitoring or in following treatment instructions are accountable only to a counselor. However, in the group format, the same nonadhering clients meet with a more forceful reaction from other group members. Group members seem to be less willing to tolerate nonadherence from each other.

Case Examples

Case 1

Ms. Y is a 36-year-old attorney who sought counseling to understand "why I'm so driven" and to get relief from her insomnia. She reports having had difficulty falling asleep most nights since she was a law student. She indicates that she is "mentally hyperactive" at bedtime and is unable to stop thinking

about significant events of the day, particularly those involving her courtroom performance. When she feels she has not been very effective in court, she believes she does not deserve to fall asleep. Any evening excitement, such as an exciting movie or a lively conversation, leaves her unable to unwind for several hours. Occasionally, in the middle of the night, she awakens and begins ruminating about the day's events. On the nights when she sleeps poorly, she feels high-strung and tense the following day. Because many of her clients are corporate executives, she has a number of dinner engagements each week. She notices that, on the days when she has had wine or a mixed drink with dinner, she invariably awakens in the middle of the night aroused and slightly sweaty. Business travel also seems to worsen her sleep. Ms. Y is unmarried and has a wide circle of friends and enjoys socializing with them. However, relaxing alone has always been anxiety-producing for her, and so, if she found herself at home alone, she would immerse herself in her work. Over the years, she has tried a variety of prescription and over-the-counter sleeping medications, which left her feeling "hung over" the next day.

Ms. Y's excessive devotion to work and productivity to the exclusion of leisure activities is suggestive of an obsessive/compulsive personality style. In addition, her long-standing problems with falling asleep and frequent midcycle awakenings with rumination are characteristic of insomnia. In this regard, Ms. Y presents with the most prevalent personality style among chronic insomniacs. Subsequently, the counselor negotiated a combined treatment of both compulsive and insomnia features with Ms. Y. The counselor emphasized a "here and now" rather than an in-depth therapeutic approach, which could further reinforce her obsessive thinking. The counselor also interpreted Ms. Y's excessive feelings of insecurity which reinforced her need for guarantees before taking any action, and the counselor encouraged her to verbalize and work through her aggressive ambivalence and other feelings.

In the course of treatment, Ms. Y learned to self-monitor her sleep pattern and use relaxation techniques to reduce her anxiety and center herself. She was advised to avoid stimulating evening activities, discontinue the use of alcohol, and reduce her intake of caffeine. She easily learned stimulus-control techniques and, with some difficulty, was able to apply thought stopping to the ruminations she experienced when she awakened in the middle of the night. Finally, she was able to decrease her night-work obligations and replace them with more pleasurable leisure activities. Within six weeks, her sleep had greatly improved and within six months of weekly sessions, she was able to terminate treatment and feel much less "driven."

Case 2

Mr. Q is a 32-year-old computer programmer who presented to an outpatient psychiatry clinic at a local hospital with complaints of difficulty falling asleep and staying asleep combined with dependence on sleeping medication. The problem began approximately 18 months earlier, at the time Mr. Q received a job promotion to supervisor. A brief three-week period of emotional turmoil ensued, with anxiety symptoms accompanying the difficulty initiating and maintaining sleep. His family physician prescribed 10 mg of Valium a day with a dose of 0.25 mg of Halcion at bedtime. Initially, he reported symptomatic improve-

ment and, as the job stress subsided, he was able to discontinue Valium. His attempts to stop the nightly Halcion, however, resulted in severe sleeplessness, nightmares, and daytime agitation. Mr. Q resumed the bedtime Halcion and, two months later, had to double the dose as the insomnia worsened.

Before the onset of the sleeping problem, Mr. Q had always preferred to stay up late to do his programming, sleeping from 3:00 A.M. to 10:00 A.M. He reported logging 6½ hours of sleep followed by a sleep latency of 15 to 30 minutes. Bouts of initial insomnia had occurred intermittently since his early teen years.

It appears that Mr. Q's delayed phase sleep pattern—3:00 A.M. to 10:00 A.M.—is a predisposing condition as well as a major component in the circumstance that initiated the insomnia. The job promotion was the precipitant or the trigger of the insomnia. Dependence on Halcion appears to have perpetuated and as well as exacerbated his sleep problem.

After an extensive physical and psychiatric evaluation, Mr. Q was put on a weaning schedule of the Halcion. The counselor assigned to work with Mr. Q described the expected withdrawal reactions and, along with the attending psychiatrist, closely monitored the gradual withdrawal of the medication over the course of two weeks. The counselor also explained how Mr. Q's delayed sleep pattern had led to the recurrence of insomnia and discussed the value of keeping regular sleep/wake patterns in light of Mr. Q's tendency to stay up late at night. In two weeks, the Halcion was successfully discontinued. For the next two weeks, Mr. Q was asked to monitor his sleep in a sleep diary and, two weeks later, Mr. Q began a course of group treatment for insomnia based on the treatment protocol developed by Lacks (1987). By the third week of the program, Mr. Q reported the return of normal sleep with no episodes of insomnia.

Prevention

Although most of the scientific knowledge about good sleep is common sense, it is surprising how often the rules for good sleep hygiene are not followed by individuals who suffer from serious insomnia. Some common suggestions are listed below.

Sleep Hygiene Principles

1. Sleep only as long you need to feel refreshed the next day.
2. Maintain a regular wake-up time, as this helps you synchronize circadian rhythms.
3. Remember that general exercise can help you relax and tends to deepen sleep; however, you should avoid strenuous exercise within three hours of bedtime.
4. Try to establish a simple routine about going to bed.
5. Watch your diet: coffee, cola, tea, and chocolate all contain stimulants.
6. Don't smoke: smoking also increases arousal and makes sleeping more difficult.
7. Keep in mind that alcohol may facilitate relaxation, but it usually results in fragmented and poor sleep.

8. Create a conducive environment for sleep; fresh air and little noise are very helpful.
9. Interrupt ruminative worry about personal or business problems by cognitive refocusing or thought stopping.

Lacks and Rotert (1986) studied the knowledge and practice of sleep hygiene of poor sleepers compared with good sleepers. They found that poor sleepers have more knowledge about sleep hygiene than good sleepers but practice it less often. Poor sleepers have more awareness of the effects of caffeine and other stimulants on sleep disruption but continue to use stimulating substances one or two nights a week.

Since shift work and jet lag represent two very common phenomena among patients who work with counselors on a variety of health concerns, we present the following primary prevention suggestions.

Prevention of Insomnia in Shift-Workers

The following preventive measures are suggested for individuals who work nights or on rotating shifts.

1. Eat meals at the same time each day to make as little change in the circadian rhythms as possible.
2. Sleep at least four hours during the same time each day.
3. When sleeping during the day, darken the room with heavy drapes or shades.
4. Experiment with ways to block out daytime noise, such as with earplugs, white-noise machines, an air conditioner, or a fan.
5. Restrict the use of stimulants. Don't drink coffee, tea, or cola drinks or smoke heavily in the hours before going to bed.
6. Try not to shift gears by changing wake/sleep schedules on weekends or brief holidays.
7. Try to reduce family stress related to shift work. Discuss the resentment your spouse and children feel about your absences at night, and enlist the family's help in finding ways and times to spend some time together each day.

The preceding preventive measures are focused primarily on the individual. We also have some suggestions about preventive measures at a *systemic level.* Some guidelines for scheduling shift rotations have been suggested recently. For routine jobs, daily shifts may be better than weekly ones. Workers should report for the day shift on Mondays, switch to evenings on Tuesdays, work nights on Wednesdays, take Thursdays off, then again work during the day on Fridays. Popular in Europe, this schedule allows employees to stay tuned to a standard time frame and to eat at least one meal a day with their families. For jobs that require more concentration or decision-making abilities, much longer shifts—of months rather than days or weeks—may be better because they allow the body clock to catch up with the time clock (Monk, 1986; Hauri, 1990).

Prevention of Jet Lag

Jet lag can hardly be avoided; however, some of its effects can be minimized. Sleep specialists suggest:

1. Begin the time shift before leaving home. The week before the trip, gradually begin going to bed and getting up earlier if traveling east or staying up later if traveling west.
2. Leave home rested; avoid last minute hassles.
3. Dress comfortably, stretch occasionally, and alternatively tense and relax muscle groups while in flight.
4. Eat lightly during the flight and for a few days afterward. Don't drink alcohol or caffeinated beverages; substitute water, soft drinks, or fruit juices.
5. Do not smoke or smoke infrequently.
6. Schedule arrival for late in the day, close to the normal bedtime at home. Spend the first day upon arrival in a quiet and relaxed manner.
7. On short trips, stay on "home time"; on longer trips, start living by the new time frame immediately; and if traveling halfway around the world, stop for one or two day's rest.
8. Rely on sleep rituals and relaxation exercise to ease into sleep. Avoid sleeping medications as they only mask rather than treat jet lag. (Hauri, 1990).

Summary

In this chapter, we reviewed biopsychosocial aspects of sleep and sleep disorders, particularly the circadian disregulation noted in chronic insomnia. Some of the theories of sleep and the methods for the assessment of and intervention in chronic insomnia were also discussed. Because primary-care physicians and sleep clinics are the usual places of referral for sleep problems, we assumed that health counselors will not ordinarily be consulted by clients who complain primarily of insomnia. More likely, clients will present with another health problem or a psychological issue, and only during the course of the assessment will the counselor find out that an intercurrent sleep problem such as chronic insomnia is present. For this reason, the treatment protocol and suggestions for assessing and intervening in chronic insomnia were geared to this treatment setting.

Relapse is considerably less of a problem for sleep disorders than it is in most of the other health counseling areas. A number of specific suggestions for the primary prevention of insomnia involved: common principles of sleep hygiene; specific recommendations about preventing or reducing the impact of jet lag; and individual and systemic guidelines for reducing the incidence of insomnia among shift-workers.

Resources

Organizations
There seem to be 12 Step groups and national organizations for every imaginable health concern except insomnia. Your local sleep clinic might be able to refer you to a local group. On the other hand, there are narcolepsy support groups as well as AWAKE groups for sleep apnea patients in most cities. They can be found by consulting the telephone directory.

Publications: Professional References

- Kales, A., & Kales, J. D. (1984). *Evaluation and Treatment of Insomnia.* New York: Oxford University Press. Of the comprehensive professional manuals, this one takes a biopsychosocial view of insomnia. There are outstanding sections on psychotherapy as well as on the behavioral treatment of insomnia. The author offers authoritative reviews of the effects on sleep of nutrition, exercise, medications, and alcohol. Included is an extensive section on psychological testing.
- Lacks, P. (1987). *Behavioral Treatment for Persistent Insomnia.* New York: Pergamon Press. A part of the popular and practical "Psychology Practitioner Guidebooks" series, this step-by-step treatment manual guides the reader through protocols for both individual and group treatment sessions. It includes a useful section on dealing with common treatment problems.

Publications: Patient Education

- Hauri, P. (1990). *No More Sleepless Nights.* New York: Wiley. Dr. Hauri is a well-regarded sleep researcher who has written a very readable account of treatment for insomnia. A unique feature of this self-help book is the emphasis on preventing and reducing the effects on sleep of jet lag and shift work.
- Hales, D. (1981). *The Complete Book of Sleep: How Your Nights Affect Your Days.* Reading, MA: Addison-Wesley; and American Medical Association. (1984). *Guide to Better Sleep.* New York: Random House. These are two of the better popular books. They are well-researched and accurate accounts of treatment that are consistently checked out of our public library. Hales's book describes a patient's experience during the course of a sleep clinic evaluation.
- Ferber, J. (1988). *Solving Your Child's Sleep Problems.* New York: Fireside. This is one of the few books that focuses on sleep disturbances among children from infants to adolescents, with specific suggestions for parents on dealing with these problems.

References

BECK, A. (1967). *Depression: Clinical, experimental and theoretical aspects.* New York: Harper & Row.

BERKOWITZ, A., & Perkins, W. (1985). Correlates of psychosomatic stress symptoms among farm women. *Journal of Human Stress, 17,* 76–81.

BOOTZIN, R. (1977). Effects of self-control procedures for insomnia. In R. Stuart (Ed.), *Behavioral self-management strategies.* New York: Bruner/Mazel.

BOOTZIN, R., & Nicassio, P. (1978). Behavioral treatments in insomnia. In M. Hersen, R. Eisler, & P. Miller (Eds.), *Progress in behavior modification.* New York: Academic Press.

CARTWRIGHT, R., & Knight, S. (1987). Silent partners: The views of sleep apneic patients. *Sleep, 10,* 244–248.

DEMENT, W. C. (1983). Signs and symptoms of sleep disorders. In J. Walsh, A. Bertelson, & P. Schweitzer (Eds.), *Clinical aspects of sleep disorders: Proceedings of a symposium.* St. Louis, MO: Deaconness Hospital.

DRUGS AND INSOMNIA: The use of medications to promote sleep. (1984). *Journal of the American Medical Association, 18,* 2410–2414.

DUNKELL, S. (1978). *Sleep positions: The night language of the body.* New York: North American Library.

FOLKARD, S. (1983). Diurnal variations. In R. Hockey (Ed.), *Stress and fatigue in human performance.* New York: Wiley.

HALES, D. (1981). *The complete book of sleep.* Reading, MA: Addison-Wesley.

HAURI, P. (1982). A sleep disorders primer. In R. Gatchel, A. Baum, & J. Singer (Eds.), *Handbook of psychology and health, Vol. 1.* Hillsdale, NJ: Erlbaum.

HAURI, P. (1989). Primary insomnia. In T. Karasu (Ed.), *Treatment of psychiatric disorders, Vol. 3.* Washington, DC: American Psychiatric Association.

HAURI, P. (1990). *No more sleepless nights.* New York: Wiley.

INSTITUTE OF MEDICINE. (1979). *Sleeping pills, insomnia, and medical practice.* Washington, DC: National Academy of Sciences.

KALES, A., & Kales, J. (1984). *Evaluation and treatment of insomnia.* New York: Oxford University Press.

KALES, A., Soldatos, C., & Kales, J. D. (1981). Sleep disorders: Office evaluation and management. In S. Arieti & H. Brodie (Eds.), *American handbook of psychiatry, Vol. 7.* (2nd ed.). New York: Basic Books.

KALES, J., & Kales, A. (1982). Rest and sleep. In R. Taylor (Ed.), *Health promotion: Principles and clinical applications.* Norwalk, CT: Appleton-Century-Crofts.

KAZARIAN, S., Howe, M., & Csapo, K. (1979). Development of the sleep behavior self-rating scale. *Behavior Therapy, 10,* 412–417.

LACKS, P. (1987). *Behavioral treatment of persistent insomnia.* New York: Pergamon Press.

LACKS, P., & Rotert, M. (1986). Knowledge and practice of sleep hygiene techniques in insomniacs and good sleepers. *Behavioral Research and Therapy, 24,* 365–368.

LARSON, J., Crane, D., & Smith, C. (1991). Morning and night couples. *Journal of Marital and Family Therapy, 17,* 53–65.

LAWRENCE, P. (1982). Behavioral assessment of sleep disorders. In F. Keefe, & J. Blumenthal (Eds.), *Assessment strategies in behavioral medicine.* New York: Grune & Stratton.

LICHSTEIN, K., & Rosenthal, T. (1980). Insomniac's perceptions of cognitive versus somatic determinants of sleep disturbance. *Journal of Abnormal Psychology, 89,* 105–107.

MONK, T., & Folkard, S. (1983). Circadian rhythms and shift work. In R. Hockey (Ed.), *Stress and fatigue in human performance.* New York: Wiley.

MONK, T. H. (1986). Advantages and disadvantages of rapidly rotating shift schedules—A circadian viewpoint. *Human Factors, 28,* 553–557.

NAUTH, R., & Rutenfranz, J. (1976). Experimental shift work studies of permanent, night, and rapidly rotating shift systems. *International Occupational Environment Health, 37,* 125–137.

ROFFWARG, H. (1979). Association of Sleep Disorders Centers: Diagnostic classification of sleep and arousal disorders. *Sleep, 2,* 1–137.

SOLDATOS, C., Kales, J., Scharf, M., et al. (1980). Cigarette smoking associated with sleep difficulty. *Science, 207,* 551–552.

SPEILMAN, (1986). Assessment of insomnia. *Clinical Psychology Review, 6,* 11–25.

WALSH, J. K. (1983). Overview of polysomography and sleep physiology. In J. Walsh, A. Bertelson, & P. Schweitzer (Eds.), *Clinical aspects of sleep disorders: Proceedings of a symposium.* St. Louis, MO: Deaconness Hospital.

WEBB, W. B. (1979). Theories of sleep function and some clinical implications. In R. Drucker-Colin, M. Shkurovich, & M. Sterman (Eds.), *The functions of sleep.* New York: Academic Press.

WEHR, T., & Goodwin, F. K. (1983). Psychology and psychopathology. In T. Wehr, & F. K. Goodwin (Eds.), *Circadian rhythms in psychiatry.* Pacific Grove, CA: Boxwood Press.

WEVER, R. (1979). *The circadian systems of man: Results of experiments under temporal isolation.* New York: Springer-Verlag.

8

Sexual Health

What we're born with, what we experience all through infancy and childhood is a sexuality that isn't concentrated on the genitals: it's a sexuality diffused through the whole organism. That's the paradise we inherit. But the paradise gets lost as the child grows up.

Aldous Huxley

The so-called sexual revolution has certainly had many positive effects on the social climate. It has paved the way for more frank and open discussion of sex and sexual problems, has made it easier to get needed information on sexual matters, and has fostered a more tolerant attitude toward behaviors that in previous times would have been condemned as unhealthy, deviant, or criminal. Unfortunately, this new openness has not solved all our problems; in fact, it has created a few new ones. A quick glance at the newspaper, an overheard conversation, discussions with friends, perhaps an examination of your own thoughts will reveal that problems, misconceptions, and fears about sex still abound (Travis & Ryan, 1988).

Research and popular books both focus on human sexuality as an experience commonly beset by one problem after another. These problems are presented in stereotypical fashion: women are lacking in physical arousal, unable to reach orgasm, or just plain uninterested in sex; men are required to endure infrequent sex, impotence, and problematic premature ejaculation.

All people in our society have been or will be involved in sexual behavior. The professional literature and public media conclusively document the confusion and distress couples feel regarding their ability to fully utilize and express their sexual potential. The extent of these widespread problems would seem to mandate that counselors develop diagnostic and therapeutic skills to meet clients' needs. Unfortunately, too few counselors have the skills to feel comfortable working in the area of sexual counseling.

Although interventions to deal with problems of sexual functioning date back to earliest recorded history, sex therapy as an independent discipline has only recently been introduced, in the early 1970s. From the beginning of this century until the latter part of the 1960s, the treatment of sexual dysfunction was approached primarily from a psychoanalytic viewpoint. Dysfunctions were viewed as the result of deep-seated personality conflicts—specifically, as a failure to resolve the Oedipal complex. This therapeutic orientation viewed unconscious conflicts as the underlying cause of sexual problems and the resolution of these conflicts as the cure. However, empirical outcome studies of analytical psychotherapy applied to sexual problems failed to demonstrate that psychotherapy was an effective intervention (Cooper, 1971; Reynolds, 1977). Later in the 1950s, learning theory and behavioral therapy were introduced and, in 1970, Masters and Johnson's *Human Sexual Inadequacy* was published. With the publication of this volume, sex counseling and therapy became established as a distinct therapeutic discipline.

It is undeniably important for counselors to be aware of the assessment issues and intervention strategies that are required in the treatment of sexual dysfunction. Yet, although we remain mindful of what might go wrong, it is equally important to be aware of ways in which we can help our clients enjoy and enhance their sexual health.

Sexuality is a basic part of our humanness. Through sexuality, we can experience a greater repertoire of communication than is otherwise available. Desire to be interconnected, unfulfilled longing, and pure ecstasy are but a few of the emotions experienced that are often difficult to put into words. Sex as a vehicle of expression is said to be the barometer of a marital relationship. When

issues of sexual health are explored, good sex is seen as more than just an expression but also as an amalgam of beliefs, attitudes, physiology, and communication. When sexuality is viewed as a communication process, we can assess the quality of the relationship by examining the satisfaction of the sexual experience. Because sexuality is a complex blend of beliefs and attitudes, physiology, and communication, this chapter will begin by exploring each of these components.

The Components of Sexuality

Beliefs and Attitudes

An undeniable force in an individual's sexuality is the ideas espoused, either directly or indirectly, by the family. These attitudes influence the "when" and "how" of sexual behaviors as well as what is acceptable and unacceptable for expression. It has often been said that when a couple gets into bed, there are actually six people present: the man, the woman, and both sets of parents.

The earliest attitudes about sexual behavior are rooted in body image (Fisher, 1989). Body images often suffer gross distortions because of the discomfort that many parents experience when discussing the body. Further distortions may also occur depending on the degree of parental acceptance of early (but phase-appropriate) masturbation. Although infants may revel in the discovery of their genitalia, the parents usually do not. Mothers and fathers may be equally uncomfortable with acknowledging the mere existence of genitals, not to mention discussing their relative functions (Fisher, 1989).

These early experiences of disappointment in the acceptance of the genitalia lead to a sense of discomfort and possibly even a sense of alienation from one's own body (Fisher, 1989). How this influences one's self-concept as a sexual being is readily apparent. One way that a healthy self-image is expressed in sexuality is in the ability to give and receive pleasure. If the self-concept of the individual is plagued by sexual embarrassment, then sexual expression is hindered. Early memories of severe disapproval or punishment for masturbation can also impede the healthy sexual feelings that develop in adolescence. How can individuals enjoy something that is wrong and still see themselves as good? The idea that sex is sinful or bad can translate into later problems with the individual's own sexual expression.

When considering personal beliefs, we must also look at cultural differences. The sexual relationships, customs, and attitudes of a particular society are an integral, functional element in that culture. Therefore, what might be sexually permissive or repressive in one culture may appear natural and normal in others (Maier, 1984).

Physiological and Biological Factors

The exploration of the physiological component of sexual health requires a thorough health screening. The screening should encompass as many variables as possible, including the client's past illnesses, current subjective state of health, body deformities, and current medications. It is also appropriate for the coun-

selor to note whether any early illnesses resulted in developmental or physical handicaps. Handicaps can have a significant impact on all the developmental processes of the individual. Disabled people are often regarded as asexual, and this cultural attitude and people's behavior toward the handicapped have seriously retarded the social and sexual development of many sick or disabled people. Whether the handicap should be of prime consideration in sexual functioning is a subjective opinion of the client. If clients do not view a particular problem as handicapping, then it will likely not impinge on their sexual identity or functioning (Maier, 1984).

Current complaints of ill health should be carefully investigated as either the cause of or a contributing factor to sexual dysfunction. For example, certain illnesses create respiratory problems that impede the flow of oxygen throughout the body, creating temporary erectile dysfunctions. Although the incident is still disconcerting, the client's fears are greatly alleviated once the temporary nature of the condition is understood.

Certain drugs induce biochemical changes in the body that result in such diverse complaints as decreased sexual drive, erectile dysfunction, premature ejaculation, and painful coitus (dyspareunia). Alcohol and illegal drugs also create sexual problems. Few research studies have been successful in identifying the medications that cause sexual dysfunction (Crenshaw, Kessler, & Hildebrandt, 1985). Counselors need to be aware of both the possible side effects of medications and the possible alternative procedures that will not affect the client's sexual functioning.

Another assessment issue is the growing incidence of infertility. Infertility is defined as the inability to conceive within a one-year period of time. The prevalence of infertility has risen dramatically in the past decade, with estimates of infertility ranging in the 15 to 20 percent range for couples in their childbearing years. Numerous factors have been cited as causally related, including increased incidents of sexually transmitted diseases, increased medication or drug usage, and increased popularity of having children later in life. Clearly, infertility will continue to be a treatment issue for counselors (Sadler & Syrop, 1987).

A process of evaluation for infertility includes a health history (which includes contraceptive usage and prior exposure to sexually transmitted diseases), a detailed list of coital frequency (and how it corresponds to the ovulatory cycle), and a complete physical examination of both partners. This may include a postcoital examination as well as a semen analysis. The actual treatment of infertility has some significant psychological implications (Reed, 1987). When couples decide to undergo infertility treatment, their whole life appears to give way to the mechanization of a treatment team. Their privacy ceases to be of concern to the physician who cares for them. The focus of the genitals ceases to be sexual and is transformed into a purely mechanical reproductive one. Sexuality is out and baby making is in. Sex ceases to be an enjoyable and spontaneous event and every sex act becomes the ultimate test of fertility. Sexuality is no longer a dimension of a relationship but has been reduced to its elemental form of reproduction. The strain that this poses on the relationship is often enormous.

Communication

Couples who are in the process of changing their sexual behavior must also change their relationship. At the heart of any relationship is the ability to communicate. Couples need to evaluate their relationship on many levels, and communication is at the core of this process.

The assessment issue is complex. Couples who request help for sexual problems often have difficulty communicating, but they may not realize it because the patterns are an established part of their overall interaction. To work on sexual issues, couples must first address the underlying purpose served by their communication process. The process of discovery could easily double the length of time that couples will need to engage in counseling. Most likely, couples will not want to waste time on this issue and will want more direct treatment of the sexual problem. The counselor may therefore need to utilize sexual exercises designed to enhance the couples' communication.

It is important to stress again that sexuality is much more than a mechanical interaction of bodies. It is actually a complex interaction of beliefs, attitudes, and communication, as well as physiology.

There is a very interesting system that assesses sexual behavior by focusing on the purposiveness of the actions, as opposed to their causes (Shulman, 1967). This strategy looks at sex from the point of view of the goal of sexual behavior and assesses the social purpose, or effect, of the sexual behavior. Social purposes are not hard to judge; behavior is either socially useful or socially useless. Destructive sexual behavior would always seem to be useless, and so, one would think, is unethical sexual behavior. Furthermore, the existence of sexual drives is taken for granted, as is the idea that sexual behavior is under the individual's control. Sex is therefore something a person does, not just something that happens to her or him. Why a person uses sex in one way rather than another is related to her or his personal opinion of sex and of life. For example, if clients see life as a competitive striving to get, to have, and to achieve, then their sexual behavior will reflect these attitudes, and they may have trained themselves over the years to use sex for personal triumph in a competitive manner.

Sex is useful when it promotes what we ordinarily consider good: social harmony, pleasure, love, and so forth. Sex is useless when it is destructive, socially isolating, produces suffering, and so on. There are at least six useful ways of using sex: (1) for reproduction; (2) for pleasure; (3) to create a feeling of belonging; (4) as a cooperative endeavor to create a feeling of sharing; (5) for the purpose of consolation; and (6) for self-affirmation. In addition, sex can be abused by using it for the following purposes: (1) to make mischief; (2) to create distance; (3) to dominate; (4) to serve; (5) to demonstrate success or failure; (6) to express vanity; (7) to get revenge; and (8) to prove abnormality (Shulman, 1967).

Assessment

The three major methods of assessing sexual dysfunction are the interview, psychometric testing, and medical evaluation.

Interview

The initial interview is used to help determine the nature of the dysfunction and whether sex therapy is an appropriate intervention. Areas for the counselor to consider in making this determination include:

1. a description of the sexual difficulty or difficulties
2. what attempts have been made to resolve these difficulties
3. a description of the current sexual activity of the couple, including coital and noncoital activities
4. an assessment of the overall quality of the relationship
5. the presence or absence of individual psychopathology
6. a medical history and physical status
7. the individual and joint motivation for treatment
8. a detailed assessment of functioning in each phase of the sexual response cycle—desire, arousal, and orgasm

A counselor will also gain information from the manner in which the responses are conveyed by observing the couple's interaction and other nonverbal communication.

If sex therapy is deemed appropriate, the next step is for the counselor to obtain a detailed history of each individual. The purpose of such an interview is to help the counselor gain information about factors that may contribute to the maintenance of the dysfunction, which will help in creating an intervention strategy. As a skilled counselor knows, additional information is gathered throughout the therapeutic process, as each individual's personality and the couple's interactive dynamics become more and more observable. Information required for adequate assessment should include a general individual history, a sexual history, a relationship history, and an assessment of current status. The general history should:

1. assemble information on the family structure and background over the past two generations
2. assess current psychopathology
3. assess individual interactive styles—how communicative and how assertive a person is, how he or she goes about getting needs met
4. identify the values, morals, and religious beliefs that guide the individual
5. identify individual life goals
6. determine the level of anxiety, both in general and in response to sexual and other life events
7. assess the questions of extramarital relationships and love for the partner
8. assess the individual's view of the world, whether there is a positive or negative focus

The individual's sexual history could also include assessment of early sexual learning, early sexual experiences, frequency of and desire for sexual activities, masturbation history and current behavior, sexual attitudes and fantasies, and gender preference.

The relationship history should include assessment of the couple's skills in conflict resolution, communication, decision making, and responsibility sharing,

as well as assessment of affection; sexual satisfaction; relationship with children and parents; ability to express anger, love, and attraction to the partner; the power structure in the relationship; and the future relationship goals (Friedman & Czekala, 1985).

Psychometric Testing

A number of paper-and-pencil tests have been developed to aid in the assessment of sexual dysfunction. Tests have been developed to identify arousal deficits as well as to isolate problem behaviors. Attitudinal tests and other instruments intended to measure sexual capability, sexual experience, pleasure, fear, anxiety, and guilt are also available. An excellent review of these instruments can be found in a special issue of *The Journal of Sex and Marital Therapy*, 1979, Volume 5, Number 3.

Medical Evaluation

Accepted clinical opinion states that almost all sexual dysfunctions are psychogenic. Recent evidence, however, suggests that the arousal and orgasm responses are vulnerable to impairment of hormonal (Spark, White, & Connolly, 1980), vascular (Karacan et al., 1978), and neurological (Karacan, Salis, & Williams, 1978) functions. All clients should be asked about their medical history and current health. A thorough evaluation by a gynecologist, urologist, or, preferably, a specialist in sexual medicine should be performed in cases of erectile dysfunction, painful coitus, subjective loss of genital sensation, reduction in intensity of orgasm, or for anyone who has a history of diabetes, alcoholism, or spinal cord trauma or takes medications that might affect sexual functioning (Schover, 1982).

For further information on the advancement in knowledge and technique regarding the physical contributions to sexual dysfunction, see Kolodny, Masters, and Johnson (1979), Krone, Siroky, and Goldstein (1983), and/or Yaffe and Fenwick (1988).

Interventions

Before discussing specific intervention strategies, we will take a look at the major concepts of modern sex therapy. Although these concepts have been chosen and developed primarily to help people who experience sexual dysfunctions, they will be of interest and value to health counselors because of their proven relevance in treating many types of relationship conflicts. The following list is developed by Humphrey (1983) and identifies the major concepts of sex therapy.

1. Sex is a natural function. In healthy partners, male and female sexual-response cycles occur as a result of normal erotic stimulation just as naturally as heavy breathing follows vigorous exercise.
2. Every human being has his or her own unique S.V.S.—Sexual Value System. If a person does not act in accordance with his or her sexual value system, conflict, guilt, and other such negative consequences will occur.

3. Sexual intercourse involves a mutual activity between two persons—hence, there is no such thing as an "uninvolved" sexual partner who can blame his or her spouse for all the couple's sexual troubles.
4. First events carry special meanings to each person, so such things as first orgasms, first acts of intercourse, and so on are especially significant events in the life of individuals and couples.
5. Sex is a medium of exchange between persons. Partners must *give* pleasures in order to *get* pleasures themselves.
6. Authoritative "command" concepts (musts, shoulds, oughts) have no place in sexual activity. For instance, an attitude of "I must have an orgasm or I'll be unhappy" places excessive pressure on sexual performance. Sexual functioning cannot be forced or ordered. An attitude of openness, neutrality, and vulnerability is necessary for one to completely "surrender" oneself sexually to one's partner.
7. Feelings are facts. For example, a man may be very upset because his wife feels that his sexual language is crude, but her feeling is a fact. He must therefore talk "appropriately" if he is going to be able to communicate sexually with her on a positive basis.
8. Intercourse does not occur in a psychosocial vacuum. What goes on outside the bedroom has a direct bearing on what goes on sexually within the bedroom.
9. Each sexual partner needs to speak for him- or herself, not for the partner. People should learn to use "I" statements to achieve this and avoid "mind reading," second-guessing, or blaming their partners. Instead of saying "you weren't turning me on," people can be taught to reframe the message by saying "I wasn't feeling turned on by you . . . ," thus acknowledging their feeling but not blaming the partner.
10. Good communications are of vital importance to the maintenance of any relationship. They are especially critical in communicating attitudes, feelings, and wishes about sexuality.
11. Good marital sexual intercourse is most likely to occur if it is engaged in regularly over the years. The adage of "use it or lose it," referring to a person's ability to respond sexually, holds true.

Most therapists use a multifaceted package of interventions that range from a psychodynamic exploration of the individual through relationship restructuring to a prescription of direct changes in sexual behavior. The following principles currently underlie most sex-therapy interventions:

1. mutual responsibility
2. elimination of performance anxiety
3. education
4. attitude change
5. improved communication
6. enhanced relationships
7. physical and medical interventions
8. behavior change

Sexual problems can be divided into two categories: primary and secondary. Primary sexual problems arise from sex-related stimuli and occur only in sexual situations. Secondary sexual problems are only one manifestation of a larger personal relationship problem. Classifying cases as primary or secondary helps the counselor determine the appropriate counseling strategy. Primary problems usually respond well to brief counseling. Secondary problems usually require intensive counseling or therapy. The major focus of health counselors, therefore, is on brief therapy. This section will describe a process that should be sufficient to alleviate many of the sexual problems that counselors encounter. It is based on psychological learning theory and can be used compatibly with all major intervention systems. Learning is emphasized as the means of changing both overt and covert sexual behavior. One to five visits of 30 to 60 minute duration are involved (Pion, Annon, & Carlson, 1982).

The Four-Levels-of-Intervention Model

A treatment model has been developed to aid counselors in helping clients with sexual problems* (Annon, 1974; Pion & Annon, 1975). The model, referred to as P-LI-SS-IT, provides for four levels of intervention, with each letter or pair of letters designating a suggested method for handling the particular sexual concerns. The four levels are: (1) *P*ermission, (2) *L*imited *I*nformation, (3) *S*pecific *S*uggestions, and (4) *I*ntensive *T*herapy.

To attempt to assess and treat each concern in exactly the same way would be inappropriate. The model, both flexible and comprehensive, provides a framework for distinguishing problems that are amenable to brief therapy from others that require intensive therapy. The first three levels can be viewed as brief therapy, as contrasted with the intensive therapy of the fourth level.

This model has a number of distinct advantages. It may be applied in a variety of settings and adapted to whatever client time is available. Theoretically, each ascending level of approach requires increasing amounts of knowledge, training, and skill on the part of the counselor. Because each level requires increased experience, the model allows professionals to gear their approach to their own particular level of competence. This also means that counselors now have a plan to help them determine when referral elsewhere is appropriate. Most important, the model provides a framework for discriminating between and among problems. How many levels that counselors will feel competent to use directly depends on the amount of interest and time they are willing to devote to expanding their knowledge, training, and skill.

The First Level of Treatment: Permission Giving

Sometimes, all that people want to know is whether they are normal or "okay," not perverted, deviant, or abnormal. They would like to find this out from someone with a professional background or from someone who is in a position of authority. Many times, clients are not bothered by their specific behavior but,

---

*This material is available in an extended version in Pion, R. J., Annon, J. S., and Carlson, J. (1982). Brief Sexual Counseling. *Counseling and Human Development, 14* (8), 1–8.

rather, by the thought that something may be "wrong" or "bad" about what they are doing or not doing. Frequently, clients just want an interested professional as a sounding board for expressing their concerns. In these cases, the counselor will probably be able to tell them that they are not alone or unusual in their concerns and that many people share them. Reassurance of normality and permission to continue doing exactly what they have been doing are often sufficient to resolve what might eventually become a major problem.

Permission giving will certainly not solve all sexual problems, but it will resolve some. It has the advantages that it can be used in almost any setting at any time (given some measure of privacy) and that the counselor needs only minimal preparation. Finally, it may be used to cover a number of areas of concern, such as thoughts, fantasies, dreams, and feelings (covert behaviors), as well as overt behaviors.

Concerns about sexual thoughts and fantasies are common. For example, both men and women periodically have sexual thoughts and fantasies about people other than their partners, about people of the same sex, or even about their own parents, brothers or sisters, sons or daughters, or friends. Letting the client know that this is not unusual may relieve some of the anxiety or guilt about being abnormal. Only when such thoughts or fantasies become persistent or begin to interfere directly in some way with other areas of functioning do they create a problem.

Permission giving may also be appropriate for handling dream concerns. Individuals may have occasional dreams involving sexual activity with a wide variety of people other than their partners. At times, the dreams may also involve sexual activity with partners of the same sex, even though the dreamer may never have had such actual experiences. Reassurance that such dreams are perfectly normal and not unusual or indicative of abnormality is usually sufficient to relieve the anxiety or guilt associated with them. Often, permission giving is also sufficient to stop the recurring dream that initially caused the anxiety.

Another common concern is the clients' anxiety over experiencing sexual arousal to what they consider to be inappropriate stimulation. Many of these concerns arise from the failure to discriminate between arousal that results from sexual thoughts and fantasies and arousal that results from direct tactile stimulation. For example, a mother who is breast feeding her baby might experience some degree of sexual arousal because of the direct tactile stimulation to her breasts. A father may experience an erection when playing with a young child on his lap. Reassurance that these are normal, involuntary responses to tactile stimulation may reduce the client's unnecessary anxiety and prevent a minor happening from developing into a major concern. Similar permission giving for such feelings can apply to horseback and motorcycle riding; tree and rope climbing; the use of tampons, douches, and enemas; or any other circumstance that involves tactile stimulation of the breasts, genitals, or anal area.

Permission giving may be applied to a wide range of sexual behaviors that the counselor recognizes as common and normal but that the client does not. Take, for example, the case of the couple who read in their favorite magazine that the average frequency of sexual intercourse for people of their age and

education is two-and-a-half times a week. Their own frequency may be eight times a week or eight times a year, but now they begin to worry whether they are normal, oversexed, or undersexed. A counselor's response that, in essence, gives them permission to continue with their own preferred frequency may be all that is necessary to relieve anxiety.

Many sexual concerns can be handled by giving the client permission to *not* engage in certain sexual behaviors unless he or she chooses to. An example might be the young woman who is receiving pressure from her partner to experience multiple orgasms or who has read or heard that every woman has the right to expect and demand them. However, she is satisfied with the one orgasm that she experiences with her partner and does not really care whether she is multi-orgasmic or not. Giving this woman permission to not experience multiple orgasms may be helpful to her. Conversely, in the case of the woman who would really like to experience multiple orgasms but is fearful or hesitant that she might then become a "nymphomaniac," giving permission to be multi-orgasmic, if she chooses to, might be a helpful approach.

Permission giving is most appropriate and helpful when used in direct relation to the client's goals. By keeping this in mind, the counselor will be able to decide what form of permission giving will be the most beneficial for a particular client.

On the surface, the basic assumption underlying the permission-giving approach may appear to be that the counselor should sanction whatever sexual thought, fantasy, or behavior that a consenting adult wishes to engage in. In a general sense, this may be correct, but such an assumption has some definite limitations. Although an individual client ultimately has to decide on his or her own behavior, a counselor's blanket permission giving may not be appropriate if the client is not making an informed choice. The counselor is responsible for informing the client of the possible adverse consequences of engaging in certain thoughts, fantasies, or behaviors.

A number of books have "given permission" for the indiscriminate use of any fantasy a person may desire while engaging in masturbation or sexual behavior with a partner. Learning theory suggests, and clinical evidence substantiates, that systematically associating thoughts and fantasies with sexual activity is a powerful means of conditioning sexual arousal to almost any stimulus (Annon, 1973). This fact has been used to therapeutic advantage. In certain circumstances, however, engaging in such activity by the uninformed may have undesired results. Informing clients of the possible consequences of their behavior and leaving the ultimate choice to them seems more appropriate than blanket permission giving.

Limitations.   The extent to which the counselor feels comfortable with and is willing to use the permission-giving approach depends in general on his or her breadth of sexual knowledge, orientation, and value system. The more knowledge that counselors have of sexual behavior in their own and other cultures, the more comfortable they feel in applying this level of treatment. Counselors' theoretical or professional orientation may also place limits on how appropriate permission giving may be for a particular thought, fantasy, dream,

feeling, or behavior. Counselors with a psychoanalytic background may wish to withhold permission giving for recurrent sexual dreams, preferring to work through such material in therapy with the client. Obviously, that is the individual counselor's choice.

We do not wish to suggest that counselors change their viewpoint to that of a learning-oriented approach. The counselor should use only those suggestions that he or she thinks are appropriate to his or her frame of reference. At the same time, however, we hope that counselors will be willing to experiment a little.

Ideally, counselors will try not to impose their personal value systems on their clients intentionally. In practice, however, this is sometimes difficult to achieve. Of course, the counselor should not give up his or her own value system. At times, the client's stated goals may come into direct conflict with the counselor's value system. When this happens, the counselor's responsibility is to clearly inform the client of this and refer him or her elsewhere.

A final important point is that of self-permission. Counselors should be able to give permission to themselves to not be experts. They must not be afraid to say they do not know the answer when they do not. No one person is an expert in this field. Theory, research, and practice in the sexual area are so far-ranging that no individual or group of individuals can be expected to know or keep abreast of even a sizable fraction of the information in this area. Counselors do what they can for their clients on the basis of their own knowledge and experience. In some cases, the most important thing a counselor has to offer is him- or herself—someone who will listen; who can communicate interest, understanding, and respect; and who will not label or judge the client.

If permission giving is not sufficient to resolve the client's concern, and if the counselor is not in an appropriate setting or does not have sufficient time or relevant knowledge and skills, the client should be referred elsewhere. Otherwise, the counselor can combine permission giving with the next level of treatment, limited information.

The Second Level of Treatment: Limited Information

In contrast to permission giving—which basically is telling the client that it is all right to continue doing what he or she has been doing—*limited information* means giving the client specific factual information directly relevant to his or her sexual concern. This may result in clients continuing to do what they have been doing, or it may result in something different.

Limited information is usually given in conjunction with permission. Each may be used as a separate treatment level, but considerable overlap exists between the two.

Common areas of sexual concern.   Providing limited information is an excellent method for dispelling sexual myths, whether they are specific ones, such as those that pertain to genital size, or more general ones, such as that men and women differ markedly in their capacity to want and enjoy sexual relations and to respond to sexual stimulation. Other common sexual concerns are about breast and genital shape and size, masturbation, intercourse during menstruation, oral-genital activities, sexual frequency, and sexual performance.

A great deal of evidence indicates that men and women are far more similar than dissimilar to each other in their capacity for and experience of sexual desire, arousal, and orgasm. Numerous cross-cultural studies from fields such as anthropology and sociology consistently reveal that cultures that encourage women to be free in sexual expression produce sexually responsive women who are as uninhibited and responsive as males. Cultures that encourage and expect women to experience orgasm yield women who do experience orgasm.

Limitations.   The extent to which counselors are willing to use limited information in handling sexual concerns depends on their breadth of knowledge in the area. How counselors offer information to their clients depends on the individual style with which they feel most comfortable and the manner of presentation that they feel will be most helpful to their clients. With a conservative-appearing, middle-aged couple who hesitantly ask if anal contact is normal, the counselor might reply, "Such activity is not considered unusual or abnormal. In fact, a recent national survey of married persons under 35 indicated that half of them experienced manual anal foreplay." With a young couple who casually ask if germs can be transferred through oral genital contact, the counselor may respond, "Yes, it is possible. The mouth has a very high bacteria count."

Whatever their style, counselors now have two strategies for approaching sexual concerns. As with permission giving, the degree to which counselors feel comfortable with and are willing to use the second level also depends on their theoretical orientation and value system. The limitations imposed by the factors discussed in the first level of treatment apply here as well.

The addition of this level of treatment may resolve some concerns that could not be handled by application of the first level of treatment alone. If giving limited information is not sufficient to resolve the client's sexual concern, the counselor has two additional options. He or she may refer the client for treatment elsewhere or, with the appropriate setting, knowledge, skills, and experience, he or she may proceed to the third level of treatment, specific suggestions.

The Third Level of Treatment: Specific Suggestions

Before counselors can give specific suggestions to clients, counselors must first obtain specific information. The assumption here is that offering specific suggestions would not be therapeutically appropriate or helpful to the client without having first obtained information about the client and his or her unique set of circumstances. If the counselor were to immediately launch into a number of suggestions after hearing the client's initial *description* of the problem (not the "label" of the problem), the counselor may not only waste the client's time (such as by offering suggestions the client has already tried) but may also further compound the problem. By suggesting inappropriate and possibly useless treatment procedures based on insufficient data, the counselor may overlook other more necessary and appropriate treatment.

The sexual-problem history.   At this stage, we recommend that the counselor elicit a sexual-problem history. This is not to be confused with a

comprehensive learning-about-sex history. The model proposed here assumes that a comprehensive learning history may not be relevant or necessary for instituting effective brief therapy. Application of the specific-suggestion approach may resolve a number of problems that filtered through the first two levels of treatment but, needless to say, it is not expected to successfully dispense with all such problems. If the third level of approach is not helpful to the client, a complete sexual history may be a necessary first step toward intensive therapy.

Guidelines for taking a sexual-problem history, which is necessary for a brief therapy approach to treatment, are outlined below.

1. Description of current problem
2. Onset and course of problem
   a. Onset (gradual or sudden, precipitating events, consequences)
   b. Course (changes over time: increase, decrease, or fluctuation in severity, frequency, intensity; functional relationships with other variables)
3. Client's concept of cause and continuation of the problem
4. Past treatment and outcome
   a. Medical evaluation (specialty, date, form of treatment, results, current medication for any reason)
   b. Other professional help (specialty, date, form of treatment, results)
   c. Self-treatment (type and results)
5. Current expectations and goals of treatment (concrete versus general)

How such a history is taken has to be adapted to the counselor's setting and the amount of time available. The problem history is easily adapted to sessions of five minutes or of several hours. Making up a form with the sexual-problem history guidelines may be helpful. The counselor could use this as a general guide while interviewing or could write the client's responses directly on the form for future reference. Either way, the form may help the counselor become comfortable and experienced with the guidelines until they are memorized.

Self-recorded problem history.   During the past few years, considerable research has been done on the use of self-recorded (audiocassette) problem histories. In this method, the couple is requested, at the time of the first interview, to prepare a tape before the next visit. The purpose of doing so is explained to the client as follows:

• To describe the problem(s) for which the person(s) is seeking help.
• To describe the possible influences that relate to or have preceded the onset of the problem.

The counselor provides an introductory letter and a guideline that outlines a satisfactory method of tape preparation, and the client is asked to read them in the office. In the letter, the client is told: (1) that the tape is a means of describing the problem and its history, (2) that listening to the tape again after the therapy is over may help give the person a measure of self-growth and understanding, and (3) that preparation of the tape at home can save treatment hours and thus lessen expenses. (The client is also assured that the counselor

will maintain the material's confidentiality and will adhere to professional standards.) We have found that permitting the client a greater amount of responsibility for history taking may actually facilitate the therapeutic process.

Once the counselor feels comfortable in obtaining the problem history from the client in whatever fashion, he or she is ready to offer specific suggestions. In contrast to permission giving and limited information, which generally do not require that clients take any active steps to change their behavior unless they choose to, specific suggestions are direct attempts to help clients alter their behavior to reach their stated goals.

Most of the suggestions that may be given can be used by a counselor who has only 10 to 30 minutes for a client interview. Furthermore, they may be used when the counselor is able to see the client on only one or a few occasions at the most. Obviously, these are minimum time limits that may be expanded and adapted to the time available, but this level of approach is intended for use within the brief therapy framework proposed. If the suggestions are not perceived as potentially helpful within a relatively brief time period, intensive therapy is probably more appropriate.

As with the methods in the previous levels of treatment, specific suggestions may be seen as a preventive measure as well as a treatment technique. For example, suggesting specific ways to avoid pain associated with genital intercourse may prevent a woman from experiencing vaginismus—painful vaginal spasms. Or a direct treatment approach to ejaculation problems may prevent the eventual occurrence of a man's erection difficulties. This level of treatment may be combined easily and advantageously with the previous two levels.

Two common sayings are helpful when applying this third level of approach. One that is particularly beneficial for clients with concerns about a particular feature of their body is, "What you do with what you have, rather than what you have, is what counts!" The second has even broader applications. Many clients who have sexual concerns tend to see each forthcoming sexual event with their partner as the "final test." If the man once again ejaculates too soon or does not obtain an erection, he often feels as though he has lost his last chance. Similar concerns are reported by women in search of orgasms. Thoughts such as, "Will it happen this time?" or "It's got to happen this time or I'll just die!" are not conducive to success in attaining such goals. Helping the client learn to say and believe that "There is always another day (another time, another occasion)" can do a great deal to modify some of the self-defeating attitudes of many clients.

This level of treatment is particularly effective for dealing with heterosexual problems involving arousal, erection, ejaculation, orgasm, or painful intercourse. The specific suggestions offered (redirection of attention, sensate focus techniques*, interruption of stimulation, squeeze technique, vaginal muscle training, and so on) depend on the information obtained in the sexual-problem history. In general, suggestions fall into three categories: (1) suggestions to the male, (2) suggestions to the female, and (3) suggestions to the couple.

---

*Sensate focus techniques are described on p. 221 in "Common Sexual Dissatisfactions and Their Treatment."

Often, the counselor sees a client who has no immediate partner available. In such cases, a number of suggestions can be made for self-stimulation procedures. The counselor may encounter other situations in which a client is involved in a relationship with a person who has a problem but who is not able or willing to come in for consultation. Assuming that the second person is open to suggestions, the client can pass along whatever suggestions he or she feels might be appropriate under the circumstances.

The most helpful suggestions are usually those that can be made to both partners together. Clients should be encouraged to have their partners come in with them. When the couple comes in together and is willing to cooperate with the treatment suggestions, the probability that mutual goals will be realized is much greater. Working with one person on a problem that involves two is always more difficult.

Limitations.   Efficient use of this treatment level depends largely on the counselor's breadth of knowledge, skill and experience, and awareness of relevant therapeutic suggestions. The limitations discussed under the other treatment levels apply here as well. For interested readers, Annon (1974) provides a detailed description of the application of suggestions to the more prevalent heterosexual problems encountered by males and females.

Readings.   Counselors might suggest that clients read material related to their concern. The counselor may use these reading materials as another means of providing permission or limited information about a certain sexual area or client concern. Readings may be used to supplement specific suggestions or promote new client-initiated procedures. Because of time limitations on either the counselor's or the client's part, the counselor may suggest readings in lieu of other specific suggestions. The counselor, of course, should not suggest any readings to clients unless he or she is well acquainted with the content and feels comfortable recommending them. Helpful materials for both clients and counselors include *The Last Sex Manual* (Pion & Hopkins, 1978), *For Each Other* (Barbach, 1982), *Falling In Love Again* (Barbach, 1990), *Taking Time for Love* (Dinkmeyer & Carlson, 1989), *Super Marital Sex* (Pearsall, 1987), and *Sexual Happiness* (Yaffe & Fenwick, 1988).

This third level of approach concludes the presentation of the brief therapy approach of the P-LI-SS-IT model. A number of sexual concerns may be treated successfully through such an approach. Those that cannot be resolved will filter through, at which point the counselor may refer the client for appropriate treatment elsewhere. If the counselor has the requisite time, knowledge, experience, and skills, he or she may proceed to the fourth level of treatment, intensive therapy.

The Fourth Level of Treatment: Intensive Therapy
We will not describe or attempt to outline the intensive-therapy approach to the treatment of persisting sexual problems. But, for the counselor who has already received training for intensive therapy, this is the appropriate time to initiate such treatment.

We believe that involving a client in an expensive, long-term treatment program without first trying to resolve the problem from within a brief therapy approach may be unethical. A number of sexual concerns may be treated successfully by such an approach if counselors are willing to apply it. Specific suggestions that may work for one client will not always be effective with another. Sometimes, interpersonal conflicts may prevent the suggestions from being carried through. When this happens, and when counselors believe they have done as much as they can from within the brief therapy approach, the time has come for highly individualized therapy.

In the model proposed here, intensive therapy does not mean an extended standardized program of treatment. By their nature, standardized programs are not of help to some people, and they may not be necessary. But many of the essential elements of some of the current standardized programs can be successfully utilized within a brief therapy approach.

In the P-LI-SS-IT model, intensive therapy is seen as a highly individualized treatment that is necessary because standardized treatment was not successful in helping the client reach his or her goals. Within the present framework, intensive therapy means undertaking a careful initial assessment of the client's unique situation to devise a therapeutic program that is unique to the individual involved.

Common Sexual Dissatisfactions and Their Treatment

There are a number of complaints about sexuality that counselors hear over and over again. These include inability to communicate about sexual likes and dislikes, lack of skill in initiating sexual activity, disagreements about the extent of foreplay or nonsexual expression of physical affection, discrepancies in the partners' desires to experiment with new sexual activities, boredom with the sexual relationship, inability to find time for sex, or differing preferences for the location or times of day for sexual activity (Schover, 1982). Each of these dissatisfactions will be discussed and treatment techniques suggested.

Difficulty with sexual communication.   "My partner and I just don't talk about sex. In our entire marriage, we've seldom said anything about it. I think I know what she likes, because after fifteen years with someone, you really get to know them; but I'm not always sure if she's turned on, and I don't know if she has orgasms. She says she does. If I want something to happen during sex, I usually just wait and see if she does it. I wouldn't know how to ask for it, as we would both be embarrassed."

This is a common story, even today when sexual freedom and performance are constantly touted. The first problem is in making sure that both partners wish to change their sexual communication. To focus on what each could gain, counselors will find it helpful to ask both partners to write down the three things they would most like to change about their own sexual behavior and the three things they would most like to change in their partner's behavior. Many clients will just write down "nothing." In that case, the counselor might explain that the goals should be small and specific. Examples might be given, such as "saying something romantic to me during intercourse," "spending more time touching my penis," or "being able to ask him to bring me to orgasm after

intercourse." These goals can later be shared with the partner as part of the communication training exercises.

If the clients have difficulty with using sexual terms, a desensitization exercise may be useful. In one session, each partner is asked to provide as many synonyms as possible for the words *penis, vagina, clitoris,* and *intercourse.* The counselor keeps a written list for each word and may model relaxed use of sexual terms by adding some slang words. Further discussion can focus on the humorous aspects of sex, any feelings of shame about the genitals, or the words that feel most comfortable to each partner and in different situations (such as in discussing sex with the counselor and in talking to each other at home).

Another in-session technique is couple-communication training (Jacobson & Margolin, 1979; Stuart, 1980; Dinkmeyer & Carlson, 1989). Partners are taught to present their points of view in the form of an "I" message such as, "When you do X, I feel Y." The other partner accurately reflects the message given and then has the opportunity to respond in the same mode. The couple is taught to ask for things that are specific ("I would like you to stroke my back gently" as opposed to "Why don't you touch me?"), positive ("I like it better when you use a harder grip on my penis" instead of "Stop touching me so lightly. It tickles!") and focused in the present ("I would like to take more time in foreplay tonight" rather than "You never give me a chance to get turned on! I don't think we've spent more than two minutes in foreplay during the last five years.") The couple begins by using these techniques to discuss a sexual topic that is not a point of conflict. The partners can then proceed to communicate about their goals for sexual behavior change. After they have had successful communications within a session, they can be assigned to have a discussion at home, which they can audiotape for the counselor.

Other homework assignments include using sensate focus exercises and gradually building in immediate feedback. Complete instructions for sensate focus may be found in Kaplan (1975) or Dinkmeyer and Carlson (1989). In the most basic version, the couple is requested to take turns being the giver and receiver of nongenital body caresses. The task of the giver is to focus on his or her own sensations as the partner's body is touched for a set period of time. The receiver also focuses on his or her own body rather than worrying about the giver's feelings. At this stage, there is no verbal or nonverbal feedback during the touching, unless the stimulation is painful. After being the receiver, each client should tell the partner the three touches they liked the best and the one kind of caress they liked the least. This feedback should specify the part of the body and the type of touch.

The next task is for the receiver to give immediate positive feedback. Again, comments should be specific. If one partner does not enjoy a caress as the receiver, the partner should ask for something that he or she liked better rather than just requesting that the giver stop the stimulation.

These steps are then repeated with the breasts and genitals also caressed. The couple is cautioned not to focus exclusively on the genitals, now that they are allowed to touch them. Some nonverbal communication techniques may also be demonstrated, such as guiding the giver's hand.

Lack of skill in initiating sexual activity. "My wife never initiates sex. It's always my job. I get tired of always being the aggressive one. It makes me wonder whether she really likes sex, even though she seems to enjoy it. It would turn me on if she let me know she was in the mood once in a while."

"He just doesn't know how to get me ready for sex. He always seems to wait until I'm busy with something else, and then he just comes up behind me and grabs me. Then he's hurt if I don't respond right away. Or else he just turns around and says, 'Let's go to bed.' "

Many clients have difficulty initiating sex or doing so in a way that evokes a positive response in their partners. Often, the place to begin treatment is with a discussion of how clients express their wishes for sex and how they know when their mates are likely to be responsive. Many clients have never identified their own sexual signals. One spouse may also have no idea how to tell whether his or her partner is feeling sexually receptive. If a wife often goes up to bed with the expectation that her husband will follow her upstairs to make love but he watches TV until midnight, it is not surprising that her frustration and anger will build up. The first step is for the couple to recognize each other's signals. The next step is to build some pleasurable strategies for sexual initiation into the couple's interaction.

Each partner should offer some suggestions in the counseling session on ways that the other partner can initiate sex. The counselor can also offer some strategies that have been successfully used by other couples, such as giving a kiss and a whisper in the ear, having dinner by candlelight, or wearing sexy apparel. Schover (1982) has given the following assignment:

> This week I would like each of you to practice initiating sex at least three times. That doesn't mean I want you to have sex six times. I just want you to think of some different ways to ask your partner for sexual activity, and to carry them out. Probably this will not lead up to having sex on most of the occasions. I want you to try something different each time you initiate, including some things that usually might make you feel silly, or embarrassed. The partner's task is to write down afterwards how you felt when your mate initiated. Say a little about the things you did and did not like about the approach (p. 61).

This assignment often brings out conflict about being assertive, both in asking for what the partner would like and in refusing the mate's requests. An assignment that Zilbergeld (1978) calls "Yes's and No's" can help the couple explore these issues further. Each partner is asked to make three requests during the week for something he or she would like but usually would not demand. In addition, each is asked to say "no" three times to something he or she does not want to do but would usually agree to do. If the couple's difficulty in assertion is mainly in the sexual area, the yes's and no's can be restricted to sexual situations. The important task for the therapist when discussing the results of these assignments is to reinforce new positive behaviors and help clients become aware of self-statements and feelings that prevent them from being assertive.

Disagreements about foreplay and nonsexual physical affection. Unlike difficulties with communication or initiation, which are seen

equally often in men and women, disagreements about the length of foreplay and the amount of nonsexual touching and cuddling in a relationship are often (but not always) gender-specific. The typical pattern is:

She: "He never really gives me time to warm up for intercourse. All he wants to do is kiss me once or twice, and maybe feel my breasts, and then he's ready. It's frustrating, because I want more touching, and more tenderness. He never even likes to sit with his arm around me in the evening. He only touches me when he wants sex."

He: "She just wants to hang on me all the time. I'm tired when I get home from work and I don't feel like hugging and kissing. I just want to read the paper after dinner. And I suppose I should spend more time on foreplay, but I get impatient for the real thing. Anyway, I'm afraid I would just come too fast if we spent more time touching first."

Munjack and Oziel (1980) provide a practical outline for counseling clients on increasing foreplay. They suggest educating the couple in the woman's slower time to arousal and in her need for more genital stimulation while limiting genital stimulation during foreplay for the man. The man can also be taught simple methods of delaying ejaculation (Zilbergeld, 1978).

In addition, some exploration of each partner's subjective experience during nonsexual and sexual touching should be undertaken. What is perceived as relaxed tenderness to one person may seem overwhelming and intrusive to the other. The counselor may find it helpful to assign 15 minutes of kissing and cuddling, with each partner asked to examine what personal thoughts occur during the experience. Then, new self-talk may replace the less productive messages. For example, a husband who finds himself thinking, "Ugh, I feel smothered. I wish I could go watch the football game," might be asked to focus on his wife's soft skin or to ask her to rub his back instead of kissing him passionately. Or he may be asked to say to himself, "I can stop this stimulation any time I wish, so I might as well try it a little longer and see if there is any part of it that I enjoy."

Again, sensate focus exercises can be a useful way for the couple to try new kinds of nongenital stimulation. The structure provided by the counselor can short-circuit arguments about how much touching is enough. The counselor might also assign kissing, hugging, and genital and nongenital touching, for a maximum of 15 minutes, outside the bedroom with some clothes on and with the stipulation that the activity will not lead to intercourse. This may help the couple rediscover some of the excitement felt while dating. This exercise also combats the stereotype that all sexual activity must be an elaborate routine of foreplay that ends in intercourse and orgasm for both partners. Another useful technique is to assign a "quickie"—a sexual session in which only a minimal amount of preparation and foreplay is included. The couple's task is to see how quickly each can get in the mood for intercourse. The ultimate goal is flexibility in choosing to have a romantic atmosphere or take all evening for sex some-times and to enjoy each other in an uncomplicated way at other times.

In this same vein, the partner who is pushing for more physical affection and/or foreplay may be asked whether there are nonsexual activities that would

serve as a substitute for these ways of demonstrating caring. Sometimes, either setting aside 15 to 30 minutes in an evening just to talk or going out on a "date" together may fulfill cravings for attention and contact that were perceived as sexual frustration.

Disagreements about the variety of sexual activities.

"We just do the same thing each time we have sex. We kiss for a few minutes, touch each other in the usual places, and then go on and start intercourse, either with him on top or with me on top. I tried to get him to read some books about sex or go to an X-rated movie, but he says he's satisfied with things the way they are. Sex is OK, but I want it to be more like what I read about."

A wish for more sexual variety can arise from a number of issues. One partner may be somewhat depressed or feel unstimulated in the nonsexual areas of life and seek diversion in the bedroom. There may be unrealistic expectations for sexual pleasure, fed by media myths. Other clients may have cherished certain sexual fantasies for many years and finally have gotten up the nerve to ask their spouses to try them out. Often, however, the sexual routine has really become rigid and boring, so that the sense of playfulness and exploration has disappeared.

When one partner wishes to try a particular sexual activity that the other finds distasteful, the counselor has a dilemma. As Munjack and Oziel (1980) point out, no one should be forced (or even coaxed) into an activity that is personally unpleasant or painful. Often the reluctance to be involved is for other relationship reasons, and the counselor can help the couple discover what the real issue is. When the desired behavior is something that one partner is ambivalent about trying, however, the partner should first identify what he or she finds negative about it.

Another area for therapeutic exploration is the couple's subjective emotional experience during sexual activity. If one or both partners are feeling bored or constrained, building in some playfulness may provide relief. The partners could be assigned to do some physical activity of their choice that would put them in a playful mood before having sex (such as taking a shower together, wrestling, tickling, or having a pillow fight) or to play at taking certain roles during sex (such as being very shy and innocent or very seductive).

Sometimes, verbally sharing a sexual fantasy with a partner may increase arousal and can substitute for activities that could have a negative impact on a relationship (such as joining a mate-swapping club or trying something that one partner finds frightening). Clients who have difficulty fantasizing may be encouraged to read anthologies of fantasies, such as *My Secret Garden: Women's Sexual Fantasies* (Friday, 1973), or the columns in such magazines as *Penthouse*. The counselor may ask each person to write his or her own sexual fantasy and then allow the partner to read it. If both partners feel comfortable with these activities, they may try telling fantasies to one another before or during sexual activity.

Disagreements about the frequency of sexual activity.

"We don't get enough sex. Our lives are so busy with work and the kids. I also think my

partner is happy with sex once a week or once every two weeks, but I'd like it more often."

Sometimes, neither partner in a couple has a real lack of sexual desire, but both disagree about the frequency for sexual activity. Zilbergeld and Ellison (1980) provide a cogent discussion of the causes of this situation and some good treatment suggestions. They point out that sex counselors have been biased in trying to increase the desire of the partner who wants sex less often rather than suggesting that the more lusty client examine the reasons for wanting sex so frequently. As was mentioned before, sometimes sexual desire may mask a longing for more affection or time shared with the partner. One assignment that may help increase nonsexual expression of affection is "Encouraging Days" (Dinkmeyer & Carlson, 1989). Both partners identify small ways that their mates can express caring, and then they are asked to increase their rates of the desired behaviors.

When it does seem important to increase a couple's frequency of sexual activity, there are exercises that aid clients in discovering what brings on a sexual mood. One exercise is having clients keep a daily "desire diary," in which is recorded all sexual feelings and thoughts, where they occurred, who was present, and what the other person's reaction was. Another exercise is to have clients list as many things as they can that make them feel more sexual. The list can include physical activities, such as playing sports, dancing, dressing certain ways, looking at erotic materials, and so on. Clients are then assigned to try several of these activities during the week. Once the clients realize which situations elicit a sexual mood, they can use their knowledge to create arousal when their partners are available.

Many couples complain that they cannot find the time for sex. Sometimes, this complaint generalizes into a situation in which the only time spent together is taken up with household tasks or child care. When asked to set aside an evening to go out on a "date" together, such a couple may insist that it is impossible to take the time off from errands or to afford a babysitter. Sometimes counseling needs to focus on a reassessment of priorities, including how the clients' current emotional distance affects the future of their relationship. Realistically, some couples may have to choose between having the added income from extra jobs and having enough time to be alone with each other. Couples with children may need to consider getting some child care or letting the children know that the parents need private time.

Other couples complain that they cannot agree on a time of day for sex. One is a "night person" and the other is a "morning person." Often, their sexual moods correspond to their periods of high energy. Some discussion and eventual compromise is needed.

Finally, some couples disagree about the location for sex. One person feels most comfortable in bed, whereas the other enjoys having sexual encounters on the living room rug, in the bathtub, and or in the backyard. The couple may need to deal realistically with one partner's concern about being "caught in the act" by children or neighbors. The couple may also need to make the environment comfortable for both partners, perhaps by putting big cushions in front of the fireplace or by having curtains around the porch.

Differences in sexual desire.   A common complaint in relationships is that one partner wants sex more often than the other does. Many people are able to reach some kind of compromise and make a satisfactory sexual adjustment. For others, however, the differences in desire continue to be a troublesome aspect of their relationship that can often lead to other distresses. It is practically impossible to state what "normal" desire is. We each have different appetites for sex, just as we do for food. Individuals have different needs for intimacy and for romance as well as for sexual contact. Differences in sexual desire can sometimes be so serious that anger and resentment carry over into other areas of a couple's life (Friedman, 1984).

For many couples, the early stage of a relationship contains sexual novelty and discovery. Once the "honeymoon" period comes to an end, couples are forced to confront each other on a wide variety of issues. The novelty of the relationship wears off, and people discover in each other imperfections and annoying habits and attitudes. The media—particularly television and men's and women's magazines—tend to present relationships in an extremely unrealistic manner. Conflict is rarely seen in any form that is comparable to people's personal experiences, and it is easy to become disappointed and unhappy when problems occur for which there is no effective resolution. It is not surprising that disappointment, disillusionment, and unhappiness often translate into a lack of desire for sex with one's partner. Imbalance of power in a relationship can also have a negative influence on sexual functioning. If one partner has all the power or makes all the decisions, the other partner may feel that the only power he or she has is to not want sex. One of the biggest stumbling blocks to a close sexual relationship is a lack of trust. People have to be willing to become vulnerable with one another to enjoy sex together.

For other individuals, low desire has nothing to do with the partner in particular but is just a general state. Perhaps the individual has had some negative experiences or has been brought up to believe that sex or pleasure in general is wrong. Others who just have a lower appetite for sex are perfectly happy when they do have sex, they just do not want it very often. Although this is not a problem for them, it may become a problem for their partner.

Sexual desire and health.   Although your sexual desire may have nothing at all to do with the state of your health, there are some cases in which health does affect sexual desire. Particularly, if your level of desire has dropped off after a period of higher desire and you cannot attribute this to any significant changes in your life, you should consider a full physical check-up to determine whether the change in desire is due to physical factors. Some health conditions and some medications have a detrimental effect on sexual desire. Depression can also cause a drop in desire, as can extreme fatigue or tension. Endocrinological problems, such as changes in the flow of particular hormones, can also affect sexual desire. It is important to inform a medical doctor about the change in desire so that the possibility of medical causes can be examined.

Suggestions for the partner with a higher level of desire.   The suggestions and questions presented in this section are *not* meant to imply that

one partner is at fault for his or her partner's more infrequent desire for sex. It is important for both partners to cooperate in finding ways to make the overall and sexual relationship more comfortable and enjoyable. Some people are able to leave their individual and relationship problems outside the bedroom door, whereas others find it difficult or impossible to want and enjoy sex if things are not going well in other aspects of their lives. Some people can use sex to make up after a fight; others can only enjoy sex if they are feeling good about themselves and about their partner.

Counselors often find it important to help the couple carefully choose the times to initiate sex. If either partner is excessively tired or rushed, it is difficult for sex to be a relaxed and enjoyable experience. It is important to make time to be together for other activities—as well as for sex—and for the sexual time to be relaxed, warm, romantic, and intimate. Couples might consider preparing for sex by putting on some soft music, lighting candles, or making some other romantic gesture that will indicate that they are thinking about and planning time together.

Communication during sex is also extremely important. It is important that the partners communicate what each likes and what feels good. When sex is placed within the context of a romantic setting, is leisurely, and has some imagination and variety associated with it, it often becomes more enjoyable for both partners.

If one partner has a lot of worries and stresses in other areas of life, he or she often finds it difficult to take time to relax and enjoy sex. The other partner can help by providing an environment that is calm and relaxing and letting his or her partner know that time together can be a haven from the stresses of everyday life. Finally, if the relationship is generally poor, if the two cannot communicate, and if they frequently argue and disagree about important issues, it may be necessary to alleviate some of these problems before the partners can become confident and relaxed enough to be sexual.

Suggestions for the partner with a lower level of desire.   Again, the suggestions here do *not* imply that there is anything wrong with an individual because he or she has less sexual desire than his or her partner. However, these suggestions may be helpful if the partners would like to resolve their different needs, have sex more frequently, or increase their desire. An important first step is to spend some time thinking about how they really feel about sex in general and about sex with their partner in particular. Is sex a neutral experience that they can take or leave, or is it something that they find aversive?

If most of one's difficulties are partner-specific, then the focus needs to be on making sex better and more enjoyable with the partner. Communication is the key to any good relationship in general and to good sex in particular. It is important for partners to tell what they want, what they would like, and what would make sex more relaxing and more enjoyable for them. Sex is a lot more than intercourse and orgasm, and if partners can communicate and share other sexual activities and other ways of being intimate, they may find their desire increasing. It is important for couples to be assertive but to not use sex as a way

of expressing anger. People need to learn to express feelings directly to their partner. If partners have difficulty trusting and being intimate with one another, they need to develop ways of increasing trust and intimacy. They need to ask what they want sexually. If both partners would like to be better lovers, they must give each other feedback on what feels good and what is most arousing. It is important to focus on the positive rather than on the negative when engaging in sexual activity. It is easy to focus on the unattractive aspects of one's partner, but this focus can be redirected. For example, rather than focusing on the "roll of fat around the waist," focus instead on "beautiful blue eyes." The choice of focus helps to determine each partner's sexual desire.

Some people find that their desire is low in general and not directly related to sex with their partner. There are several questions that can be used to help explore the role of sex in their life. For example:

"Are you under a good deal of stress?"

"Are you willing and able to take time for yourself and look toward your own needs and pleasures?"

"Are there things in your life that are making you feel depressed?"

"When you do engage in sexual activity, do you enjoy it and wonder why you do not pursue it more often but then find yourself reluctant to initiate or accept your partner's initiation?"

Life stress and depression are frequently incompatible with sexual desire and often explain why one partner's desire is lower than the other's.

Taking time for oneself and for one's own pleasure is an important component in the enjoyment of sexual activity. Sometimes, "old messages" intrude and keep people from enjoying their own sexuality. For example, if one partner learned that sex was wrong, dirty, or immoral when he or she was young, it may be difficult for the individual to give up the feelings associated with those messages, even though those beliefs are no longer held. Reminding oneself that those "old messages" need not currently influence one's life can often have a strong impact on changing sexual desire. Sex should be fun and not a chore. Counselors should try to help give the couple permission to have fun and to play, so that the couple can then start treating sex as a playful activity. This focus on play often makes a significant difference in treating clients with low desire.

What both partners can do.   It is unfair to assume that the partner with lower desire has to make all the changes in the relationship. Compromise, with both partners making changes, is necessary to make any relationship work. Frequently, it seems that the partner with higher desire wants sex all the time. However, in many cases, if sex occurred more frequently, the partner with higher desire would lower the number of requests. The actual frequency of sex will determine who has to make the most changes. Clearly, if one partner wants sex once a week and the other wants it every day, it should be possible to compromise on two or three times per week. However, if one partner wants sex once a week and the other partner wants it once a year, compromise may be more difficult.

Working together, both partners can increase their communication and try to resolve other issues in their relationship so that sexual activity is not used to act out their power struggles, control conflicts, and anger. Frequently, who initiates sex and how sex is initiated and refused are issues for many couples. If one partner tends to turn down sex because of the way it is initiated, it is important for the partner to say so. However, when refusing an invitation for sex, the individual needs to let the partner know that it is not a rejection of him or her but simply a statement about how the partner is feeling at the time. By making another date for sexual activity or making a point to initiate sex at some later time, the refusing partner can help prevent feelings of anger and frustration in the other partner. Communication and compromise can go a long way toward improving a couple's sexual relationship. It is important that both partners learn to focus on what *they* can do to make things better, rather than on what their partner should do.

Sometimes sexual desire disappears because of other issues in the relationship. For example, if there is conflict over having or not having children or over who is responsible for contraception, sexual desire may decrease. Again, if these issues can be discussed openly and a compromise reached, sexual desire may return.

Psychosexual Disorders and Their Treatment

Male Sexual Dysfunction

There are three main types of male sexual dysfunction: erectile dysfunction, premature ejaculation, and retarded ejaculation.

Erectile dysfunction.   The term *erectile dysfunction* refers to the on-going inability of a male to have or maintain an erection throughout intercourse. This dysfunction may be primary or secondary. In primary dysfunction, the man has never been able to sustain an erection long enough to complete intercourse. Secondary erectile dysfunction, also known as impotence, applies to the man who enjoyed the ability to gain and sustain an erection for intercourse before but is currently experiencing difficulties.

McCarthy and Perkins (1988) suggest an eclectic therapeutic approach to secondary erectile dysfunction. Techniques such as stop/slash intromission (described in the section on retarded ejaculation) and sensate focus have been successfully employed (Brown & Field, 1988). Counseling can help the individual overcome the underlying dynamics of secondary sexual dysfunction.

Premature ejaculation.   Another common male sexual dysfunction is premature ejaculation. Two variations of this dysfunction have been observed. If the man reaches an orgasm and loses his erection before inserting his penis into the vagina, this is known as "too early orgasm." If the man can achieve vaginal penetration but experiences orgasm very quickly or significantly earlier than his partner climaxes, this is known as "too quick orgasm."

It is important to note that there is a subcategory called situational pre-

mature ejaculation, which is temporary and can occur for a variety of reasons. For example, if a man is enjoying sexual experience after a long period of abstinence, he may ejaculate too quickly. These types of situations are to be placed in a separate category from the individual who has continuous problems with premature ejaculations. Although disquieting, these experiences are normal and occur with relative frequency for all males (Kaplan, 1979).

Retarded ejaculation.   The third type of male sexual dysfunction is *retarded ejaculation*, and it is relatively uncommon. Although the male is able to reach orgasm through masturbation, he is unable to climax through any form of vaginal stimulation. Some researchers, such as Kaplan (1979) and Newcomb and Bentler (1988), take issue with the whole concept of retarded ejaculation. They argue that if a man is able to achieve orgasm through a form of stimulation other than vaginal, then the only dysfunction that exists is psychodynamic.

Much has been written about the remediation of male sexual dysfunction by Masters and Johnson (1970). Their literature on the effectiveness of the "squeeze technique" is widely written about. Other methods in the treatment of male sexual dysfunction have made a concerted effort to include the partner in the treatment plan; the most popular current form is the stop/slash technique. When the man is about to reach orgasm, his partner stops stimulation. As soon as the urge to ejaculate subsides, the man and his partner continue stimulation. This technique enjoys wide approval from counselors because it focuses on the couple instead of treating the man as an instrument to be acted upon. McCarthy and Perkins (1988) also suggest that couples are more receptive to this intervention than to others because of the role of the woman as an active agent of change. This heightens the sense of unity within the couple and prevents the focus from being placed on the male as the identified "patient." Another common and effective behavioral technique is to prohibit intercourse and substitute touching exercises. This technique allows the partners to learn to listen to their bodies and get in touch with what feels pleasurable to them (Dinkmeyer & Carlson, 1989). Since many men are apt to move toward intercourse shortly after gaining an erection, this series of nondemand exercises allows the man to experience a wider range of sensation and arousal patterns. Sensate focus also enjoys a high degree of use as a relaxation technique.

Female Sexual Dysfunction

There are three main sexual dysfunctions that are present in women: dyspareunia, orgasmic dysfunction, and vaginal spasms.

Dyspareunia.   Painful intercourse, or *dyspareunia*, occurs during the arousal phase. The lack of vaginal lubrication or the presence of vaginal infection are the predisposing factors. Although painful intercourse can be experienced by men, it is much more common for women. The most common antecedent for women is insufficient vaginal lubrication. Many times, this dysfunction is further complicated by the inability of the woman to articulate specifically what she wants sexually. This communication problem can be

explored through counseling. Psychoeducation, along with assertiveness training, can also be valuable for helping the woman learn to express her needs.

Orgasmic dysfunction.   Primary *orgasmic dysfunction* occurs when a woman has never experienced orgasm, as opposed to secondary anorgasmia, in which the woman previously was orgasmic but currently is experiencing difficulties. Women who masturbate to orgasm but are unable to achieve orgasm through a partner's stimulation fall into this category. Another category of female orgasmic dysfunction is classified as random. This describes women who experience orgasm but only on an occasional basis. For the purposes of remediation, anorgasmia and dyspareunia share some common elements.

Practical suggestions are that the couple practice touching exercises and abstain from intercourse for a predetermined amount of time. This in and of itself may allow the woman to relax and lubricate sufficiently. Other techniques include additional stimulation of the genital area. Oral stimulation paired with manual stimulation can be an effective arousal technique (Kaplan, 1979). The point of this intervention is that the partners are to experiment and discover what works for them.

It is essential that counselors be aware of sexual stereotypes. Often, the importance of the female orgasm is diminished as unnecessary to female fulfillment (Masters & Johnson, 1970). Masters and Johnson's (1970) data indicated that what women really wanted from sex was closeness and love. What counselors now see is that women want those things plus an orgasm (McCarthy & Perkins, 1988).

Vaginal spasms.   Clinically known as vaginismus, *vaginal spasms* are the spastic contractions that prevent the insertion of the penis into the vagina. This dysfunction is quite rare, occurring in approximately one-quarter of one percent of the population. But another associated problem, functional vaginismus, occurs with greater frequency. The difference is that "true" vaginismus actually prevents the intromission of the penis, whereas lesser versions of vaginismus create extreme discomfort but do allow penetration to occur.

Treatment for vaginismus is similar to the desensitization process used in phobias (Masters & Johnson, 1970). The woman is first led through guided imagery activities, whereby she learns to relax when envisioning intercourse. Then the counselor suggests a series of exercises to be implemented at home, either alone or with a spouse. The woman or her partner insert into her vagina first one finger and then two fingers, gradually increasing the dilation of the vaginal muscles. This exercise then proceeds to the insertion of a vibrator until the vaginal muscles are sufficiently relaxed to accommodate the man's penis.

An important consideration in the treatment process is the possible interplay of emotional factors. Earlier traumatic experiences such as rape or incest may have led to the symptom cluster known as vaginismus. Sprei and Courtois (1988) indicate that in the case of early trauma, intensive counseling is indicated to dissipate the factors that precipitated the vaginismus. Behavioral interventions only alleviate the symptoms. Another possible contributory feature is the in-

dividual's faulty sexual beliefs and attitudes. The best course for remediation of misconceptions is psychoeducation, through which the counselor is able to help the client both identify and explore faulty beliefs.

Treatment Adherence and Relapse Prevention

Treatment adherence can be increased when counselors use brief therapy that employs the use of contracts. Masters and Johnson (1970) utilize a brief, intensive therapeutic model that includes a contract stipulating that the couple will be seen every day for two weeks, at which point the treatment ends. The contract enforces the notion that the couple and not the counselor is responsible for the couple's continuing growth toward sexual health. Self-responsibility is an important and often underutilized component of therapy. Self-responsibility has been emphasized throughout this book and is at the heart of effective sexual therapy.

The essential components of relapse prevention and treatment adherence are part of the therapeutic process. Effective psychoeducation may be one of the best strategies to prevent relapse. Current research is considering the most effective forms of psychoeducation that can be utilized (McCarthy & Perkins, 1988). We have found that the utilization of sexual intimacy activities, such as those in Dinkmeyer and Carlson's *Taking Time for Love* (1989), is helpful.

Activity #1: Be informed. In this exercise, couples read books and watch films together.

Activity #2: Touch. Couples are taught how to use intimate focus, a technique very similar to sensate focus.

Activity #3: Learn to pay attention to your sex life.

Activity #4: Make time for sex.

Activity #5: Continue to court each other.

Activity #6: Fantasize.

Activity #7: Learn how to say yes or no to sexual activity.

Activity #8: Avoid falling into rigid or boring routines.

Activity #9: Learn to give positive feedback.

Activity #10: Feel fit and sexy.

Activity #11: Take responsibility for your own sexual pleasure.

Summary

This chapter described brief strategies that apply a biopsychosocial understanding to the creation of sexual health. The extent of sexual problems is widespread and, unfortunately, counselors are often unprepared (or uncomfortable) working in this area. Through the counselor's use of the P-LI-SS-IT model with psychoeducational supplements, many concerns can be alleviated.

Resources

Treatment

It is often difficult to locate a counselor, and it may seem to be an overwhelming task. In most states, anyone can hang out a shingle that says "therapist" and can advertise and begin counseling. It is important to be sure that a professional counselor who has training in sexual counseling is consulted. It might be helpful to contact the appropriate certifying organization for each of the various professions. Marriage and family therapists are clinically certified by the American Association of Marriage and Family Therapy (AAMFT, 1717 K Street, NW, Room 407, Washington, DC 20006). Social workers are certified by the National Association of Social Workers (NASW, 7981 Eastern Avenue, Silver Springs, MD 20910). Psychologists are members of the American Psychological Association (APA, 1200 17th Street, NW, Washington, DC 20036). Sex therapists are certified by the American Association of Sex Educators, Counselors, and Therapists (AASECT, 435 North Michigan Avenue, Suite 1717, Chicago, IL 60611-4067), as well as by the American Board of Sexology (2113 S Street, NW, Washington, DC 20008). The American Psychiatric Association (1700 13th Street, NW, Washington, DC 20009) certifies psychiatrists. Professional counselors are certified by the American Counseling Association (ACA, 5999 Stevenson Avenue, Alexandria, VA 22304). These organizations are good sources of referrals to counselors in your area. If you cannot locate a local chapter, write to the national headquarters and ask for the name of a qualified person in your area.

One thing to consider when referring the client to a treatment facility is its location. Although Masters and Johnson are well regarded, they are not easily accessible to everyone. The easiest and most reliable way to refer a client is to consult the nearest major medical center in your location. The chances are excellent that if they do not have a sexual treatment program, they will know how to link you up with one.

Here is a partial list of the facilities that offer treatment within the continental United States.

- *Johns Hopkins University, Sexual Disorders Clinic, Meyer Building, Room 101, 600 North Wolfe Street, Baltimore, MD 21205: Fred S. Berlin, M.D., Director.* This clinic offers treatment of sexual dysfunctions as well as a comprehensive program for sex offenders. Johns Hopkins also participates in ongoing research on the effects of medications on sexual behavior.
- *Kinsey Institute for Sex Research in Sex, Gender, and Reproduction, 313 Morrison Hall, Bloomington, IN 47405: June Reinisch, M.D., Director.* The Kinsey Institute always has ongoing research of gender-based differences in attitudes to sexuality as well as beliefs and attitudes. Although the clinic currently does not offer direct treatment as one of its services, the Kinsey Institute is an excellent referral service for those based in the heartland of the United States.
- *Masters & Johnson Institute, 24 South Kings Highway, St. Louis, MO 63108: Virginia Johnson Masters, Director.* The clinic offers both direct service (which it is well noted for), as well as an excellent research facility. The direct service

component is an intensive two-week program that employs behavioral techniques aimed at remediation of the dysfunction within the brief time-limited program.

Publications

- Barbach, L. (1990). *Falling in Love Again.* Los Angeles: Venus Group. This is a multimedia program that helps couples who have sexual problems. The kit consists of an hour-and-a-half videotape, a pair of identical manuals—one for each partner—and two audiocassettes. The program is designed for couples who are having common problems.
- Barbach, L. (1976). *For Yourself: The Fulfillment of Female Sexuality.* New York: Anchor Press/Doubleday. This book made a significant contribution by giving women permission to enjoy their sexuality. Although dated, this book remains an important contribution to women's understanding of their own sexuality.
- Comfort, A. (1988). *The Joy of Sex.* New York: Pocket Books. This book is designed to help couples alleviate the boredom in their sexual experiences. Replete with a smorgasbord of new positions for intercourse, this book is much more than a "how to" book; it celebrates the overall experience of our sexuality.
- Dinkmeyer, D., & Carlson, J. (1989). *Taking Time for Love: How to Stay Happily Married.* Englewood Cliffs, NJ: Prentice-Hall. This book is a solid resource guide for those who wish to enrich their marriage with their partners. Written by two psychologists, this book will show you how to enrich your relationship in just a few short minutes a day.
- Pearsall, P. (1989). *Super Marital Sex.* New York: Doubleday. This book is also much more than a guide to sex; it is a guide to attaining satisfaction in the overall relationship of the couple.
- Ortiz, E. T. (1989). *Your Complete Guide to Sexual Health.* Englewood Cliffs, NJ: Prentice-Hall. This book is designed for Planned Parenthood of San Diego and Riverside Counties and provides a complete guide to reproductive health. High school and college students will find this book useful, as it provides practical information on sex and birth control.
- Yaffe, M., & Fenwick, E. (1988). *Sexual Happiness: A Practical Approach.* New York: Henry Holt. A thorough guidebook on how to achieve and maintain sexual happiness.

References

ANNON, J. S. (1973). The therapeutic use of masturbation in the treatment of sexual disorders. *Advances in Behavior Therapy, Vol. 4* (pp. 199–215). New York: Academic Press.

ANNON, J. S. (1974). *The behavioral treatment of sexual problems. Vol. 1: Brief therapy.* Honolulu, HI: Enabling Systems, Inc.

ANNON, J. S. (1975). *The behavioral treatment of sexual problems. Vol. 2: Intensive therapy.* Honolulu, HI: Enabling Systems, Inc.

BARBACH, L. (1976). *For yourself: The fulfillment of female sexuality.* New York: Anchor/Doubleday.

BARBACH, L. (1982). *For each other: Sexual intimacy.* New York: Doubleday.

BARBACH, L. (1990). *Falling in love again*. Los Angeles: Venus Group.

BROWN, R. A., & Field, J. R. (Eds.). (1988). *Treatment of sexual problems in individual and couples therapy*. Baltimore: PMA Press.

COOPER, A. J. (1971). Treatments of male potency disorders: The present status. *Psychosomatics, 12,* 335–344.

CRENSHAW, T. L., Kessler, J. M., & Hildebrandt, S. E. (1985). Alcohol, antihypertensives, and sexual dysfunction: A common problem. *Medical Aspects of Human Sexuality, 19*(3), 165–168.

DINKMEYER, D., & Carlson, J. (1989). *Taking time for love: How to stay happily married*. Englewood Cliffs, NJ: Prentice-Hall.

FISHER, S. (1989). *Sexual images of the self: The psychology of erotic sensations and illusions*. Hillsdale, NJ: Erlbaum.

FRIDAY, N. (1973). *My secret garden: Womens' sexual fantasies*. New York: Trident Press.

FRIEDMAN, J. M. (1984). Differences in sexual desire. In *Innovations in clinical practice: A sourcebook, Vol. 3* (pp. 464–467). Sarasota, FL: Professional Resource Exchange.

FRIEDMAN, J. M., & Czekala, J. (1985). Advances in sex therapy techniques. In *Innovations in Clinical Practice: A Sourcebook, Vol. 4* (pp. 187–200). Sarasota, FL: Professional Resource Exchange.

HUMPHREY, F. G. (1983). *Marital therapy*. Englewood Cliffs, NJ: Prentice-Hall.

JACOBSON, N. S., & Margolin, G. (1979). *Marital therapy: Strategies based on social learning and behavior exchange principles*. New York: Brunner/Mazel.

KAPLAN, H. S. (1975). *The illustrated manual of sex therapy,* (2nd ed.). New York: Brunner/Mazel.

KAPLAN, H. S. (1979). *Disorders of sexual desire and other new concepts and techniques in sex therapy*. New York: Simon & Schuster.

KARACAN, I., Salis, P. J., & Williams, R. L. (1978). The role of the sleep laboratory in diagnosis and treatment of impotence. In R. L. Williams, & I. Karacan (Eds.), *Sleep disorders: Diagnosis and treatment*. New York: Wiley.

KARACAN, I., Ware, J. C., Dervant, B., Altinel, A., Thornby, J. I., Williams, R. L., Kaya, N., & Scott, F. B. (1978). Impotence and blood pressure in the flaccid penis: Relationship to nocturnal penile tumescence. *Sleep, 1,* 125–132.

KOLODNY, R. C., Masters, W. H., & Johnson, V. E. (1979). *Textbook of sexual medicine*. Boston: Little, Brown.

KRONE, R. J., Siroky, M. B., & Goldstein, I. (Eds.). (1983). *Male sexual dysfunction*. Boston: Little, Brown.

MAIER, R. (1984). *Human sexuality in perspective*. Chicago: Nelson Hall.

MASTERS, W. H., & Johnson, V. E. (1970). *Human sexual inadequacy*. Boston: Little, Brown.

McCARTHY, B. W., & Perkins, S. (1988). Behavioral strategies and techniques in sex therapy. In R. Brown, & J. Field (Eds.), *Treatment of sexual problems in individual and couples therapy*. Baltimore: PMA Press.

MUNJACK, D. J., & Oziel, L. J. (1980). *Sexual medicine and counseling in office practice: A complete treatment guide*. Boston: Little, Brown.

NEWCOMB, M., & Bentler, P. (1988). Behavioral and psychological assessment of sexual dysfunction: An overview. In R. Brown, & J. Field (Eds.), *Treatment of sexual problems in individual and couples therapy*. Baltimore: PMA Press.

PEARSALL, P. (1987). *Super marital sex*. New York: Doubleday.

PION, R. J. (1975). Diagnosis and treatment of inadequate sexual response. In J. Sciarra (Ed.), *Gynecology and obstetrics, Vol. 2*. New York: Harper & Row.

PION, R., & Annon, J. (1975). The office management of sexual problems: Brief therapy approaches. *Journal of Reproductive Medicine, 15*(4), 127–144.

PION, R. J., Annon, J. S., & Carlson, J. (1982). Brief sexual counseling. *Counseling and Human Development, 14*(8), 1–8.

PION, R. J., & Hopkins, J. (1978). *The last sex manual*. New York: Wyden Press.

PION, R. J., & Wagner, N. N. (1971). Diagnosis and treatment of inadequate sexual responses. In R. David (Ed.), *Davis' gynecology and obstetrics, Vol 2*. New York: Harper & Row.

REED, K. (1987). The effects of infertility on female sexuality. *Pre- and Peri-Natal Psychology, 2*(1), 57–63.

REYNOLDS, B. S. (1977). Psychological treatment models and outcome results for erectile dysfunction: A critical review. *Psychological Bulletin, 84,* 1218–1238.

SADLER, A. G., & Syrop, G. H. (1987). The stress of infertility: Recommendations for assessment and intervention. *Family Stress Journal, 1*(1), 1–17.

SCHOVER, L. R. (1982). Enhancing sexual intimacy. In *Innovations in Clinical Practice: A Sourcebook, Vol. 1* (pp. 53–66). Sarasota, FL: Professional Resource Exchange.

SHULMAN, B. H. (1967). The uses and abuses of sex. *Journal of Religious Health, 6,* 317–325.

SPARK, R. F., White, R. A., & Connolly, P. B. (1980). Impotence is not always psychogenic: New insight into hypothalamic-pituitary-gonadal dysfunction. *Journal of the American Medical Association, 243,* 750–753.

SPREI, J., & Courtois, C. (1988). The treatment of women's sexual dysfunction arising from sexual assault. In R. Brown, & J. Field (Eds.), *Treatment of sexual problems in individual and couples therapy.* Baltimore: PMA Press.

STUART, R. B. (1980). *Helping couples change: A social learning approach to marital therapy.* New York: Guilford Press.

TRAVIS, J. W., & Ryan, R. S. (1988). *Wellness workbook* (2nd ed.). Berkeley, CA: Ten Speed Press.

YAFFE, M., & Fenwick, E. (1988). *Sexual happiness: A practical approach.* New York: Henry Holt.

ZILBERGELD, B. (1978). *Male sexuality.* Boston: Little, Brown.

ZILBERGELD, B., & Ellison, C. R. (1980). Desire discrepancies and arousal problems in sex therapy. In S. R. Leiblum, & L. A. Pervin (Eds.), *Principles and practice of sex therapy.* New York: Guilford Press.

PLEASE SEND ME A $50.00 CHEQUE FOR EACH FRIEND WHO ENROLS.

My Name

Address

City Prov.   Postal Code

Student Number   YYY410

PLEASE SEND COURSE INFORMATION TO ACQUAINTANCE(S) LISTED BELOW

Name   Age

Address   Apt.

City Prov.   Postal Code

Course of Interest

- Accounting
- Air Conditioning/Refrigeration
- Aircraft Maintenance & Repair
- Animal Care Specialist
- Appliance Servicing
- Art
- Auto Mechanics
- Bicycle Mechanics
- Bookkeeping
- Business Management
- Catering/Professional Cooking
- Child Psychology
- Computer Programing
- Computer Spreadsheets/Lotus
- Cosmetology/Esthetics
- Creative Writing
- Dental Administrative Assistant
- Desktop Publishing
- Early Childhood Education
- Electrician
- Electronics Technician
- Fashion Design & Merchandising
- Firearms Repair
- Fitness & Nutrition

What we request, through our Student Referral Program, is the name, address, and subject of interest for each of your relatives or friends whom you think might be interested. Why do we want this information? So that we can send them the same information package you received from us (or a similar one, if their field of interest is different).

We will keep your name and theirs linked together in our computer. If we end up receiving an enrolment from any of the persons whose names you have submitted, you will automatically be flagged for a special thank-you from us — a $50.00 cheque or credit to your account! That is **$50.00 for EACH enrolment.** If more than one friend decides to enrol, you get more than one cheque. When your friend becomes a student in good standing for a period of ninety days, you will receive your reward. There is no limit, and no other condition.

If they choose not to join immediately, they may change their minds once they see you

UNIVERSAL CAREER INSTITUTE

The UCI Student Referral Program...

A UNIQUE OPPORTUNITY TO:

- *Earn money*
- *Help a friend*

EARN $50

Dear Student,

Advertising is a necessary but expensive part of our school. We have to let a large number of people know what we do so that those who need our services, and are ready to make a commitment to their future, can link up with us.

By far the most beneficial form of "advertising" comes from word-of-mouth recommendations from our students. Not only are stud

9

Chronic Pain

Pain is perfect misery, the worst of evils, and excessive, overturns all patience.

Milton

Pain has been defined as a sensory and emotional experience of discomfort associated with actual or threatened tissue damage or irritation (Sanders, 1985). Nearly everyone reports the experience of pain sometime throughout the course of life. (According to Karoly and Jensen (1987), pain is the most pervasive symptom in medical practice, the most frequently stated "cause" of disability, and the single most compelling force underlying a person's decision to seek medical care. The purpose of this chapter is to survey the various factors and methods in assessing and treating clients with chronic pain. As with other health-counseling issues, our approach emphasizes a biopsychosocial perspective. This chapter reviews various theories of pain; individual and group intervention strategies for managing pain; and issues of relapse, adherence, and prevention. Since the two most common chronic pain syndromes are headaches and back pain, our discussion is directed to these two complaints.

Before proceeding further, an important distinction must be made; pain is usually characterized as either acute or chronic. Whether it is mild or severe, and whether the cause is known or unknown, the duration of acute pain is of only a few day's duration. Sufferers expect relief through some kind of medical intervention, and the health-care provider expects pain to decrease as the affected area heals. Whether it is sunburn, toothache, or postsurgical pain, acute pain can be either recurrent or progressive. With intermittent pain, such as in arthritis, there are pain-free intervals. With progressive acute pain, such as in cancer, the pain is ongoing and increases in intensity.

Chronic pain and the chronic-pain syndrome are characterized by disability and suffering of over six months' duration that are disproportionate to detectable, undetectable, or remedial disease. Chronic-pain syndrome is benign but correctable, and so it excludes the pain of cancer. It may be initiated by acute trauma or disease, such as back injury or heart attack, or it can develop in association with an intermittent disease, such as angina or rheumatoid arthritis (Sternbach, 1968). The most common forms of chronic-pain syndrome are low back pain and headache (Blackwell, 1989).

Chronic back pain originates with injury to soft tissue or to bony structures, and the frequency of occurrence of back pain is high. Svensson and Anderson (1982) estimate that 50 to 80 percent of the population will have back complaints. Most of these back-pain problems resolve themselves within a matter of days or a few weeks; however, many do not. Hult (1954) found that approximately 20 percent of the population is incapacitated for periods ranging from three weeks to six months, and 4 percent is incapacitated for more than six months. Johnson (1978) reports similar findings from a worker's compensation sample, suggesting that chronic back pain affects about 4 percent of the population.

Headache is even more common than back pain. It has been estimated that as many as 80 million Americans—one-third of the population—suffers from headaches. Americans lose in excess of 700 million work days a year at a cost of $65 billion in health-care costs. In addition, Americans spend over $2 billion a year on over-the-counter headache remedies. For many of us, headaches are minor occurrences that can be relieved with aspirin or ibuprofen. However, not all headaches are alike, and some may be so frequent and severe that the

sufferer is unable to function in daily activities. In reviewing several epidemiological studies of headache, Blanchard and Andrasik (1985) concluded that headaches severe and chronic enough to interfere with daily functioning affect approximately 20 percent of the American population. And, since approximately 7 percent of visits to general medical practitioners are precipitated by headache complaints, the authors conclude that headache is a major health problem in the United States.

Biopsychosocial Aspects of Pain

Biological Factors

Both anatomical and biochemical structures and processes are involved in the experience of pain. This section reviews the biological aspects of pain by tracing the neurological pathways that convey painful stimuli to the brain as well as the pathways that provide pain relief. It also briefly describes the body's own endogenous opiates—natural pain relievers present in the nervous system—that provide pain relief.

Painful tissue inflammation releases various chemicals that stimulate certain nerve endings that respond to pain stimuli and signal injury. These nerve endings, or receptors, are called nociceptors. While the nerve-stimulation process is still in the "periphery," pain may be alleviated with aspirin, or anti-inflammatory agents like Motrin or Advil. These medications are analgesic in part because they reduce tissue inflammation.

Whether it originates from pressure, heat, or inflammation, pain is carried by two types of peripheral nerve fibers. A delta fibers are small, thinly myelinated nerve fibers that convey sharp or prickling sensations from the skin and mucus membranes. C fibers are small, unmyelinated nerve fibers that convey nearly all painful sensations from the viscera (internal organs) and other tissues. Painful transmissions along A delta and C fibers may be dampened by stimulating A beta fibers, the larger, myelinated sensory fibers nearby. This analgesic effect may be why individuals instinctively massage the area around an injury.

The "gate-control" theory of pain is based on this observation of nerve fibers (Melzack & Wall, 1965). Essentially, the gate-control theory postulates that stimulation of A beta fibers, which are the larger, heavily myelinated nerve fibers, inhibits pain transmission by the small fibers that have little or no myelination. This theory will be further discussed later in this chapter.

Periphery nerve fibers carry pain impulses that originate at the spinal cord. These fibers synapse, or connect, either immediately upon stimulation or after ascending a few segments of the spinal cord. At each synapse, the fibers release Substance P, which basically acts as the neurotransmitter in the spinal cord. After the synapse, a second neuron crosses to the other side of the spinal cord and moves to the brain along an ascending track.

Not all peripheral nerves synapse in the spinal cord and carry pain up to the brain. Some synapse into short neurons, called interneurons, that block nerve receptors and provide analgesia. A corresponding descending spinal cord tract originates in the lower brain stem. It has an analgesic effect on the

ascending tracts through the release of seratonin. It has been known for some time that an increase in seratonin produces analgesia, and a decrease in it intensifies pain. Brain stem structures also produce short, analgesic brain-stem tracts, which, when stimulated electrically, release endogenous opiates that produce analgesia or euphoria.

Endogenous opiates are amino acid chains within the central nervous system that create effects similar to those of morphine and other opiates. Experiments and clinical trials have shown that when endogenous opiates are administered, they produce the same effects as morphine: analgesia, mood elevation, sedation, and respiratory depression. Other endogenous opiates are located in the brain, the brain stem, and the spinal cord. The so-called runners' high, the painlessness of the injured football player, and the effectiveness of placebos are all believed to result from endogenous opiates secreted when individuals are under high levels of stress.

In summary, pain is transmitted from A delta to C peripheral nerve fibers upward through ascending pain pathways to regions of the brain stem. The body's own analgesic system includes the brain stem and descending pathways that release endogenous analgesics and opiates (Melzack & Wall, 1982).

In addition to the anatomical and biochemical processes just described, there are a number of secondary factors that contribute to the experience of pain. High fatigue and subsequent low stamina enhance sensitivity to or decreased tolerance of pain, which, in turn, initiate a vicious cycle of decreased activity and increased perception of pain. Similarly, the physiological effects of alcohol or other substances can further complicate the experience of pain and can seriously hamper rehabilitative efforts. Finnaly, there is considerable variability in the threshold of pain among individuals that cannot be accounted for entirely by social and psychological variables.

Psychological Factors

In addition to biological factors, a number of psychological factors influence the experience of pain. A pain-prone personality has been postulated to explain the development of chronic-pain syndrome. Engel (1959) noted that pain had both symbolic and functional significance in the sufferer's life. Symbolically, pain represents sublimated aggression, guilt, torment for sin, or a lost love object. Functionally, pain can serve to relieve repressed conflict or fulfill dependency needs. Blumer and Heilbronn (1982) profiled 234 chronic-pain sufferers in a 10-year study. Characteristic profiles of pain-prone personalities comprise two components: the clinical features and the psychological features. Clinical features are the overt symptoms, beliefs, and behaviors, such as continuous pain, desire for surgery, denial of emotional and interpersonal difficulties, idealization of family relationships, excessive activity prior to the onset of pain, excessive passivity after the onset of pain, and major depressive disturbances (such as insomnia). The psychological features focus on intrapsychic dynamics. These include concealment and denial of conflict, infantile needs to be dependent and cared for, marked passivity, inability to cope with anger and hostility, and guilt complexes. Many of these chronic-pain sufferers had family models of pain and disability in their early life. Many were from families whose members were alcoholic or had depressive disorders. In short, Blumer and

Heilbronn concluded that the pain-prone personality can be categorized as a "depression spectrum" disorder, which predisposes the individual to chronic pain.

Currently, there is little support for this position (Turk & Holzman, 1986; Anderson, Bradley, Young, et al., 1985). Other evidence suggests that people with chronic pain become depressed because of the stress they experience from being unable to change their situation. This sense of helplessness then leads to depression (Melzak & Wall, 1982).

Although Engel, Blumer, and Heilbronn all framed their discussion in psychodynamic terms, the behavioral perspective has become the dominant force in chronic-pain management. The behavioral perspective assumes that chronic pain can lead to behavioral and emotional deficits that serve to maintain pain and associated behaviors. The behavioral perspective emphasizes the measurement of observable behavior and the operant reconditioning of the autonomic nervous system.

In addition, chronic-pain sufferers have been shown to be predisposed to alexithymia, which means they have relatively restricted emotional vocabularies and a tendency to communicate their distress in somatic terms (for example, "I've got a terrible headache" instead of "I'm really afraid and worried"), which can further exacerbate their experience of pain (Blackwell, 1989).

Social Factors

There are a number of social factors, including the concept of the "sick role" and the influences of spouse, family, friends, and culture, that can shape both the experience of chronic pain and its treatment. Shared beliefs and reward systems can play a crucial role in the client's own attributions and behaviors. An overly solicitous spouse can systematically encourage the client to adopt a sick role, seek further medical treatment, or pursue litigation. In all cases, illness rather than wellness behavior is being reinforced. Health-care professionals can also reinforce illness behavior by ordering excessive diagnostic evaluations and treatment regimens that reinforce the client's perception that he or she has a serious, undiscovered disease that must be identified and treated. Finally, society reinforces chronic pain behavior through financial compensation for injury or disability. Litigation frequently places the individual in the position of needing to remain in the sick role in order to qualify for compensation (Blackwell, Galbraith, & Dahl, 1984).

Theories of Pain

A number of theories of pain have been proposed over the past 90 years. Of these, we will review three of the most well known: the specificity theory, the pattern theory, and the gate-control theory.

Specificity Theory

The specificity theory proposes a rather mechanistic view of pain perception. It states that the body has a separate sensory system for perceiving pain. This system contains its own special receptors for detecting pain stimuli, its own

peripheral nerves and pathways to the brain, and its own specific centers for processing pain signals. Thus, when a noxious event stimulates a pain receptor, this signal travels to the pain center in the brain.

Pattern Theory

On the other hand, pattern theory proposes that there is no separate system for feeling pain and that the receptors for pain are shared with other senses. According to this mechanistic view, individuals experience pain when certain patterns of neuroactivity reach excessively high levels in the brain. These patterns occur only with intense stimulation. Since strong and mild stimuli of the same sensory modality (such as light, sound, touch, and taste) produce the different patterns of nerve activity, being hit with a bat is experienced as painful and being hugged and kissed is not.

Gate-Control Theory

Although both the specificity and the pattern theories contain features that are supported by research, neither theory adequately explains pain perception (Melzack & Wall, 1982). A less mechanistic and more holistic alternative to the specificity theory was developed by Melzack and Wall (1965; 1982). Their theory proposes that a neural mechanism in the spinal cord acts as a "gate" that can facilitate or inhibit the flow of nerve impulses from peripheral fibers to the central nervous system. When the amount of information that passes through the gate exceeds a critical level, the neural areas responsible for pain experience and response are then activated. There are a number of conditions that open and close this hypothesized gate. For example, physical conditions, such as an extensive injury or inappropriate activity level; emotional conditions, such as too much anxiety, tension, or depression; and mental conditions, such as a focus on pain or on boredom are conditions that have been found to open the gate. On the other hand, physical factors, such as suppressing medications or counter-stimulation through heat or massage; emotional conditions, such as happiness or optimism, relaxation or rest; and mental conditions, such as intense concentration or involvement in distracting activities have been shown to close the gate and reduce the experience of pain.

According to this theory, sensory input is subjected to the moderating influence of cognitive, affective, and behavioral factors before it provokes pain perception. Thus, a central control mechanism is proposed to account for alterations in pain perception produced by psychological factors and intervention techniques. Psychological factors can modulate pain by altering the person's appraisal of the threat, ability to control the quality of the noxious stimuli, and level of emotional arousal. Furthermore, psychological interventions that reduce cognitive and affective factors can prevent the development of pain, obliterate it entirely, or reduce its intensity.

Although the postulated anatomical and biochemical basis for the gate-control theory are speculative and have been criticized (Weisenberg, 1977), its biopsychosocial perspective has received considerable support (Turk, Meichenbaum, & Genest, 1983).

Melzack and Wall's theory of pain has focused attention on the concept that

pain is not a function of a particular system; rather, each specialized portion of the entire nervous system contributes to the pain experience. Practically speaking, the gate-control theory has redirected our thinking about cognitive processes. Basically, pain can be treated not only by trying to cut down sensory input—such as by anesthetic blocks, surgical interventions, electrical stimulation, and the like—but also by influencing motivational and cognitive factors as well.

Not surprisingly, the gate-control theory has stimulated a significant amount of research and has received strong support from the findings of many of these studies (Winters, 1985; Melzack & Wall, 1982). Finally, the gate-control theory suggests that psychology has much to offer both in understanding and in treating pain, and it provides a biopsychosocial explanation of the phenomenon of pain.

Assessment

The emphasis of any assessment procedure will depend on the purpose of the assessment. Broadly speaking, three main aims in the assessment of chronic pain are: (1) to determine the client's suitability for treatment; (2) to determine the client's strengths and deficits so that the program can be tailored to his or her needs; and (3) to evaluate change over the course of treatment. Unfortunately, very little is known about which patients are likely to respond quickly to specific psychological, biological, or social interventions. Thus, at this stage in the development of health counseling, it is not possible to list a number of guidelines on client suitability. However, we can offer the counselor a number of considerations about the overall client assessment process.

A comprehensive, biopsychosocial assessment involves data from four different sources: (1) the health counselor's observation and interview data; (2) the client's self-report on various inventories, grading forms, and questionnaires; (3) the information provided by a spouse or other significant person; and (4) the associated physiological theories. Each of these four sources will be elaborated in the following sections.

Health Counselor's Perspective

The health counselor's impression of the client's pain will come primarily from the interview and from direct behavioral observation. Ideally, the clinical interview should involve the client as well as significant others, such as spouse, family members, or friends with whom the client spends much time. If treatment is to be successful, both counselor and client must arrive at a "meeting of the minds" regarding the meaning or model of pain for the client. The initial interview should therefore involve considerable information giving and education about pain mechanisms. Clients with a long history of pain are likely to have been given different and sometimes conflicting explanations of their problem by other health professionals. It is important, then, to discuss these and any worries that the client may have about his or her condition. Clients will also have their own theories about the physical and psychological bases of their pain,

which they may never have shared with others for fear of being labeled "crazy." A health counselor's failure to explore these issues at the beginning of the interview may render any detailed inquiries about pain factors or personal history of limited value. Once a shared model of pain has been established, it is much easier to take a case history.

To treat chronic pain effectively, a counselor needs a detailed description of the client's pain symptoms and history. (For example, various kinds of headache pain are described in Table 9-1.) The client is queried about the presentation of pain as well as what the client takes or does to relieve it (Blackwell, Galbraith, and Dahl, 1984). It is suggested that the following ten areas be targeted in the assessment interview.

1. The history of the pain problem, including when it started, how it progressed, and when help was first sought for it.
2. The client's explanatory model or beliefs about the cause of the pain.
3. The pain syndrome and the pain's impact on the client's current life-style, interpersonal relationships, hobbies, and work.
4. The client's previous history. This includes how the client approached and coped with stressors before the onset of the chronic pain. Also included are family structure, social supports, recreational and exercise patterns, diet, and vocational patterns.
5. The client's current recreational interests, exercise patterns, diet, family structure, social supports, and vocational activities.
6. The social context of pain episodes; what happens in the family before an attack, and what the response of family members is when pain occurs. It is important also to inquire as to whether the client knows anyone else who has a pain syndrome. Finally, it is important to inquire about early childhood models of illness behavior.
7. The factors that seem to trigger attacks or make them worse.
8. How the client typically tries to cope with the pain, and what he or she fears most about the problem.
9. The use of prescription medications for pain; the use of nonprescription medications (such as medications that have been prescribed to a family member or a friend); the use of over-the-counter medications; and the use of alcohol, caffeine, nicotine, and other addicting substances.
10. The client's expectations of treatment: what the client thinks will help the pain, what results the client hopes to receive from treatment, and what expectations the client has of the counselor as the professional and of him- or herself as the client. In other words, what is the client's receptivity and capacity for treatment?

Professionals who work with chronic-pain sufferers have found that it is useful to conduct a separate interview with the client's spouse or partner to clarify any issues and determine how the client's pain affects the spouse and how the spouse responds to the client. Then, a joint spouse/patient assessment interview is held to observe and assess marital and interpersonal dynamics (Turk et al., 1983).

Since individuals tend to exhibit pain behaviors when they are in dis-

Table 9-1. Common Types of Headaches

Headache Type	Symptoms	Precipitating Factors
Tension headaches	"Hatband" distribution, associated with tightness of scalp or neck; nonthrobbing pain, dull, frequently bilateral. Degree of severity remains constant.	Hidden depression; emotional stress.
Common migraines	Lightheadedness; blurred vision; ringing in ears; severe, one-sided, throbbing pain, often accompanied by nausea, vomiting, dizziness, tremor, sensitivity to sound and light, cold hands, hot and cold flashes.	Excessive hunger, change in weather or altitude, excessive smoking, use of oral contraceptives, flashing or bright lights, foods containing tyramine or other vasoactive substances.
Classic migraines	Same as common migraine, except for warning symptoms, which may include the smelling of strange odors, visual disturbances, hallucinations, and numbness in arms or legs. Preliminary reaction subsides within a half-hour and is followed by severe pain.	Same as for common migraine.
TMJ headaches	TMJ (tempomandibular joint) dysfunction can occasionally produce a muscle contraction–type of pain, sometimes accompanied by a "clicking" sound on opening the jaw. Infrequent cause of headache.	Stress, jaw clenching, and malocclusion (poor bite)
Cluster headaches	Tearing of eyes, excruciating pain around or behind one eye, flushing of face, nasal congestion. Attacks occur every day for weeks or months, then disappear for up to a year. Pain frequently develops during sleep and may last for several hours. Ninety percent of cluster victims are male.	Excessive smoking, ingestion of alcoholic beverages.
Caffeine headaches	These are actually caffeine-withdrawal headaches: throbbing headaches caused by rebound dilation of the blood vessels several hours after consumption of large quantities of caffeine.	Caffeine.
Hypertension headaches	"Hatband" or generalized-type pain. Pain is most severe in the morning, then diminishes as day goes on.	Severe hypertension (over 200 systolic and 110 diastolic).

comfort, it is possible to assess their pain by observing and assessing their behavior. An individual with intense pain behaves differently than someone with moderate pain, just as an individual with headache pain tends to behave differently from a person with low back pain. The observant counselor will note the range of the client's affect and behavior, noting the appropriateness of both with regard to the content of the interview. The counselor also asks the client to walk, pick up an object on the floor, remove his or her shoes while sitting, or perform several exercises such as trunk rotations, toe-touches, and sit-ups. During the exercise, the health counselor rates such pain indices as wincing and grimacing, sighing, or rubbing the painful areas. This behavioral assessment could also be compared with the client's self-ratings of these movements (Karoly & Jensen, 1987).

Client Self-Reports

One of the more obvious ways of measuring people's pain is to ask them to describe their discomfort, either in their own words or by filling out a form, rating scale, or questionnaire.

Pain-intensity rating forms are useful for revealing the course of pain over time, the fluctuations in pain intensity, and the times when medications are needed and used. It is common in pain clinics to have all clients complete a pain diary. The pain diary is designed to provide information concerning the times, places, and presence of others during pain episodes; and the thoughts and feelings that the client has before, during, and after severe pain episodes. In addition, the pain-allaying techniques or the things the client does to cope with the pain are also noted in the diary.

A number of formal rating scales have been used to assess the chronic-pain client. The Profile of Mood States (POMS) has a range of scales to assess different emotional states—such positive mood states as vigor as well as such negative mood states as depression. The Beck Depression Inventory is useful for illiciting some of the cognitive components of depression and pain. The MMPI is perhaps the most widely used formal instrument in clinical practice with pain clients.

Chronic-pain clients frequently display a characteristic MMPI profile with elevated scores on scales 1, 2, and 3, which measure hypochondriasis, depression, and hysteria. (This triad is often referred to as the psychosomatic V.) It is important to note that the validity of these three scales is reduced when organic disease is present. Scale 1 suggests a deep-seated conviction that something is wrong in the body, and scale 3 reflects the tendency to somatize. An increased awareness of symptoms may also be related to previous experience of disease or similar symptoms in a relative or a loved one. Pain and depression, as measured by scale 2, frequently coexist, and they appear to amplify each other. Among chronic-pain clients, depression may either occur simultaneously with the pain symptoms or follow the onset of pain by several weeks or months. Clinicians have also noted that some chronic-pain patients have elevated scores on scales 8 (schizophrenia) or 9 (mania) on the MMPI. This elevation usually suggests that the experience of pain is being influenced by cognitive distortions or defects in information processing rather than indicating true schizophrenia or a bipolar disorder. These elevations on scales 8 and 9 are particularly likely to occur when

the client's symptoms are vague or ambiguous (Blackwell, Galbraith, & Dahl, 1984).

One of the most direct and simple ways to assess pain is to have the clients rate some of their discomfort on a self-rating scale (Karoly & Jensen, 1987). Two types of self-rating scales to measure pain intensity are commonly used. The visual analog scale is a 10-centimeter line with endpoints of "no pain" and "worst pain ever," and the client marks a point on the line that describes the pain's intensity at a given moment. The category rating scale also uses a line, but it is divided into sections with designations such as "no pain," "mild," "discomfort-ing," "distressing," "horrible," and "excruciating." The client checks the sections that correspond to the pain experience.

Because these self-rating scales are relatively quick and easy to use, pa-tients are asked to rate their pain frequently, usually on an hourly basis. Repeated ratings reveal how the pain changes over time and what patterns occur in the timing of severe pain. For example, pain may be more severe in the evening on certain days and not on others, or when certain other people are around.

Unlike the POMS or the Beck Depression Inventory, which assess general mood states, the McGill Pain Questionnaire (MPQ) primarily assesses the affec-tive (emotional) component of the pain experience itself. The MPQ consists of 78 pain adjectives separated into a total of 20 subclasses. The test instructs the individual to select from each subclass the best word to describe his or her pain. Each word in each class has an assigned value based on the degree of pain it reflects. Melzack (1975) developed the instrument based on his belief that pain involved three broad categories: affective (emotional/motivational), sensory, and evaluative. Subsequently, of the 20 subgroups, some describe sensory experiences, such as prickling, hot, scalding; others describe affective qualities, such as sickening, fearful, punishing, cruel; and others describe evaluative aspects of pain, such as annoying, miserable, troublesome. The MPQ yields both a pain-rating index and a present-pain-intensity score. The MPQ has a number of strengths and weaknesses as an instrument for assessing chronic pain. The MPQ does differentiate among categories of pain, such as headache, arthritis, cancer, and phantom-limb pain. However, it also requires that the client have an extensive English vocabulary. For instance, it includes words such as "taut" and "lancinating," and it requires the patient to make a fine distinction between such words as "throbbing," "beating," and "pounding." Thus, the MPQ may not be particularly useful across all cultural and subcultural groups, and it cannot be used with individuals under the age of 12.

Spouse or Partner Information

Assessment of a client's everyday activities, especially those within the home, can provide significant information to the health counselor. It is useful to know how much time the client spends in bed, how often the client complains of dis-comfort, how much help he or she seeks, and how often the person walks with a limp. Family members or significant people in the client's life may be the best individuals to make these everyday assessments of pain behaviors.

As in other treatment programs, we have found it useful for the client's

spouse or partner to fill out a diary for a two-week period. This pain diary is designed to record episodes when the spouse is aware that the client's pain is very severe. The spouse records the date and time, as well as where the episode occurred, and describes the observed behaviors that suggest that the client was in pain. Spouses then indicate what they had thought and felt while observing the client and what response they made to help. They rate their actions' effectiveness on a scale ranging from "did not help at all" to "seemed to stop the pain completely." This diary provides additional data that, when compared to the client's own diary, can be of help when dealing with interpersonal issues that influence the pain experience.

Physiological Measures

A biological approach for assessing pain involves taking measurements of physiological activity. The most common physiological measure for assessing pain is the electromyograph (EMG). The EMG measures the electrical activity in muscles, which reflects their tension. Because muscle tension has been associated with various pain states such as headache and low back pain, clinicians assumed that EMG recordings could provide objective evidence for the presence or absence of pain. In fact, headache sufferers do show different EMG patterns when they have headaches than when they do not (Blanchard & Andrasik, 1985). Biofeedback technology is, in large part, based on EMG recordings. Unfortunately, more research is needed to verify that EMG recordings provide a useful measure of pain.

Another physiological measure is the electroencephalograph (EEG). When a client's sensory system detects a stimulus, such as a clicking sound, the signal to the brain produces a change in EEG voltage. Electrical changes produce evoked potentials that show up on the EEG recording as sharp peaks in the graph. Research has demonstrated that pain stimuli produce evoked potentials that vary in size with the intensity of the stimuli, decrease when patients take analgesics, and correlate with the individual's subjective report of pain (Chapman, Cassey, Dubner, et al., 1985). It should be noted that, even though these psychophysiological measures provide objective assessments, these measures may be affected by other factors, such as attention, stress, and diet. Accordingly, these psychophysiological measures are best used as adjuncts to direct observation, self-report, and other standard assessment approaches.

Treatment Planning and Interventions

Because chronic pain is multiply determined, and because most chronic-pain sufferers believe that they are victims of organic illness, the health counselor does well to approach treatment issues in both a comprehensive and judicious fashion. Engel (1959) emphasizes that the key to successful treatment resides in investigating the manner in which pain disrupts the client's personal, social, family, and occupational life and disregards the artificial separation between what could be classified as biological, psychological, or social.

A simple task in treatment planning is to help the client reframe his or her

problem without challenging the reality of the pain experience. Implicit in this change is the transfer of responsibility from health counselor to client. Accomplishing this reframing requires skill and tact because chronic-pain clients are highly sensitive to suggestion that their suffering is imagined, exaggerated, or psychological in nature. Initially, then, pain should be discussed as a source rather than as a product of stress, and it is helpful to have the clients explain how their pain keeps them from performing their normal daily activities. As a result, the health counselor can work with the client to develop strategies to achieve specific goals while the client is learning to tolerate the pain. In short, the biological basis of painful experience is emphasized in the early phase of treatment. Similarly, the health counselor should not expect the client to relinquish what he or she gains from the sick role until he or she has begun to develop coping skills for pain tolerance and alternative sources of gratification.

The question of whether pain sufferers would be better served by a course of inpatient treatment must be considered. Indications for inpatient treatment include serious substance dependency, severe physical disability, multiple somatic complaints that require medical evaluation, and overwhelming environmental influences, such as an overly solicitous spouse. By contrast, patients with localized pain, less severe limitations, and cooperative relatives can usually be managed as outpatients (Blackwell, 1989).

Because chronic pain is a multiply determined condition, it is not unreasonable to conclude that a multimodal intervention will be needed for successful treatment. Much of the success reported in the pain-management literature is attributed to the fact that several treatments are used in combination or in sequence. These treatments include a wide range of biological, psychological, and social interventions.

Biological Interventions

Depending on the severity of the chronic-pain sufferer's symptoms, biological treatment interventions may be necessary to produce at least a partial relief of pain and suffering. Thus, the health counselor will need to work collaboratively with the client's neurologist or primary-care physician. Unfortunately, biological interventions may unduly encourage the client's hope of a magical cure instead of increasing the client's autonomy and commitment to learning to live with and adapt to pain. In this section, we will review a number of the common biological interventions that can serve as useful adjuncts to psychosocial interventions.

Psychotropic medications.   Antipsychotic medications, such as Thorazine and Stelazine, and tricyclic antidepressants such as Imipramine and Nortriptyline, appear to have an opiate-sparing effect in some patients with pain. It appears that these medications bind to opiate receptors and interact with enkephalins to produce pain relief. Drugs like Valium and Librium appear to lower pain thresholds and are seldom used clinically because of their dependency-producing potential. Antidepressants are preferred because chronic-pain sufferers frequently become depressed. Approximately 60 to 80 percent of patients with chronic pain benefit to some degree from treatment with any

tricyclic antidepressant. Other medications that are sometimes used with pain patients include carbamazepine (Tegretol), clonazepam (Klonopin), clondine (Catapres), and propranolol (Inderal).

Physical rehabilitation.   Many inpatient and day-hospital pain programs include a stepwise plan of physical retraining to help reverse the effects of muscular atrophy, fatigue, and lack of stamina that normally discourages activity in patients with chronic pain. Specific goals or quotas are set for patients to reach whatever activity level is required to restore functional independence at home or on the job.

Sensory stimulation.   Massage, heat, cold, vibration, acupuncture, and various forms of electrical stimulation have a place in the biological treatment of chronic pain. Transcutaneous nerve stimulators (TENS) are lightweight units that stimulate the skin through electrodes and offer effective pain relief when there is skin sensitivity or nerve damage. Acupuncture is now regarded as a form of low-frequency stimulation that produces some relief in about 60 percent of patients, particularly those with musculoskeletal conditions.

Relaxation training and biofeedback.   Because muscular contractions or vascular dilatation is believed to worsen certain forms of pain, biofeedback may be a useful treatment. This is particularly the case with headache patients for whom there is EMG evidence of an abnormal level of activity in response to stressful stimuli. Studies have indicated that generalized relaxation training may be a simpler, less expensive, and equally effective form of treatment as biofeedback is (Blanchard & Andrasik, 1985). Nevertheless, temperature-regulation or thermic biofeedback, in which the patient learns to increase and decrease body temperature in their fingertips, is the mainstay of treatment for migraine sufferers in many headache clinics.

Drug detoxification.   Approximately one-third of chronic-pain patients use no addicting substances, approximately one-third are dependent on narcotics alone, and about one-third are addicted to both narcotics and sedatives. Chronic-pain patients who are physiologically dependent need to be weaned from these medications by a tapered withdrawal over a 10- to 14-day period. When there is also psychological dependence, which is often the case with drugs such as Valium, self-regulated reduction is negotiated with the patient, who may be asked to set goals, keep records, and give positive reinforcement for abstinence.

Nerve blocks and neurosurgery.   Nerve blocks are used for both diagnosis and treatment and are specifically indicated for pain that is caused by injury to the sympathetic nervous system. Neurosurgical techniques are usually the treatment of last choice. Some patients with chronic pain have benefited from neurosurgical techniques, but it is unclear whether this can be attributed to the techniques, to relief of severe depression or extensive personality change.

Psychological Interventions

Psychological interventions have been found to be quite effective in influencing the clients' tolerance of pain as well as their willingness to complete a treatment program. Yet, psychological interventions are often difficult to implement initially because chronic-pain clients typically resist psychological concepts. We will discuss a number of the most common psychological interventions in this section.

Operant techniques.   The aim of operant techniques is to increase the frequency of wellness behaviors and decrease that of pain and illness behaviors. The client must come to accept that the aim of treatment is not to remove pain but, rather, to help clients cope with it and resume normal activities despite it. Reinforcement, shaping, and extinction techniques are utilized extensively. Generally, the client is given no attention for pain behavior or for requests for pain medication but is provided considerable social reinforcement for wellness behaviors. Physical therapy and exercise quotas are developed to increase the patient's activity level. Each day the quotas are increased, and progress is charted visually. Attention or some other positive reinforcer is made contingent on successful daily completion of the quota (Winters, 1985).

Cognitive techniques.   Cognitive techniques are various methods by which individuals learn to distract or distance themselves from pain. Imagery and cognitive restructuring are used to reframe the experience of pain or to replace it with more pleasant thoughts or sensations. These cognitive techniques appear to work best in pain of mild to moderate intensities (Holzman, Turk, & Kerns, 1986).

Hypnosis.   Hypnosis and posthypnotic suggestion are methods by which some clients can learn to evoke images or metaphors to distract them from or to reframe pain sensations. It appears that hypnosis alone is seldom effective, and therefore hypnosis is used in combination with other psychological interventions.

Individual counseling.   Clients who have chronic pain often possess psychological characteristics and defensive styles that limit the usefulness of traditional individual counseling interventions. The presence of alexithymia (difficulty feeling or expressing emotions), overcritical superego, and defense mechanisms such as denial, rationalization, projection, or suppression make it difficult to engage these clients in treatment. Therefore, counseling goals and strategies must be tailored to the client's needs and style. The major goals of counseling are to increase self-awareness, build ego support, and enhance coping skills. Self-awareness can be fostered through cognitive learning and pattern recognition techniques that, over time, allow the client to become aware of the linkages between feelings, autonomic (involuntary) arousal, and painful sensations. Strategies for strengthening healthy defenses, enhancing coping skills, and supporting the ego in the here-and-now have been found useful with

the chronic-pain sufferer. In time, some clients become more verbally skilled and able to internalize the counselor's benign, nonjudgmental qualities and develop trust. This then makes it possible for the client to discuss deeper-seated conflicts, explore face-saving avenues to escape psychological predicaments, and relinquish the secondary gains of pain (Blackwell, 1989).

Group therapy.   Group approaches have been particularly effective with chronic-pain clients in inpatient, day-hospital, and outpatient settings. The therapeutic factors of cohesiveness, altruism, universality, hope, guidance, and identification are particularly pertinent to pain sufferers. Since loneliness and helplessness are often accompaniments of chronic pain, the group process helps chronic-pain clients feel understood and empowered. In addition to giving support, groups also provide invaluable opportunities for modeling wellness behavior. Once norms that affirm wellness and coping behaviors are established, the group itself becomes a powerful reinforcer of change (Pearce & Erskine, 1989).

Social skills training.   Clients with chronic pain often lack the ability to assert themselves to get their needs met. Instead, they use illness behavior to control or avoid situations and to solicit attention and care from others. Assertiveness training, problem-solving training, and role playing are methods used to help clients express their needs more directly. Other social skills may be lacking in communication, vocational, or sexual areas that are also amenable to specific social-skills training (Turk & Holzman, 1986).

Social Interventions

Social interventions are useful for reducing the influence of the environmental, communicative, and behavioral aspects of pain. Generally speaking, social interventions require the cooperation and involvement of the family, the community, or governmental agencies. Couples and family therapy, peer-support groups, social security disability, or worker's compensation and reentry planning are some examples of points-of-entry for social interventions (Blackwell, 1989).

Couples and family therapy.   Since relatives play a significant role in shaping a client's behavior in response to pain, relatives may be willing to learn alternate ways of helping the client develop a more healthy adaptation to their pain. As treatment progresses, couple or family sessions are scheduled to reward and encourage healthy new behavior while ignoring the pain behaviors (Pearce & Erskine, 1989).

Peer support groups.   As in support groups for overeaters, cancer patients, and the like, groups for chronic-pain sufferers can provide an inexpensive and effective method of producing sustained encouragement and support. Owing to their emphasis on mutual problem solving and acceptance of personal responsibility, peer groups have been unusually effective in helping pain sufferers cope with their difficulties and learn or reinforce healthy skills (Pearce & Erskine, 1989).

Compensation and disability payments.   Another consideration in treatment planning is the role that financial reward plays in perpetuating pain behaviors. An important step in rehabilitation is the settlement of lawsuits or disability claims. Yet, it is unrealistic to assume that pain behavior will be resolved by financial settlement. Because chronic pain is multiply determined, removing a single source or reward is unlikely to produce a dramatic change. As Fordyce (1985) implies, social security disability payments have unintentionally and unfortunately reinforced the sick role in many chronic-pain sufferers.

Reentry planning.   Because chronic-pain clients often display anxiety, a reappearance of somatic symptoms, and complaints at the time of discharge or at the end of outpatient treatment, reentry planning is crucial. Planning for reentry into social and occupational roles means that stressors need to be anticipated and the client prepared for brief relapses. The counselor should also confer with employers and shop stewards if job changes or accommodations are indicated.

Chronic-Pain Control in a Group Format

Pearce and Erskine (1989) offer a group approach to chronic-pain control based on cognitive, behavioral, psychoeducational, and group techniques. The groups consist of 8 to 10 male and female chronic-pain clients. Each group meets once a week for seven successive weeks. Each session begins with group education and cognitive pain-control training, which lasts for one hour and is followed by one half-hour of relaxation and stress management. This is followed by 45 minutes of physical therapy or exercise and a 15-minute coffee break, which provides an opportunity for patients to socialize informally. The last hour focuses on life-style restructuring and general goal setting. Each of these four treatment components will now be described briefly.

Group education and cognitive pain-control training.   The group begins with a detailed explanation and rationale for the cognitive-behavioral approach for the basis of the course. This establishes the validity of the various group components and begins to shift the client's focus from passive helplessness toward active responsibility. Presentations are made to outline the gate-control theory and the notion of pain as a multiply determined, multi-dimensional phenomenon. Clients are asked to make free associations with the word *pain,* and the adjectives are categorized into three sections: physiological, subjective, and behavioral manifestations. In this way, a multidimensional view of pain is reinforced. The rest of this first session and the next two focus on techniques aimed at altering the subjective component of pain. Distraction and reframing are two such techniques. Each technique is illustrated and in-dividualized for each group member. These individual members choose a technique or techniques that will be practiced daily at the first sign that pain intensity is on the increase. Specific homework assignments are given and checked at subsequent sessions (Pearce & Erskine, 1989).

Relaxation and stress control.   Progressive relaxation and self-in-duced relaxation are both taught to and practiced by chronic-pain clients.

Self-hypnotic relaxation training has been found to be useful, and clients prac- tice by listening at home to a tape recording of a counselor's instructions. The ultimate goal of this training is for clients to learn to achieve deep states of relaxation without cues from either the group counselor or the tape (Turk et al. 1983).

Exercise therapy.   This part of the session is structured around a core of exercises that involve all the major muscle groups and is designed to promote increased flexibility and stamina. Every client is given a booklet in which he or she can write down individualized, weekly homework goals and record the progress made. Specifically, the group aims to decrease the level of fear sur- rounding movement and activity and to increase the patient's level of physical activity and fitness. In addition, the exercises alert clients to posture problems and the benefits of good posture while improving the patient's body image.

Analgesic reduction and life-style restructuring.   Goal setting is the basic technique utilized for reducing the use of analgesics, and eliminating avoidance behavior over a wide range of activities: self-care work, social interac- tion, and leisure pursuits. A case for discontinuing analgesics is made by emphasizing the potential advantages of alternative methods of pain control. For those clients who are on medication, reassurance is given that a gradual reduc- tion rather than an immediate cut-off of medication is the aim. Long-term goals to change medication intake and life-style are then negotiated individually. Once formulated, these goals are specified in clear and specific language. In the group, each client's goals are shared and written on a large sheet of paper. The chart is referred to in future sessions so that individual progress is constantly monitored. Each week, individual homework tasks related to the goals are set and then checked the following week. Clients are warned about vicious cycles between avoidance behavior and certain cognitions. Clients often expect pain to increase on exposure to some feared stimuli, or, because of past experiences, they believe that they will be incapable of controlling pain. Exposure to the feared stimuli through graded tasks (that progress from less to more fearful) provides an invaluable way of testing and challenging these cognitions and thereby improving self-efficacy. The group itself acts as a powerful reinforcer once norms about task completion are established. Finally, issues of relapse are discussed.

Although there is some evidence (Pearce & Erskine, 1989) that group treatment of chronic pain is effective, more research is needed to establish this conclusion. Pearce and Erskine (1989) offer some indications and con- traindications for group treatment. The indications for groups are broad: the client should be an adult with significant chronic disability for which all con- ventional physical treatments have been tried and have failed. Excluded are individuals who have a history of severe mental illness, a terminal disease, or strong suspicions about the efficacy of psychologically based approaches.

Chronic-Pain Control in an Individual Format
Effective individual health counseling with chronic-pain clients can be done. Turk et al. (1983) and Holzman et al. (1986) give detailed accounts of individual

cognitive-behavioral and psychoeducational treatment of pain sufferers. Usually, six to ten individual weekly sessions are scheduled. These individual sessions with a health counselor can be scheduled back-to-back with sessions with a physical therapist, who focuses on the graded exercise component. Or the health counselor can incorporate both the cognitive-behavioral and psychoeducational interventions along with the exercise training.

Pearce and Erskine (1989) outline a typical program with six to ten weekly sessions. In the first session, psychoeducation is utilized to reframe pain problems, and the client is introduced to long-term goal setting and homework to monitor the intensity of pain and the tension level. The second session is devoted to relaxation training, analysis of homework, and identification of major stressors. Goal setting to increase exercise and physical activity levels is also addressed. In the third session, the patient begins to learn stress inoculation, and goals are adjusted for increased exercise and physical activity. In the fourth session, specific cognitive pain-control techniques are taught, practiced, and assigned for homework, and goals are set again to increase physical and social activities. In the fifth session, previously learned cognitive-control techniques are monitored and new ones taught. Once again, goal setting increases both physical and social activities. In session six, all techniques previously learned are reviewed. A discussion about relapse prevention and the importance of planning follow-up sessions are held. Finally, additional goal setting is established.

Relapse Prevention

To prevent relapse once treatment has been completed, Marlatt and Gordon (1985) recommend a series of techniques for use with clients. These include: (1) identification of individual high-risk situations; (2) development of coping skills for high-risk situations; (3) practice in coping with potential lapses; (4) development of cognitive coping strategies for use immediately after a lapse; and (5) development of a more balanced life-style. Discussion about preventing relapse is a usual part of the last stage of treatment. In their work with chronic-pain clients, Turk et al. (1983), convey to clients that there are likely to be times when the client's pain may, in fact, increase. If this occurs, the patient is urged not to panic or to "catastrophize." Instead, the health counselor encourages the patients to use a relapse-prevention strategy and the skills that have been worked on in treatment. This is particularly important to ensure that any setbacks are not viewed as failures of counseling or of the client him- or herself.

Turk and his colleagues believe that the discussion of relapse must be done in a delicate fashion. On the one hand, the counselor does not want to convey an expectancy of treatment failure but on the other hand, the counselor does want to anticipate and include in treatment the client's possible reaction to the likely recurrence of pain. Turk suggests two techniques. First, the counselor reanalyzes with the client reactions that have followed previous relapses. Second, the counselor can suggest to the client the types of thoughts and feelings that imaginary pain clients might have had upon reexperiencing pain

and what they might have done to cope with them. The counselor can mention that he or she does not know whether the client will have such feelings or thoughts but that it is worthwhile to determine the client's own possible reactions to similar situations.

Case Examples

Case 1

Ms. C is a 32-year-old married female referred by her neurologist for a combination of muscle contractions and migraine headaches. She reported that her headaches of 15 years' duration had recently worsened. Ms. C added that she was ingesting an alarming amount of narcotic analgesics and was fearful of becoming a drug addict.

She denied any difficulties in her personal life but expressed a great deal of puzzlement about the exacerbation of her pain symptoms over the past several months. She indicated that her physician recently placed her on Elavil, a tricyclic antidepressant, but she did not believe she was depressed, and she thought the Elavil was another form of analgesic. Upon further inquiry, it was learned that Ms. C had experienced two recent deaths in her extended family: her maternal grandmother and maternal aunt. She admitted that both had been very close to her. Also, she returned to university studies after several years' absence to finish a degree. Her husband was completing his last year of medical school. The C's had two children, aged 6 and 4, and Ms. C's return to school had unbalanced the family's homeostasis. She found herself facing a variety of conflicts. In addition to doing her schoolwork, she insisted on maintaining her household responsibilities. Although she found it increasingly difficult to meet all these obligations, she was unable to make any demands on her husband.

A mutual agreement about treatment was reached in which Ms. C's goals were to reduce and eliminate her medication under the guidance of her prescribing neurologist; to reduce her narcotic analgesics under the guidance of her prescribing physician; and to decrease family conflicts and increase her self-efficacy. Within six weeks, Ms. C had been weaned completely from her narcotic analgesics. At the same time, she made steady progress in relaxation training and in temperature-regulation biofeedback. Ms. C proved she was adept at learning self-regulatory skills, and she experienced considerable reduction in her headaches.

She also discovered, as a result of keeping her headache diary, that some of her headaches were strongly associated with interactions with her rather dominating husband and with the male instructor in one of her courses. Treatment to explore these problems and their similarities included specific assertiveness training that focused on dealing with her instructor. As this problem improved, Ms. C noted improvement in her relationship with her husband. Next, Ms. C was assisted in analyzing and changing her perfectionistic and unrealistic expectations for herself by cognitive reappraisal and the use of positive, coping self-statements. The counselor also pointed out that all the changes in her family situation and the deaths of her grandmother and aunt had

failed to make any impression on her. The counselor helped her to see that her headache pain masked much of the grief and unhappiness in her life. Subsequent sessions focused on other issues, and Ms. C was able to recall that her first migraine headache occurred in adolescence when one of her close friends died in a car accident.

In all, Ms. C met with the counselor for ten sessions and set up a follow-up appointment after three months. At the last contact, Ms. C described herself as being more in control of her headaches and better able to handle emotional upsets. Her headaches were much less frequent and, when present, were significantly reduced in duration and intensity. Her medication had been completely eliminated and, although she continued in her university courses, her expectations for her household responsibilities became more realistic.

Case 2

Mr. F is a 51-year-old construction worker who incurred a work-related injury involving his right hip and lower back for which he was awarded worker's compensation. A predictable pattern of seeking medical help, blaming physicians for their inability to cure him, and facing limited prospects of returning to work ensued. Subsequently, he neglected his family responsibilities, lost interest in sex, and began consuming large quantities of tranquilizers and narcotic analgesics to control his pain. He was irritable and impatient with his wife and children. He denied his problems by attempting to undertake tasks that could not possibly be completed, such as painting his house. His wife assumed the major responsibility for running the affairs of the family, which involved assuming a mediating role between her husband and the two children.

Mr. F began group treatment similar to that described by Pearce and Erskine (1989) and, by the seventh session, had not only learned cognitive skills to sufficiently distract himself from his pain but was also able to be weaned from all his addictive medications. After the group treatment, he followed through with the counselor's referral to the state Division of Vocational Rehabilitation (DVR). Subsequently, he began a job-retraining program, which would conceivably lead to employment in a less physically demanding job.

Prevention

There are a number of preventive measures that chronic-pain clients or potential chronic-pain clients can utilize. We will briefly discuss two: one for clients with back pain, and the other for those who suffer from migraine headaches.

Exercise is a major factor in the prevention of back pain. First, it can strengthen abdominal muscles and thus relieve excess demands on the back muscles. Any number of exercises, including graduated sit-ups, have been recommended. Most communities have hospitals or clinics that offer a "back college" for people to learn appropriate exercises, posture, and bending movements tailored to the back-pain sufferer. Orthopedic specialists and physical therapists can recommend such programs.

Exercise also can help relieve muscle tension when it develops in response to stress. Such exercise can consist of brisk walking, jogging, rope skipping, tennis playing, or other appropriate sports. When an individual feels tension mounting, simply walking about for 5 or 10 minutes—even indoors—can help considerably in relieving muscle tension.

Preventive measures for migraine sufferers are many. Often, modifying one or two aspects of a stressful life-style can result in reduced headache symptoms. Although there is much debate among headache experts regarding the importance of diet, many headache patients have benefited from restricting foods that contain tyramine and other substances that relax or contract blood vessels, as well as decreasing their caffeine intake. Clients can also be prescribed a "migraine diet" (Diamond & Ebstein, 1982). This diet recommends that no more than two caffeine-containing beverages be consumed per day. Smoking has also been considered a precipitating factor in headaches. Therefore, clients are encouraged to stop smoking or at least limit their intake to one-half pack of cigarettes a day. Specific foods that have been found to trigger migraine headaches are chocolate, aged cheese, onions, yogurt, canned figs, avocados, hotdogs, bacon, dry soup mixes, chicken livers, fermented sausage, Chinese food (which contains MSG), citrus fruits, tea, bananas, nuts, and alcohol. Diamond has found that these food substances tend to lower the migraine threshold and can precipitate a migraine attack. Clients are counseled to stay on this elimination diet for at least two months, and any improvement in the client's headache condition is an indication that at least some of the foods are implicated. The client can then add one of the restricted foods in intervals of two days to two weeks to note any improvement or deterioration in the pattern of the attacks.

Finally, headaches can be avoided by refraining from oversleeping on weekends. It seems that sleeping late increases levels of carbon dioxide in the blood, which decreases blood sugar levels and precipitates headaches.

An aspect of prevention not often recognized concerns events that turn otherwise short-term problems into long-term ones. The case of chronic back pain is such an example. For back-pain sufferers, both medical-care strategies and public policies have operated to make the condition persist longer than need be the case. As Fordyce (1985) points out, the striking increase in long-term and permanent disability as a result of Social Security Disability Insurance (SSDI) came into being in the mid-1950s. Although these benefits were not intended to be automatic or to continue indefinitely, once awarded, these benefits have not often been terminated. Fordyce notes that the rate of awards of SSDI for back pain is increasing at a rate of more than ten times the growth of our population. The award rate also indicates that eligibility for wage replacement, duration of benefits, and percentage of wages replaced all seem to encourage the persistence of the disability.

In short, public policy and those physicians who make disability determinations appear to have unwittingly reinforced chronic-illness behavior as well as the disincentive to return to normal functioning at home, in relationships, and on the job. A systematic approach to prevention of chronic pain would truly call for a reevaluation of the SSDI criteria.

Summary

This chapter reviewed the biopsychosocial factors involved in the experience of chronic pain. It described various theories and emphasized that the gate-control theory of pain is a biopsychosocial formulation. Several biological, psychological, and social—particularly behavioral—methods of assessment of chronic pain were described, as were several biological, psychological, and social intervention methods. Intervention strategies for both the group and individual treatment of chronic pain conditions were elaborated. A discussion of relapse and adherence was followed by case examples involving the two most common forms of chronic pain: headache and back pain. A section on prevention measures with chronic pain completed this chapter, with a reference to a specific public policy that actually reinforces rather than prevents chronic pain. In the following section are resources for further study and references.

Resources

Organization

The National Migraine Foundation is an organization for laypersons that sponsors research in headaches and serves as a research center. It publishes a quarterly newsletter that provides articles of interest for the headache sufferer. The address is 5252 N. Western Avenue, Chicago, IL 62625.

Publications: Professional References

- Turk, D. C., Meichenbaum, D. H., & Genest, M. (1983). *Pain and behavioral medicine: A cognitive-behavioral approach.* New York: Guilford. Considered the basic reference for psychological clinicians, this book ably reviews the issues in pain and pain management and emphasizes the cognitive-behavioral perspective in the assessment and intervention of pain in various treatment formats and settings.
- Blanchard, E. B., & Andrasik, F. (1985). *Management of chronic headaches: A psychological approach.* New York: Pergamon Press. This short book, in the popular and useful "Psychology Practicioner Guidebooks" series, offers a step-by-step approach to the assessment and management of common headache presentations from a cognitive-behavioral perspective. The section on biofeedback is excellent. Both authors have extensive experience working in pain and headache clinics.
- Diamond, S., & Dalessio, D. J. (1987). *The practicing physician's approach to headaches.* (5th ed.). Baltimore: Williams & Wilkins. Though the title suggests that this book is for physicians or is basically medical in orientation, it is not. Health counselors will find this reference indispensable, as the authors achieve an expert and practical synthesis of biological and psychological treatments. Dr. Diamond is perhaps the leading medical expert on headaches, and the book is a best-seller.
- Melzak, R., & Wall, P. D. (1982). *The challenge of pain.* New York: Basic Books. The authors offer a very readable account of the biopsychosocial aspects of pain, highlighting their gate-control theory. A classic book in the field.

Publications: Patient Education

- Diamond, S., & Epstein, M. F. (1982). *Coping with your headaches.* Madison, CT: International Universities Press. Dr. Diamond is a preeminent medical headache specialist, and this book is part of the patient education program at the world famous Diamond Headache Clinic. This book is very readable and comprehensive, from analgesics, biofeedback, diet, and life-style to temperature training.
- Bresler, D., & Trubo, R. (1986). *Free yourself from pain.* New York: Fireside Press. Readily available in bookstores and libraries, this book was first published in 1981 and offers the patient an accurate view of the modern pain clinic—the UCLA Pain Clinic—and numerous self-management methods that the patient can incorporate into a pain-free life-style.

References

ANDERSON, K., Bradley, L., Young, L. et al. (1985). Rheumatoid arthritis: Review of psychological factors related to etiology, effects, and treatments. *Psychological Bulletin, 98,* 358–387.

BLACKWELL, B. (1989). Chronic pain. In H. Kaplan, & B. Sadock (Eds.), *Comprehensive textbooks of psychiatry* (5th ed.). Baltimore: Williams & Wilkins.

BLACKWELL, B., Galbraith, H., & Dahl, D. (1984). Chronic pain management. *Hospital and Community Psychiatry, 35,* 999–1008.

BLANCHARD, E. G., & Andrasik, F. (1985). *Management of chronic headaches: A psychological approach.* New York: Pergamon Press.

BLUMER, D., & Heilbronn, M. (1982). Chronic pain as a variant of depressive disease: The pain-prone patient. *Journal of Nervous and Mental Disorders, 170,* 381–406.

CHAPMAN, C., Cassey, K., Dubner, R. et al. (1985). Pain measurement: An overview. *Pain, 22,* 1–31.

DIAMOND, S., & Ebstein, M. (1982). *Coping with your headache.* Madison, CT: International Universities Press.

ENGEL, G. (1959). Psychogenic pain and the pain-prone patient. *American Journal of Medicine, 26,* 899–918.

FORDYCE, W. E. (1985). Back pain, compensation, and public policy. In J. Rosen, & L. Solomon (Eds.), *Prevention in Health Psychology.* Hanover, VT: University Press of New England.

HOLZMAN, A., Turk, D., & Kerns, R. (1986). The cognitive-behavioral approach to the management of chronic pain. In A. Holzman, & D. Turk (Eds.), *Pain management: A handbook of psychological treatment approaches.* New York: Pergamon Press.

HULT, L. (1954). The Munkfors investigation. *Acta Orthopedia Scandinavia, 42,* 174–175.

JOHNSON, A. (1978). *The problem claim: An approach to early identification.* Dept. of Labor and Industries, State of Washington.

KAROLY, P., & Jensen, M. (1987). *Multimethod assessment of chronic pain.* New York: Pergamon Press.

MARLATT, G., & Gordon, J. (1985). *Relapse prevention.* New York: Guilford Press.

MELZACK, R. (1975). The McGill Pain Questionnaire: Major properties and scoring methods. *Pain, 1,* 277–299.

MELZACK, R., & Wall, P. (1965). Pain mechanisms: A new theory. *Science, 150,* 971–979.

MELZACK, R., & Wall, P. (1982). *The challenge of pain.* New York: Basic Books.

PEARCE, S., & Erskine, A. (1989). Chronic pain. In S. Pearce, & J. Wardle (Eds.), *The practice of behavioral medicine.* Oxford: BPS Books/Oxford University Press.

SANDERS, S. (1985). Chronic pain: Conceptualization and epidemiology. *Annals of Behavioral Medicine, 7,* 3–5.

STERNBACH, R. A. (1968). *Pain: A psychophysiological analysis.* New York: Academic Press.

SVENNSON, H., & Anderson, G. (1982). Low back pain in 40–47-year-old men: Frequency of

occurrence and impact on medical services. *Scandinavian Journal of Rehabilitation Medicine, 14,* 47–53.

TURK, D., & Holzman, A. (1986). Commonalities among psychological approaches in the treatment of chronic pain: Specifying the meta-constructs. In A. Holzman, & D. Turk (Eds.), *Pain management: A handbook of psychological approaches.* New York: Pergamon Press.

TURK, D., Meichenbaum, P., & Genest, M. (1983). *Pain and behavioral medicine: A cognitive-behavioral perspective.* New York: Guilford.

WEISENBERG, M. (1977). Pain and pain control. *Psychological Bulletin, 84,* 1008–1044.

WINTERS, R. (1985). Behavioral approaches to pain. In N. Schneidmen, & J. Tapp (Eds.), *Behavioral medicine: The biopsychosocial approach.* Hillsdale, NJ: Erlbaum.

10

Coping with Illness

In the midst of winter I finally learned that there is within me an invincible summer.

Albert Camus

Programs designed to promote health and prevent illness have become more and more prevalent in recent years. An increasing variety of strategies has been implemented, encouraging people to engage in health-protective behaviors and training them in the skills they need to achieve wellness. The resulting life-style changes have helped countless individuals maintain their health and reduce their risk for the development of serious health problems.

Reality tells us, however, that everyone is subject to illness at some time in his or her life. Whether the illness is chronic or acute, mild or life-threatening, some degree of adaptation has to occur. The general goals of health counseling for people faced with illness include the following:

- Helping individuals and their families cope with illness-related crisis.
- Helping people cope with anxiety-provoking medical treatments.
- Helping people adhere to medical regimens that may require lifelong behavioral changes.
- Helping social systems adapt to the special needs of people with health problems.
- Working to prevent or minimize the long-term effects of illness.

A biopsychosocial approach can help us achieve these goals.

Biopsychosocial Factors in Coping with Illness

Each biological illness affects and is affected by psychological and social factors. The individual's psychosocial well-being may be challenged—even jeopardized—by his or her physical illness. At the same time, the person's ability to mobilize personal and social resources can have major implications for his or her success in combatting or coping with the disease or disability.

The client dealing with an illness or disability faces a number of tasks that must be performed effectively for adaptation to occur (Moos & Tsu, 1977). First, the individual must cope with the physical aspects of the health problem. He or she may have to deal with pain, discomfort, or disability, while at the same time being forced to make personal and social adaptations to a major life change. Medical treatments may also be invasive or uncomfortable, requiring still more adaptive efforts. The individual's psychological well-being must be preserved; emotional balance and a new, but satisfactory, self-image have to be sought. While these intrapersonal tasks are being addressed, new interpersonal challenges develop. The individual must forge new relationships and accept the reality of changes in the existing social network. Health-care professionals become a new part of the social network, and communication concerning medical issues become a necessity. Finally, some clients need to cope with the loss of good health, the loss of physical abilities, and—probably most importantly—the loss of a sense of certainty about the future.

The interaction of biological, psychological, and social factors has a major impact on the process of adaptation, whether the problem being faced is acute or chronic. The sudden onset of an illness may throw an individual into a crisis situation, requiring new ways of behaving and altered perceptions of the world.

His or her success in coping with this crisis can have long-term implications for both physical and mental health. Focusing attention narrowly on the physical aspects of the newly diagnosed disease, without equally intense regard for psychological and social variables, may jeopardize the individual's stabilization or recovery.

Coping with a chronic illness is an equally complex challenge. An illness is considered chronic if it involves some type of long-term disability that is irreversible. The health problem can be stabilized and controlled, but the affected individual cannot expect to return to the level of health enjoyed before the onset of the illness. Chronic illnesses are becoming more and more widespread in today's society. Improvements in medical care bear at least some of the responsibility for this phenomenon.

> Better emergency treatments allow many patients to now survive the initial critical stages of acute illnesses or trauma (e.g., stroke, accident, or heart attack). Patients live with the effects of these acute illnesses and trauma and thus face chronic illness from which they will never recover. . . . Thus better medical care, coupled with demographic trends that produce an increase in the elderly population, contributes to an increase in chronic illness (Friedman & DiMatteo, 1989, p. 222).

In addition to helping people survive the acute phases of illnesses, improvements in medical techniques also tend to prolong the lives of individuals with chronic diseases so that they need to cope with their conditions for longer periods of time than was true in the past (Kendall & Turk, 1984). Now, millions of people find themselves trying to cope with unrelenting health problems. Among the special problems they face (Friedman & DiMatteo, 1989) are the need to be vigilant in checking for signs that medical problems may reappear or accelerate; the need to manage treatment regimens that may be complex, time consuming, uncomfortable, and demanding; the need to control symptoms; and the need to manage social relationships that have been jeopardized by the uncertainty of the prognosis and the behavioral limitations brought on by the illness. Because the individual's experience of the illness is as salient as the physical symptoms, "the biopsychosocial model proposes that medical diagnosis should *always* consider the interaction of biological, psychological, and social factors in order to assess a person's health and to make recommendations for treatment" (Schwartz, 1982, p. 1047).

Assessment

If we are to help people cope effectively with illness, we need to recognize that the medical examination and the diagnosis are only the first steps in assessment. Successful treatment planning requires a clear understanding of the kinds of personal, behavioral, and social factors that might affect the client's success in managing the illness and limiting its effects. Williamson, Davis, and Prather (1988) suggest several assessment techniques that can help in treatment planning for people affected by certain health disorders.

For example, behavioral assessment has obvious relevance for clients with

coronary heart disease. Behavioral risk factors, including the Type A behavior pattern and such life-style-related behaviors as eating habits, exercise regimen, and smoking and drinking behaviors, play a part in the origins and control of heart disease. Once a medical diagnosis has been made, procedures for assessing these behavioral factors can be implemented. The Type A personality profile, which involves time urgency, aggressiveness, hostility, competitiveness, and restlessness, can be measured through use of a structured interview (Rosenman et al., 1964), the Jenkins Activity Survey (Jenkins, Rosenman, & Friedman, 1967), or the Framingham Type A Scale (Haynes, Feinleib, Levine, Scotch, & Kannel, 1980). These data, along with information regarding the client's participation in health-risk activities, can help in treatment planning by identifying behaviors that should be targeted for change.

Personality and behavioral factors may also affect outcomes for cancer patients, so interviews and inventories that measure psychological characteristics and emotional states can be useful. Because the cancer diagnosis is very stressful and because the side effects of its treatments are often severe, a number of psychological and physiological symptoms can appear. The Psychological Adjustment to Cancer Scale (DiClemente & Temoshok, 1986), the Health Survey (Frank-Stromborg & Wright, 1984), and symptom checklists (McCorkle & Young, 1978) can give some indication of the physical and psychosocial changes associated with the cancer diagnosis.

Williamson and his colleagues cite asthma as an additional example of a disease with strong psychosocial components. Careful assessment can help identify the role of emotional factors in precipitating or exacerbating attacks and pinpoint the psychological effects of symptoms. The Asthma Symptom Checklist (Kinsman, Dahlem, Spector, & Staudenmayer, 1977) measures subjective reports of asthmatic symptomatology, and the Asthma Problem Behavior Checklist (APBC) (Creer, Marion, & Creer, 1983) identifies specific behavior problems that may exacerbate asthma and that should be addressed. The APBC also illuminates issues related to family systems, which appear to play a major role in affecting the severity of the disease.

Assessment Tools

Efforts to develop specialized, disease-specific assessment tools continue. Just as promising, however, are efforts to develop and validate instruments that address more general health issues. Among the instruments that can be helpful in a biopsychosocial assessment are the following.

Health and Daily Living Form (Moos, Cronkite, Billings, & Finney, 1984).   The HDL Form is a 200-item instrument that can be self- or interviewer-administered. It assesses health-related functioning, social functioning and resources, family functioning and home environment, children's health and functioning, life-change events, and coping responses. It is one of the few instruments that takes life circumstances and events outside of the treatment milieu into account.

Psychosocial Adjustment to Illness Scale (Derogatis, 1977). The PAIS self-report assesses the client's adjustment to his or her illness. The instrument yields a score for overall adjustment to the illness as well as subscores in several related domains.

Health Locus of Control Inventory (Wallston, Wallston, & Devellis, 1978). The Health Locus of Control Inventory assesses the individual's attributions concerning health outcomes. Given the importance of the cognitive factor of control in individual health behaviors, this inventory can help the counselor anticipate problems in the client's progress.

Millon Behavioral Health Inventory (Millon, Green, & Meagher, 1982). The MBHI was designed for use with clients who are dealing with medical problems. This self-administered instrument yields scores on a number of variables associated with health behaviors and outcomes. Eight scales identify coping styles, six measure the existence of psychosocial stressors associated with illness, and six assess emotional factors that might be associated with psychosomatic illnesses or complications. The scales were designed to assess the presence of factors that are shown by research to relate to health outcomes (such as chronic tension, recent stress, pre-illness pessimism, social alienation). Several scales were designed for use with patients diagnosed with allergy, gastrointestinal problems, or cardiovascular disease. These scales compare the client's responses with those of patients whose illnesses have been complicated by psychosocial factors or whose course of treatment was unsatisfactory.

Symptom Check List-90 (revised) (Derogatis et al., 1983). This 90-item check list has been used with patients in medical settings, although it was originally designed for use with psychiatric patients. Clients are asked to record the degree of difficulty they currently feel regarding each problem.

The use of these assessment instruments, as well as others that might focus more directly on an individual client's needs, can lead the way toward treatment planning that addresses issues beyond the medical diagnosis. Ideally, patient evaluation in any medical setting should take into account personal and environmental dimensions as well as biological factors (Schwartz, 1982).

Treatment Issues and Strategies

A client who is coping with an illness may need assistance in making emotional, behavioral, and social adaptations. Health-counseling strategies can address each of these needs, whether services are provided in a medical setting or in the context of ongoing personal counseling. In the sections that follow, we review some promising approaches and discuss some pressing issues related to illness. It is, of course, far beyond the scope of this chapter to address any more than a small sampling of the health problems with which people are forced to cope in

contemporary society. For this reason, we will use specific illnesses only as examples to illustrate various types of intervention.

Dealing with Psychological Reactions to Illness

The onset of serious illness represents one of the most disruptive crises an individual can endure. When an illness has been diagnosed, the client must ready himself or herself to cope with what may be a staggering number of separate problems. Among the many nagging questions—some conscious and some unconscious—for which the client must seek answers are the following:

• Will I be completely incapacitated?
• Do I face a life of pain?
• Will I be able to make the changes that the doctor has said I have to make?
• Will I have to be dependent on others to take care of me?
• What will this mean for my family and my relationships with family members?
• Can I still see myself as a sexual being?
• How will this affect my relationships with friends and colleagues?
• Will I be able to participate in any kind of recreation?
• Will I have to give up my job or my career plans?
• Will my family and I be wiped out financially?
• Will I be completely isolated?
• Is this my fault?
• Is there a God?
• Will I live?

These questions become particularly intense in the context of the anxiety and fear brought about by diagnosis of a life-threatening illness. Consider, as an example, the plight of the individual whose illness has been diagnosed as Acquired Immune Deficiency Syndrome (AIDS).

Persons with AIDS (PWAs) can be expected to go through stages of adaptation that are similar to those experienced by people who have received diagnoses of other life-threatening illnesses (Macks & Turner, 1986; Mandel, 1986; Mejta, 1987). At the earliest stage, when the diagnosis is first received, a client may respond with denial or with such strong emotions as shock, anxiety, depression, fear, and anger. As the reality of the diagnosis becomes engrained in the person's perceptions, he or she may continue to experience these emotions and may also develop feelings of worthlessness, self-devaluation, social withdrawal, and isolation; suicidal ideation may intensify. As the individual moves toward an acceptance of the diagnosis, he or she might become ready to take more responsibility for participation in decisions and behaviors related to treatment. If the PWA is able to deal with fears and concerns about impending death, he or she can make emotional and practical preparations.

But not all clients move in an orderly way through these stages. Recognizing the existence of the stages can help the counselor become aware of the individual client's issues. Often, however, clients move in and out of stages in reaction to changes in symptoms or treatments (Mejta, 1987).

The adjustment of a client diagnosed with AIDS is further complicated by the effects of prejudice, discrimination, and blame. The phenomenon of blam-

ing the victim for bad outcomes in his or her life is exacerbated by our society's view of people who have AIDS.

> This tendency, prodded by panic, fear, and misinformation about AIDS and already existing prejudices toward groups particularly at risk for contracting AIDS, is especially strong when attributing responsibility or blame for contracting AIDS. Furthermore, it lays the groundwork for unfounded prejudices and discriminatory behaviors toward those with or at risk for AIDS. The stress already experienced by persons at risk or with AIDS is exacerbated by society's reactions toward them (Mejta, 1987, p. 2).

Thus, people may be denied social support at the time in their lives when they need it most. They may be targets of prejudice and irrational hatred at the point when their self-esteem is at its lowest point. They may be forced to cope with such practical problems as job discrimination and lack of funds for medical treatment at the very time when their energy should be focused most directly on self-care.

Coping processes are also complex and challenging for HIV-positive persons. People who have been tested and whose blood shows antibodies to the human immunodeficiency virus (HIV) may be as highly stressed as PWAs.

> This seems to be a result of feeling like one may be a walking time bomb—knowing one is not completely healthy and yet not having any serious signs of illness. People who are HIV-positive carry similar stressors to people with AIDS, yet they must also live with the uncertainty of it—when and how their infection will progress (Cramer, 1989, p. 63).

Counseling interventions for clients who have been diagnosed with AIDS or whose blood tests have shown them to be HIV positive should include helping them come to terms with the diagnosis and its meaning, helping them improve the quality of their lives, and helping them feel more in control of their lives and their illness (Mejta, 1987; Namir, 1986).

> Psychological interventions should be sensitive to the individual's feelings, reactions, and experiences related to the AIDS diagnosis, the process of adjusting to it, and self-reported concerns and needs. Typically, both emotional and practical support is needed (Mejta, 1987, p. 5).

Assisting clients with the illness crisis may involve helping them sort out the kinds of coping mechanisms that are most likely to be useful. Active, problem-focused coping behaviors are generally considered to be healthier than passive efforts that focus on emotional adaptation or distancing from the problem. In fact, however, when situations are beyond an individual's control, denial or resignation may be healthy options. The counselor has to be sensitive to the client's perceptions of the situation, offering support for the individual's efforts to make the decisions affecting his or her own destiny. Whether the client's need is for practical problem-solving assistance or for an opportunity to vent emotion, the counselor needs to be able to adapt.

Coping with Aversive Medical Procedures
Clients also vary in the kinds of coping styles they use to deal with such anxiety-provoking situations as surgery or other aversive medical procedures.

These variations are associated both with personality differences and with differences in the demands of a particular situation. Some patients use a vigilant coping style, seeking information and taking active steps to maintain control of the situation, while others use an avoidant style in their efforts to lower their anxiety. Which of these coping styles is more adaptive may depend on the nature of the situation.

> Presumably, non-anxious avoidant patients are naturally using strategies related to cognitive distraction, which facilitate their adaptation to surgery. . . . Whether this natural style is beneficial or detrimental may depend on whether distraction or related avoidant methods hold up during or after the actual stressful event. We would suggest that with low level or slowly rising pain, or when other anxiety-elevating stimuli are not too intrusive, this strategy is indeed an effective one. Generally speaking, a vigilant or monitoring style would be clearly preferable only where aversive stimuli or external threats cannot be ignored, either because they are too intense or because the threat demands some action requiring rehearsal or planning (Mathews & Ridgeway, 1984, p. 256).

The success of the health-counseling process depends on the counselor's sensitivity to the needs and coping styles of the individual client. Even given this assumption, however, the counselor can develop general strategies to help clients prepare for medical procedures.

Mathews and Ridgeway (1984) reviewed a number of experimental studies that focused on the effects of processes used to help patients prepare psychologically for surgery. The types of *preparation* measured were categorized as (1) procedural information (describing pre- and postoperative procedures, whether to reassure or to forewarn the individual), (2) sensation information (telling patients what they are likely to feel), (3) behavioral instructions (telling patients what they should do after surgery or during a medical procedure in order to facilitate recovery), (4) modeling (providing information through methods such as filmed models), (5) relaxation (using hypnosis or other methods so the patient can reduce anxiety and cope with pain), and (6) cognitive coping training (encouraging the client to identify fears or worries and counter them with positive self-statements). The measures used to assess *recovery* included (1) the patient's performance of such recovery-relevant behaviors as ambulation, (2) clinicians' ratings of recovery or adjustment, (3) length of stay from surgery to discharge, (4) amounts of analgesics and other medications, (5) self-reported mood, (6) self-reported pain, and (7) physical indices, including medical complications.

This meta-analysis led Mathews and Ridgeway to state that psychological preparation for surgery was clearly associated with positive outcomes in terms of the recovery variables measured. Despite some individual differences, such as the likelihood that patients already using avoidant coping styles with some success might find unsought information disruptive, they were able to generalize that "the evidence clearly favors the efficacy of sensation information, behavioral instructions (including relaxation), and cognitive coping methods in promoting recovery" (Mathews & Ridgeway, 1984, p. 256). Cognitive strategies were found to be most consistently effective, but the successful methods probably interact with one another. Cognitive methods may help give the client a

sense of the possibility of control, which in turn motivates him or her to use relaxation methods and follow other behavioral instructions. Sensation information, too, may enhance patients' sense of control by helping them avoid the anxiety and alarm associated with unexpected sensations; again, cognitive preparation may play an important role.

Some differences exist between the outcomes sought from preparatory strategies for surgery and the results desired when clients are being prepared for other procedures. Although other medical procedures may be painful or aversive, "physical recovery variables are less relevant and the main targets of psychological intervention are the reduction of anxiety during the procedure itself and facilitation of the patient's active cooperation" (Mathews & Ridgeway, 1984, p. 248). Cognitive-behavioral strategies have proven equally successful in achieving these goals.

For example, Kendall, Williams, Pechacek, Graham, Shisslak, and Herzoff (1979) reported on the use of cognitive-behavioral strategies in preparing patients for cardiac catheterization. Kendall and his associates compared the effectiveness of a cognitive-behavioral treatment and a patient-education treatment for reducing the stress of patients undergoing this diagnostic procedure. Their design also included the use of two control groups: one that received attention and one that was treated in accordance with current conditions. The cognitive-behavioral strategy used was an adaptation of stress inoculation (Meichenbaum, 1985), which involves helping people deal with stressful situations through preparation, skills training, and application and practice. Kendall and his colleagues trained cardiac catheterization patients to identify aspects of the situation that they found stressful and identify and apply the cognitive coping strategies that they found most helpful in lessening their anxiety. Cognitive and behavioral coping techniques were practiced in response to stress cues. The results of the study indicated that the peoople who received this cognitive-behavioral intervention adjusted to the procedure more effectively than did patients in any of the other groups.

> Physicians and technicians independently rated the patients' behaviors during catheterization, and these ratings indicated that the patients receiving the cognitive-behavioral treatment were best adjusted—that is, least tense, least anxious, most comfortable. . . . The patient education group was rated as better adjusted than the two control groups but significantly less well adjusted than the cognitive-behavioral group (Kendall & Turk, 1984, p. 399).

Evidence has also been accumulating to indicate that cognitive and behavioral strategies may also be useful in preparing people for other medical procedures, including endoscopy, sigmoidoscopy, electromyography, and dental surgery (Caplan, 1982, p. 187).

Treatment Adherence Issues

One of the most important functions of health counseling is to help clients develop the kinds of self-management skills that they can use to work toward their own health goals. When clients are forced to cope with illness, they frequently need to engage in new behaviors to stabilize their condition or move

toward optimal health. Chronic illnesses provide a special challenge in this regard, forcing clients first to learn new health-oriented behaviors and then permanently integrate these behaviors into their life-styles. Although treatment regimens may be clearly delineated, clients are affected by a number of factors that can complicate their behavior-change attempts. For the counselor, the effort to encourage clients to adhere to treatment regimens can be frustrating.

Adherence to medical regimens involves such behaviors as staying in treatment programs, keeping appointments, taking medication as prescribed, making suggested life-style changes, performing home-based therapies correctly, and avoiding health-risk behaviors (Meichenbaum & Turk, 1987).

People jeopardize their health, their recovery, and even their lives by failing to adhere to medical advice concerning appropriate behaviors; yet nonadherence is normative. Approximately one-third to one-half of all medical patients fail to follow through on the regimens that have been prescribed for them (Stone, 1979; Meichenbaum & Turk, 1987), and levels of adherence are even poorer for certain medical problems. The people who are most likely to follow through on recommended behaviors are individuals whose illnesses are serious and acute and who show distressing, overt symptoms. Clients whose illnesses are chronic and of long duration show very low adherence rates, as do individuals whose treatment regimens are complex. For instance, Stone (1979) cited studies showing that patients whose diabetes had lasted for more than twenty years had much higher rates of dosage errors than patients whose diabetes had been diagnosed less than five years earlier. Furthermore, the number of dosage errors made by diabetes patients increased with the number of different drugs involved. Adherence rates are lowest when no symptoms are present, especially when regimens are essentially preventive.

Although the nature of the illness and the form its treatment takes are important factors that affect adherence, additional variables also come into play, including the individual's beliefs about the threat posed by noncompliance and the benefits of adherence (Janz & Becker, 1984), the nature of the relationship between the individual and the health-care provider (Stone, 1979), and the client's perceptions concerning the quality of the care provided by the clinical setting.

Meichenbaum and Turk (1987) suggest that there are a number of possible reasons for nonadherence. Sometimes, clients really do not understand what they are supposed to do. Frequently, they lack the skills, resources, or self-confidence needed to carry out the treatment protocol. They may believe that the regimen is too demanding, too difficult, or too unpleasant to carry out. They may not think that carrying out the required behaviors will make enough difference to make the effort worthwhile. Sometimes, the problem lies in the relationship between the client and the helper or in shortcomings of the health care system.

Traditionally, medical transactions have been based on the assumption that it is the role of the physician to decide the course of treatment, and it is the role of the client to take the responsibility for complying. This type of transaction has been ineffective in assuring compliance. In fact, "physicians systematically overestimate the extent to which their patients adhere to their recom-

mendations" (Stone, 1979, p. 48). Health counseling can play an important role as an adjunct to the medical transaction. Clients' performance of behaviors that conform to medical recommendations can be improved through psychoeducational and counseling approaches designed to solidify self-management.

One important aspect of a self-management approach is recognition of the client's role in determining the goals and methods of the treatment. Although health-care professionals may have expert knowledge of the positive and negative aspects of various regimens, they are not necessarily aware of the individual client's values and priorities. Selection of a regimen to which a client can be expected to adhere depends on a combination of the helper's knowledge about the illness and its treatment and the client's self-knowledge.

> Rational selection of a course of treatment requires that the patient take (and the health professional give) some responsibility when the treatment course is being selected. The health care professional must be willing to take advice from the patient, who, after all, is the only person who really knows what manner of treatment he or she will be able and willing to follow (Friedman & DiMatteo, 1989, p. 98).

If the client is to be held responsible for carrying out a course of action, he or she must be involved in selecting it. Although involving the client in negotiating the goals and methods of the regimen is time consuming, this involvement increases the likelihood of adherence far beyond what could be expected if the client were simply instructed in or advised about appropriate behaviors.

The clients' commitment to a health-enhancing regimen is an important first step in their long-term adherence. Ideally, clients can develop intervention plans that they can use to develop new, health-oriented behaviors. And once clients have set realistic behavioral goals, they can learn to monitor their performance of these health-oriented activities. A behavioral contract—either with others or with themselves—can be used by clients to identify desired levels of performance and schedule personally designed reinforcements. Because individuals differ in the kinds of rewards they find reinforcing, each client needs to identify his or her own reinforcers. Reinforcement can then be made contingent on completion of the specific activity as contracted. As this plan is implemented, clients can continue to maintain careful records so that improvements in their performance levels can be identified. At the same time that clients maintain their reinforcement schedules, they can also attempt to identify and manipulate the internal and environmental cues that are associated with their health-oriented behaviors. This approach establishes a collaborative relationship between client and counselor, with the counselor's efforts concentrated on (1) helping the client select realistic and measurable goals, (2) coaching the client in his or her use of self-management techniques, (3) supporting the client's efforts, and (4) providing feedback to ensure that prescribed behaviors are implemented correctly.

The sense of self-efficacy that accompanies self-management training increases the likelihood of long-term adherence. Self-efficacy is also enhanced by training in the specific skills that are associated with the practice of health-associated behaviors. Carrying out new behaviors may require the develop-

ment of skills that have not previously been part of the individual's repertoire. Informing a client about the need to change behaviors does not encourage adherence unless the individual has specific knowledge about the new behaviors, possesses the skill to implement the behaviors, and believes in his or her ability to carry out the recommended action. The client's ability to adhere to treatments may depend on his or her opportunity to participate in carefully designed training sessions. If these sessions are carried out in group settings, the client may enjoy the added benefit of mutual support.

Cardiac rehabilitation provides a good example of the importance of a behavioral self-management approach. People who are recovering from myocardial infarction (MI) are faced with the need to make major life-style changes at the same time that they are trying to cope with the stress of their illness. If rehabilitation is to be successful and recurrences prevented, patients need to: (1) change such health-risk behaviors as smoking, high-cholesterol diet, and lack of physical activity; (2) alter Type A behavioral patterns; and (3) learn how to manage stress without eliciting heightened cardiovascular responses (Langosch, 1984). Several projects have demonstrated success in bringing about behavioral changes and thereby avoiding multiple acute episodes. For instance, the Recurrent Coronary Prevention Project (Thoresen & Eagleston, 1985) focused on altering Type A behavioral responses through group interventions using discussion, modeling, relaxation training, and practice. Clients learned how to alter the cognitions, behaviors, and environmental and physiological factors associated with the Type A personality.

> In the cognitive area, treatment covered such topics as self-instructional training, evaluation of basic beliefs, active listening skills, and mental relaxation. Behaviorally, participants learned to alter certain speech patterns (such as interrupting others), psychomotor actions (such as excessive or abrupt emphatic gesturing), and other physical activities (such as reducing hurried walking [and] fast eating, and increasing smiling and complimentary comments). . . . The basics of social problem solving were used to help participants alter stressful environmental factors, such as revising work routines cooperatively with a supervisor or scheduling time to practice relaxation. Physiologically, participants were informed how biochemical processes appear to function in chronic stress reactions. . . . The feelings of anger, irritation, aggravation, and impatience . . . were equated with potential increases in a variety of biochemical and cardiovascular variables (Thoresen & Eagleston, 1985, pp. 60–61).

These interventions were found to have a positive impact on rehabilitation. Participants had significantly fewer repeat infarctions than did those in a control group. The best results in terms of recurrence were shown by the clients who had shown the most substantial changes in their behaviors.

Razin (1984) also reported good results for a cardiac stress-management training program that focused on psychosocial rehabilitation for a group of post–MI patients. The program's weekly sessions included: (1) discussion of risk factors and their modifiability; (2) progressive relaxation training; (3) cognitive-behavioral approaches to stress management, including the use of stress diaries and "self-talk" practice; (4) work on modification of Type A behaviors, including

the use of videotapes to provide feedback on individual behaviors; and (5) anger-management training. Favorable results were reported for behavioral, physiological, and self-report measures.

An interesting aspect of Razin's study was the active involvement of spouses who participated with the patients in the training program. This approach reflects an important trend in the health field. Regardless of the particular disease or disability being addressed, family members are always deeply affected. Any attempt to help an individual cope with illness brings with it the need to work with his or her family as well.

Illness and the Family

Of course, the illness of a family member has a major impact on the family unit as a whole.

> Few health professionals or family scholars challenge the proposition that illness or impairment in a family member has adverse effects on family functioning. Most agree that families of ill people generally function more poorly than families in which all the members are healthy. With the onset of an illness, the family's social life contracts and becomes primarily family centered. Within this circumscribed existence, the patient often becomes the focus of the family, with other family members forced into the background. . . . The more severe and long lasting the illness or impairment, the greater the potential for family disruption (Turk & Kerns, 1985, p. 15).

Illness can be highly disruptive to a family's functioning, but many families do manage to cope with this stress and even become more cohesive in the process. Families that have shown a general ability to function well can continue to do so even in the wake of a serious health crisis. A family that is functioning effectively can cope with the disruption of illness and, at the same time, play an important role in supporting and assisting the affected family member. Family-focused interventions should have a dual emphasis: (1) supporting and strengthening family units as a means for enhancing the adaptation of the individual patient, and (2) helping the family system as a whole maintain its functionality despite illness-related crises or challenges. Most efforts have tended to focus on the family's role in helping the affected individual achieve health stabilization or improvement.

A good example of a chronic illness that can act as a major family stressor is diabetes mellitus.

> Despite medical advances, following the diagnosis of diabetes the patient and family still must adapt to a radically altered life. There are continuing stresses such as living with the foreboding of a shortened life span for the patient; the specter of severe complications that may result in coronary disease, blindness, stroke, amputation, or other major physical handicaps; apprehension over unpredictable occurrence of insulin reactions or life-threatening crises related to ketoacidosis; and pervasive concern over ability to handle these crises. At best, there are daily problems of fitting a personal and family lifestyle around monitoring and regulating the diet, exercise, and medication of the diabetic patient (Hamburg, Elliott, & Parron, 1982, p. 147).

The family as a whole must make major adaptations, as would be the case with any serious illness. In the case of diabetes, an additional challenge is created by the urgent need for adherence to a complicated medical regimen involving a high degree of self-care. The individual affected with this disease has major health-related tasks to perform, including careful, long-term self-assessment and adherence to self-administered medical regimens that can be complex. "The diabetic patient really needs to be his or her own physician" (Hendrick, 1985, p. 521). For an affected individual, compliance to treatment may involve monitoring blood sugar levels; making decisions concerning insulin injections; using oral medications; and maintaining such ongoing health behaviors as a carefully regulated diet, a weight-control regimen, and an exercise program. The family's success in adapting to the challenges of the disease may have a major effect on the individual's success in self-treatment.

The family plays an especially important role in adherence for children.

> The family is an important ingredient in treatment. If the diabetic's parents are educated about the disease, offer help and support, encourage independence, stress a "health-care" orientation to the disease . . . and in general focus on the child rather than the disease, normal family development and interaction should ensue. However, this optimum level of behavior is extremely difficult to achieve. . . . Obsessive concern with diabetic control by parents can result in either rebelliousness or in almost overcompliance by a child, neither extreme a healthy one. On the other hand, denial of or uninvolvement with the diabetes by parents can be disastrous (Hendrick, 1985, p. 127).

As the health counselor works with the diabetic child to enhance the likelihood of adherence to treatment regimens, he or she should also work with other family members. Although knowledge of the disease is important, awareness of the challenges of self-care may have even greater significance. The more that family members understand about the nature of the self-care skills required, the more they will be able to help and support the child's efforts. Family members may also need assistance in examining their own reactions to the child's health problems so that they can balance positive concern with recognition of the child's need for control. This process is further complicated by the need to make changes in response to the child's development. As Johnson (1985) points out, the disease of younger children is best controlled through active parental involvement and "giving the youngster too much responsibility too early may prove disastrous" (p. 225). In contrast, adolescents show better results if they control their own regimens. Families may need ongoing help and support if they are to adapt to constant changes in the disease itself and in the patient's psychosocial needs.

One helpful approach is to provide this assistance in the context of family support groups, which can furnish mutual nurturance along with skill development. This type of intervention may be especially useful in helping families cope with illnesses that tend to exacerbate feelings of helplessness. For example, family support groups have been used for dealing with such health problems as adult cancer (Dunkel-Schetter & Wortman, 1982; Euster, 1984), childhood cancer (Chesler & Yoak, 1984), Alzheimer's disease (Kapust & Weintraub, 1984;

Kerns & Curley, 1985), spinal cord injuries (Eisenberg, 1984), and multiple sclerosis (Pavlou, 1984), all of which tend to be intensely crisis-provoking.

Case Example

Forty-eight-year-old Mark T. was told after his bypass surgery that he would have to make major changes in his life-style. Mark was a hard-driving executive, dedicated to his work but also intensely involved in competitive sports. In his youth, he had concentrated on team sports: football and hockey. Now, his focus was on handball and golf; his country-club trophies provide evidence of his success.

Mark's wife, Ellen, was desperately concerned about his health. She felt that the bypass surgery had given him a new chance for longevity. She thought that this experience, which had come as a surprise after what they had thought was a routine check-up, should have jolted him into reality and forced him in the direction of more health-oriented behaviors. She tried to help him maintain a low-cholesterol diet; in fact, she and their two teen-aged children had begun to eat differently because of her attempts to prepare healthful meals that Mark might enjoy. She became more and more upset because, despite her efforts, Mark failed to bring his cholesterol under control. She knew that he ate correctly at home but consumed whatever he wanted at restaurant lunches and during business travel. She also realized that, although her reminders had stopped him from smoking in the house, he continued to "sneak" cigarettes at his office. Mark insisted that he was, in fact, healthy and that his continued athletic success proved it. He worked as hard as he ever had and tended to lose his temper when Ellen confronted him.

Mark was referred for health counseling by the coronary rehabilitation unit because follow-up checks showed no change in his cholesterol levels or in his stress tests. The Jenkins Activity Survey indicated a clear tendency toward a Type A behavior pattern. Mark's wife indicated that this result was accurate and that time urgency, competitiveness, and restlessness continued to be his most obvious characteristics both at work and in his leisure time.

The counselor's first intervention for Mark and Ellen T. involved short-term counseling for the couple. The focus of this counseling process was placed on the question of responsibility for Mark's health-risk behaviors. Ellen had become overly responsible for his behavior; the more responsibility she took, the less Mark accepted. As long as this pattern of interaction continued, Ellen felt frustrated and powerless and Mark ignored the problem. The couples counseling helped bring this process to Mark and Ellen's awareness so that both could begin to interrupt their circular pattern. Ellen tried to turn the responsibility for his health back over to Mark, although she was able to do this only through the support of a group of women whose husbands had had either myocardial infarctions or surgery.

Mark was referred to a training group that focused on helping heart patients regain their health through behavioral changes. He and the other participants learned behavioral self-management strategies to change Type A

patterns and eliminate such high-risk behaviors as smoking and eating foods high in cholesterol.

The educational component of the program helped Mark identify the differences in effect between aerobic exercise and the kind of sports involvement to which he was accustomed. In reality, however, Mark was a highly educated person who already possessed this information on a cognitive level. Individual counseling helped him explore his reactions to the health crisis he had endured and understand that his denial of the need to change his behavior was in part related to his reluctance to face the fact of his mortality.

Prevention

Efforts to prevent illnesses generally need a broad focus because of the difficulty of identifying a single, linear relationship between a definitive cause and a specific disorder. Health problems result from the interplay of numerous factors, and the same high-risk behaviors can place people in jeopardy for a number of disorders. Health-promotion programs that encourage self-management, enhance people's sense of control over their health, and support the development of new behaviors tend to serve a preventive function that is not necessarily associated with a specific disease.

Some illnesses do have a clear enough relationship with specific behavioral risk factors to make the design of preventive programs a realistic endeavor. For example, increasing success is being reported for community-based programs aimed at the prevention of heart disease. The Stanford Three Community Study (Farquhar, Maccoby, & Solomon, 1984; Farquhar et al., 1977) examined the results of an educational program that was aimed at two communities and used a third, comparable community as a control group. Citizens of Gilroy, California, received education through mass media, including television and radio programming, newspaper advertisements and stories, billboards, and mailing of printed materials. In Watsonville, the mass media program was supplemented by more intensive instruction for groups of people at high risk. Citizens of Tracy, California, received no education programs. Both Gilroy and Watsonville residents showed general improvement in comparison with the no-treatment community. The success of the program in bringing about changes in risk behaviors led to an expansion of the project to include five cities. A comparable effort in Finland also brought about clear behavior changes (Puska et al., 1980). Residents of North Karelia, Finland, received a comprehensive program aimed at improving hypertension detection and treatment, reducing smoking, changing dietary habits, and generally lowering mortality rates. In comparison with residents in the control community of Kuopio, North Karelia residents showed a greater decrease in smoking, an improvement in average cholesterol levels, and a decrease in blood pressure.

Such comprehensive campaigns can also be adapted for the prevention of other diseases that are associated with specific risk factors. New cases of AIDS, for example, can be prevented through efforts to change risk behaviors that have been very clearly identified.

The strategy of prevention of HIV transmission through education and the modification of behaviors is clearly the most hopeful approach to the prevention of AIDS. Educating persons with information that leads to changed behaviors that reduce or eliminate high-risk, unprotected sexual encounters constitutes effective prevention. Safter sexual practices, particularly if one partner has been infected, reduce the likelihood of transmission. Educating intravenous drug users about the use of clean needles and techniques for sterilizing needles and injection paraphernalia can reduce this form of transmission between IV drug users and thereby reduce the infection of IV drug users' sexual partners and many of the babies born within this social network (Albee, 1989, p. 19).

Clearly, a combination of wellness-oriented health-promotion programs and comprehensive efforts to address identified risk behaviors provides the most promising available avenue to illness prevention.

Summary

Coping with an illness can be a major challenge to the well-being of the individual and his or her family. Dealing with a sudden, acute illness can throw an individual into a crisis situation that requires new ways of behaving and of perceiving oneself and the world. Chronic illness can be equally challenging, as people try to cope with unrelenting health problems over long periods of time.

Helping a client cope with illness requires careful assessment, and a number of general and disease-specific tools are currently available. Based on information about the individual and the illness, the counselor can focus on several health-related issues, including: (1) helping the client deal with his or her psychological reactions to the illness, (2) helping the client cope with aversive medical procedures, and (3) enhancing the client's ability to adhere to recommended treatments. Emphasis should also be placed on working with the client's family, since the functionality of the family system can have a major impact on the individual's coping success and treatment adherence.

Resources

Organizations

Clients may benefit by contacting centers that provide information about the specific disease. Examples include the following:

- American Burn Association
  New York Hospital—Cornell Medical Center
  525 E. 68th Street
  New York, NY 10021

- American Cancer Society
  90 Park Avenue
  New York, NY 10016

- American Lung Association
  1740 Broadway
  New York, NY 10019

- National AIDS Information Hotline
  1-800-342-AIDS

- National Cancer Institute
  Information Clearinghouse
  9000 Rockville Pike
  Bethesda, MD 20205

Self-Help Groups

People dealing with health problems frequently find self-help groups highly beneficial as a means for obtaining emotional and social support. Self-help groups, each focused on a specific illness, are available in most communities. Among them are the following:

- AMEND (for mothers experiencing neonatal death)
- Candlelighters (for parents of children with cancer)
- Compassionate Friends (for bereaved parents)
- Epilepsy Foundation
- Heart to Heart (a visitation program for people with problems related to coronary heart disease)
- Make Today Count (for persons with cancer and their families)
- Muscular Dystrophy Association
- Phoenix Society (for burn victims)
- Reach to Recovery (for women who have had mastectomies)
- Spina Bifida Association
- United Cerebral Palsy
- United Ostomy Association

References

ALBEE, G. W. (1989). Primary prevention in public health: Problems and challenges of behavior change as prevention. In V. M. Mays, G. W. Albee, & S. F. Schneider (Eds.), *Primary prevention of AIDS: Psychological approaches* (pp. 15–20). Newbury Park, CA: Sage.

CAPLAN, R. M. (1982). Coping with stressful medical examinations. In H. S. Friedman, & M. R. DiMatteo (Eds.), *Interpersonal issues in health care* (pp. 187–206). New York: Academic Press.

CHESLER, M. A., & Yoak, M. (1984). Self-help groups for parents of children with cancer. In H. B. Roback (Ed.), *Helping patients and their families cope with medical problems: A guide to therapeutic group work in clinical settings* (pp. 481–526). San Francisco: Jossey-Bass.

CRAMER, D. (1989). The HIV-positive individual. In C. D. Kain (Ed.), *No longer immune: A counselor's guide to AIDS* (pp. 55–76). Alexandria, VA: American Association for Counseling and Development.

CREER, T., Marion, T., & Creer, P. (1983). Asthma Problem Behavior Checklist: Parental perceptions of the behavior of asthmatic children. *Journal of Asthma, 20,* 97–104.

DEROGATIS, L. R. (1977). *Psychological Adjustment to Illness Scale.* Baltimore: Clinical Psychometric Research.

DEROGATIS, L. R., Morrow, G. R., Fetting, J., Penman, D., Piasetsky, S., Schmale, A. M., Henrichs, M., &

Carnrike, C. (1983). The prevalence of psychiatric disorders among cancer patients. *Journal of Behavioral Medicine, 7,* 171–189.

DiCLEMENTE, R. J., & Temoshok, L. (1986). Psychological adjustment to having cutaneous malignant melanoma as a predictor of follow-up clinical status. In *Proceedings of the Seventh Annual Society of Behavioral Medicine Meeting* (p. 13). New York: Plenum Press.

DUNKEL-SCHETTER, C., & Wortman, C. B. (1982). The interpersonal dynamics of cancer: Problems in social relationships and their impact on the patient. In H. S. Friedman, & M. R. DiMatteo (Eds.), *Interpersonal issues in health care* (pp. 69–100). New York: Academic Press.

EISENBERG, M. G. (1984). Spinal cord injuries. In H. B. Roback (Ed.), *Helping patients and their families cope with medical problems: A guide to therapeutic group work in clinical settings* (pp. 107–129). San Francisco: Jossey-Bass.

EUSTER, S. (1984). Adjusting to an adult family member's cancer. In H. B. Roback (Ed.), *Helping patients and their families cope with medical problems: A guide to therapeutic group work in clinical settings* (pp. 428–452). San Francisco: Jossey-Bass.

FARQUHAR, J. W., Maccoby, N., & Solomon, D. S. (1984). Community applications of behavioral medicine. In W. D. Gentry (Ed.), *Handbook of behavioral medicine* (pp. 437–478). New York: Guilford Press.

FARQUHAR, J. W., Maccoby, N., Wood, P. D., Alexander, J. K., Breitrose, H., Brown, B. W., Haskell, W. L., McAlister, A. L., Meyer, A. J., Nash, J. D., & Stern, M. (1977). Community education for cardiovascular health. *Lancet, 1,* 1192–1195.

FRANK-STROMBORG, M., & Wright, P. (1984). Ambulatory cancer patients' perception of the physical and psychosocial changes in their lives since the diagnosis of cancer. *Cancer Nursing, 7,* 117–130.

FRIEDMAN, H. S., & DiMatteo, M. R. (1989). *Health psychology.* Englewood Cliffs, NJ: Prentice-Hall.

HAMBURG, D. A., Elliott, G. R., & Parron, D. L. (1982). *Health and behavior: Frontiers of research in the biobehavioral sciences.* Washington, DC: National Academy Press.

HAYNES, S., Feinleib, M., Levine, S., Scotch, N., & Kannel, W. (1980). The relationship of psychosocial factors to coronary heart disease in the Framingham Study. III. Eight-year incidence of coronary heart disease. *American Journal of Epidemiology, 111,* 37–58.

HENDRICK, S. S. (1985). Behavioral medicine approaches to diabetes mellitus. In N. Schneiderman, & J. T. Tapp (Eds.), *Behavioral medicine: The biopsychosocial approach* (pp. 509–531). Hillsdale, NJ: Erlbaum.

JANZ, N. K., & Becker, M. H. (1984). The health belief model: A decade later. *Health Education Quarterly, 11* (1), 1–47.

JENKINS, C., Rosenman, R., & Friedman, M. (1967). Development of an objective psychological test for the determination of the coronary-prone behavior pattern in employed men. *Journal of Chronic Diseases, 20,* 371–379.

JOHNSON, S. B. (1985). The family and the child with chronic illness. In D. C. Turk, & R. D. Kerns (Eds.), *Health, illness, and families: A life-span perspective* (pp. 220–254). New York: Wiley.

KAPUST, L. R., & Weintraub, S. (1984). Living with a family member suffering from Alzheimer's disease. In H. B. Roback (Ed.), *Helping patients and their families cope with medical problems* (pp. 453–480). San Francisco: Jossey-Bass.

KENDALL, P. C., & Turk, D. C. (1984). Cognitive-behavioral strategies and health enhancement. In J. D. Matarazzo, S. M. Weiss, J. A. Herd, N. E. Miller, & S. M. Weiss (Eds.), *Behavioral health: A handbook of health enhancement and disease prevention* (pp. 393–405). New York: Wiley.

KENDALL, P. C., Williams, L., Pechacek, T. F., Graham, L., Shisslak, C., & Herzoff, N. (1979). Cognitive-behavioral and patient education interventions in cardiac catheterization procedures: The Palo Alto medical psychology project. *Journal of Consulting and Clinical Psychology, 47,* 49–58.

KERNS, R. D., & Curley, A. D. (1985). A biopsychosocial approach to illness and the family: Neurological diseases across the life span. In D. C. Turk, & R. D. Kerns (Eds.), *Health, illness, and families: A life-span perspective* (pp. 146–182). New York: Wiley.

KINSMAN, R., Dahlem, N.., Spector, S., & Staudenmeyer, H. (1977). Observations on subjective symptomatology, coping behavior, and medical decisions in asthma. *Psychosomatic Medicine, 39,* 102–119.

KRANTZ, D. S., & Glass, D. C. (1984). Personality, behavior patterns, and physical illness: Conceptual

and methodological issues. In W. D. Gentry (Ed.), *Handbook of behavioral medicine* (pp. 38–86). New York: Guilford Press.

LANGOSCH, W. (1984). Behavioural interventions in cardiac rehabilitation. In A. Steptoe, & A. Mathews (Eds.), *Health care and human behaviour* (pp. 301–324). London: Academic Press.

MACKS, J., & Turner, D. (1986). Mental health issues of persons with AIDS. In L. McKusick (Ed.), *What to do about AIDS* (pp. 111–124). Berkeley: University of California Press.

MANDEL, J. (1986). Psychosocial challenges of AIDS and ARC: Clinical and research observations. In L. McKusick (Ed.), *What to do about AIDS* (pp. 75–86). Berkeley: University of California Press.

MATHEWS, A., & Ridgeway, V. (1984). Psychological preparation for surgery. In A. Steptoe & A. Mathews (Eds.), *Health care and human behaviour* (pp. 231–259). London: Academic Press.

McCORKLE, R., & Young, K. (1978). Development of a symptom distress scale. *Cancer Nursing, 1,* 373–378.

MEICHENBAUM, D. (1985). *Stress inoculation training.* New York: Pergamon Press.

MEICHENBAUM, D., & Turk, D. C. (1987). *Facilitating treatment adherence: A practitioner's guidebook.* New York: Plenum Press.

MEJTA, C. L. (1987). Acquired Immune Deficiency Syndrome (AIDS): Implications for counseling and education. *Counseling and Human Development, 20*(2), 1–12.

MILLON, T., Green, C., & Meagher, R. (1982). *Millon Behavioral Health Inventory manual.* Minneapolis: National Computer Systems.

MOOS, R. H., Cronkite, R. C., Billings, A. G., & Finney, J. W. (1984). *Health and Daily Living Form Manual.* Palo Alto, CA: Social Ecology Laboratory, Veterans Administration and Stanford University Medical Centers.

MOOS, R. H., & Tsu, V. D. (1977). Overview and perspective. In R. H. Moos (Ed.), *Coping with physical illness.* New York: Plenum.

NAMIR, S. (1986). Treatment issues concerning persons with AIDS. In L. McKusick (Ed.), *What to do about AIDS* (pp. 87–94). Berkeley: University of California Press.

PAVLOU, M. (1984). Multiple sclerosis. In H. B. Roback (Ed.), *Helping patients and their families cope with medical problems. A guide to therapeutic group work in clinical settings* (pp. 331–365). San Francisco: Jossey-Bass.

PUSKA, P., Tuomilehto, J., Nissinen, A., Salonen, J., Maki, J., & Pallonen, U. (1980). Changing the cardiovascular risk in an entire community: The North Karelia project. In R. M. Lauer, & R. B. Shekelle (Eds.), *Childhood prevention of atherosclerosis and hypertension* (pp. 441–451). New York: Raven Press.

RAZIN, A. M. (1984). Coronary artery disease. In H. B. Roback (Ed.), *Helping patients and their families cope with medical problems: A guide to therapeutic group work in clinical settings* (pp. 216–250). San Francisco: Jossey-Bass.

ROSENMAN, R., Friedman, M., Straus, B., Wurm, M., Kositchek, R., Hahn, W., & Werthesson, N. (1964). A predictive study of coronary heart disease: The Western Collaborative Group Study. *Journal of the American Medical Association, 189,* 103–110.

SCHWARTZ, G. E. (1982). Testing the biopsychosocial model: The ultimate challenge facing behavioral medicine? *Journal of Consulting and Clinical Psychology, 30,* 240–253.

STONE, G. C. (1979). Patient compliance and the role of the expert. *Journal of Social Issues, 35*(1), 34–59.

THORESEN, C. E., & Eagleston, J. R. (1985). Counseling for health. *Counseling Psychologist, 13*(1), 15–87.

TURK, D. C., & Kerns, R. D. (1985). The family in health and illness. In D. C. Turk, & R. D. Kerns (Eds.), *Health, illness, and families: A life-span perspective* (pp. 1–22). New York: Wiley.

WALLSTON, K. A., Wallston, B. S., & Devellis, R. (1978). Development of the Multidimensional Health Locus of Control (MHLOC) scales. *Health Education Monographs, 6,* 160–170.

WILLIAMSON, D. A., Davis, C. J., & Prather, R. C. (1988). Assessment of health-related disorders. In A. S. Bellack, & M. Hersen (Eds.). *Behavioral assessment: A practical handbook* (3rd ed.) (pp. 396–440). New York: Pergamon Press.

III

Conclusion

11

Toward a Wellness Perspective

To oversimplify the matter somewhat, it is as if Freud supplied to us the sick half of psychology and we must now fill it out with the healthy part.

Abraham Maslow

In the previous chapters, we have focused on a number of health-related behaviors and problems. Each of the issues we have addressed has its own body of literature, but somehow a common chord is always struck. One client may be working to eliminate a health-risk behavior such as smoking or drug use; another may be building a more positive life-style by embarking on a program of improved nutrition or exercise; still another may be searching for a way to cope with illness or pain. In each case, the counselor's most important task is to facilitate the client's ability to take responsibility for his or her own health.

Self-responsibility and self-regulation are at the heart of the concepts of wellness and good health. As early as 1947, the World Health Organization defined health as the state of complete physical, mental, and social well-being—not merely the absence of disease and infirmity. Most people would agree that an assessment of an individual's state of health would have to consider such factors as diet, exercise, coping abilities, and freedom from addictions. An individual might be free of a diagnosed medical illness but still be considered basically unhealthy because of his or her life-style. The presence of a healthy life-style—of true wellness—depends on the individual's willingness to take responsibility for his or her health rather than seeing health solely as a matter of good luck or fortunate genetic history. Wellness depends on the individual's choice to adopt a healthy life-style.

Self-Responsibility

Hundreds of millions of people remain unaware that they have a degree of accountability for their own well-being. We live in a society that encourages us to know more about the structure and function of an automobile than we know about the workings of the human body. People persist in looking "out there" for answers, formulas, and fortunes, only to discover that they have truer answers within themselves. Many fables recount adventures of young seekers who travel the world in search of a noble truth or a priceless treasure. After years of weary searching, pain, and hardship, the aged pilgrim finally returns home, only to find the object of the search in his or her own backyard.

These stories apply as much to our desires for health and wholeness as they do to the finding of treasures. Attempts to locate the doctor or the expert with a magical solution to our problems end in frustration. Looking within and assuming responsibility for what we find is a necessary condition for growth.

From our earliest years, we have been taught that somebody else knows what is best for us. As a society, we have given up personal power in many ways. To the teachers in our schools we have given the responsibility for telling us what we need to know and when and how to learn it; to professional mechanics, the decisions about the upkeep of our cars and machinery; to professional politicians, the right to use our money and direct the military power of our country. Similarly, we have entrusted our medical professionals with the responsibility for our health, giving them the power to determine what our minds and bodies need.

Initially, the general attitude of "Tell me what to do and I'll do it" or "You

do it for me" seems easier than taking responsibility ourselves. We appreciate that the training of the specialists gives them a special skill. Certainly, experts are necessary in all aspects of life. The problem is not the presence of experts but the fact that we tend to shift the responsibility to someone outside ourselves.

To take care of one's own life and well-being implies calculated risks. It involves a recognition that there are choices and a willingness to live with the consequences of those choices. For instance, a person facing an important deadline may place himself or herself under prolonged stress, neglecting his or her diet and forgetting an exercise program. These behaviors are choices that are largely under the individual's control. If the stress-linked behavior is short term, the individual will probably bounce back easily. Occasionally, however, he or she might find that these choices have brought on a cold or another condition requiring bed rest. Is he or she responsible for the condition? At least to a certain extent, yes. Without conscious awareness, he or she may have created the condition that weakened the body and made it an environment for "dis-ease." If the individual is self-responsible, he or she may see the cold not as a bit of bad luck but as an important message that the body requires rest.

Taking *responsibility* for choices that may result in unwanted health outcomes does not mean taking the *blame* for illness. With blame, people berate themselves for not learning a lesson, burden themselves with guilt, and create still more stress. With responsibility, people accept that they had a part in engineering their life situation and that they can change it as well. This process allows individuals to open themselves up to the valuable lessons that their own behaviors can teach them.

Self-Regulation

People can make the concept of self-responsibility a reality through self-regulation, which involves taking control of physiological and psychological processes. Self-regulation makes possible the kinds of meaningful changes that are likely to persist over time.

The self-care literature in health and medicine commonly assumes that, if people have education and encouragement, they will be able to maintain their own well-being. The assumption is made that people are able to act in personally responsible ways. However, as the previous chapters have made clear, self-management requires a number of skills that are not necessarily part of everyone's behavior repertoire. People need to be taught how to be more caring and more responsible for their own health and well-being, especially when the social environment commonly promotes irresponsible or nonhealthy behavior. Health counselors understand that, if clients are going to be able to control their own actions, thoughts, and emotions and at the same time manage their social and physical environment, they will need to build a number of complex skills.

According to Green and Shellenberger (1991), the ingredients of self-regulation include (1) information and knowledge, (2) decision making, (3) commitment, (4) goals, (5) maintainence of commitment, (6) willpower, (7) self-knowledge, and (8) skill acquisition. Information and knowledge help

individuals *begin* the process of change by teaching them why change is desirable and by giving them understanding of the consequences they can expect from their choices. Life-style changes depend, however, on the decisions that are made. In fact, self-regulation is possible only with effective decision making. Individuals need to understand that life-style decisions are made every day, whether or not they are aware of them.

Once a decision in the direction of health has been made, goal setting and commitment go hand in hand. Maintaining a healthy life-style takes a commitment to put the energy and time into accomplishing a goal. In order to be committed people, our clients need to believe that a particular goal is valuable enough to be worth the effort. They also need to believe that their goals are achievable. Goal setting involves the establishment of realistic goals that can be achieved through a series of intermediate goals. People tend to stay committed to change and to maintain wellness behavior when the goals of the behavior are specific and attainable (Bandura, 1986). Commitment can be enhanced through a variety of techniques, including contracting, making environmental changes, substituting healthy for unhealthy activities, developing stress-management skills, seeking social support, and providing rewards for accomplishing goals (Green & Shellenberger, 1991).

Willpower also plays a role in self-regulation, allowing people to persevere in the face of internal and external conflicts. Self-knowledge complements knowledge about the physical world, allowing people to make use of their awareness of such factors as motivations, feelings, rationalizations, expectations, values, and self-talk. Finally, self-regulation involves the acquisition of behavioral, cognitive, and physiological skills. The more skills people have in their repertoires, the greater will be the chance that they can use them in achieving their goals.

Our clients' abilities at self-regulation depend on the strategies we use to help them develop these new behaviors. Goldfried (1980) identified two basic strategies that cut across the commonly used counseling and psychotherapeutic methods: promoting corrective action and providing direct feedback. Corrective action refers to methods or techniques that essentially prompt the client to behave or act differently. Direct feedback involves providing specific and immediate information to people about their performance. Mahoney (1991) adds a third strategy: social modeling or observational learning. Mahoney's assumption is that observing the desired behavior in a systematic fashion is a very powerful and efficient technique. These three procedures are combined in Bandura's (1977) strategy of "participant modeling." In this strategy, a client observes a demonstration of some facet of a desired performance, coupled with an opportunity immediately to practice what is observed while receiving guidance and support. Various kinds of feedback on the adequacy of the performance are provided, and suggestions and additional aids to improve performance are added as needed.

Effective use of this skill-building approach clearly depends on the counselor's own ability to model desirable health behaviors. If we are to help our clients become self-regulators, we must ourselves be self-regulators. If wellness is to become part of our clients' lives, it must also be part of our own.

The Self as an Instrument

Counselors and other helping professionals are unique in that they use themselves as the primary instruments of change. Surgeons use scalpels, carpenters use tools, and pilots use aircraft, but counselors have to rely on themselves as the vehicle through which they carry out their art.

Values, beliefs, personality, habits, moods, and physical conditions influence one's counseling effectiveness. Clients learn more from how counselors act than they do from what counselors actually say. When we think of former teachers or counselors, we tend to remember what kinds of people they were more clearly than we remember the specifics of what they taught. We remember what they were like: strong or weak, caring or cold, sharing or aloof, healthy or sick, happy or sad. Certainly, counselors who have been focusing narrowly on psychological issues alone need new information to make the transition to a more holistic approach. Still, the route to improved counseling lies more in our selfhood than in the information we are able to impart.

The missing link in many medical and educational situations is the ability to make information meaningful and personalized. Counselors can provide this essential ingredient if they themselves possess self-understanding, positive health, and effective counseling strategies. A counselor is, of course, much more than a dispenser of information. A counselor is a human being with needs, abilities, beliefs, and goals. Counselors have the responsibility for creating facilitative relationships with their clients. Counselors must be able to use their own personalities and talents to help their clients—and themselves—grow.

The primary tools that counselors have to work with are themselves. These tools, like the tools of any good craftsperson, need care and attention to ensure their maximum usefulness. Counselors who live their own lives in rich, fulfilling ways enhance their potential for helping their clients as well.

Effective counseling interactions depend on the participants' ability to know what to expect from each other. Such relationships are unhealthy when counselors talk one way and act another. Clients are rightly confused when counselors with brimming ash trays on their desks try to inculcate the importance of health-oriented behaviors. Inconsistency may puzzle clients, making them uncertain whether to believe the counselor's words or the counselor's actions. Because authenticity is such an important quality for helpers, counselors need to come to grips with their own feelings, thoughts, and actions in the realm of health. To change others, counselors may first have to examine themselves. As counselors develop healthy life-styles and habits, they increase their effectiveness. Health counseling can be accomplished most effectively if it comes from counselors who are doing what they are saying and who find wellness of sufficient importance to seek its benefits for themselves.

References

BANDURA, A. (1977). *Social learning theory.* Englewood Cliffs, NJ: Prentice-Hall.
BANDURA, A. (1986). *The social foundation of thought.* Englewood Cliffs, NJ: Prentice-Hall.

GOLDFRIED, M. R. (1980). Toward the delineation of therapeutic change principles. *American Psychologist, 35,* 991–999.

GREEN, J., & Shellenberger, R. (1991). *The dynamics of health and wellness: A biopsychosocial approach.* New York: Holt, Rinehart & Winston.

MAHONEY, M. J. (1991). *Human change processes: The scientific foundations of psychotherapy.* New York: Basic Books.

MAHONEY, M. J., & Thoresen, C. E. (1974). *Self-control: Power to the person.* Pacific Grove, CA: Brooks/Cole.

WORLD HEALTH ORGANIZATION. (1947). Constitution of the World Health Organization. *Chronicle of the World Health Organization, 1,* 29–43.

Author Index

Subject Index

TO THE OWNER OF THIS BOOK:

We hope that you have found *Health Counseling* useful. So that this book can be improved in a future edition, would you take the time to complete this sheet and return it? Thank you.

School and address: _____

Department: _____

Instructor's name: _____

1. What I like most about this book is: _____

_____

2. What I like least about this book is: _____

_____

3. My general reaction to this book is: _____

_____

4. The name of the course in which I used this book is: _____

_____

5. Were all of the chapters of the book assigned for you to read? _____

   If not, which ones weren't? _____

_____

6. In the space below, or on a separate sheet of paper, please write specific suggestions for improving this book and anything else you'd care to share about your experience in using the book.

_____

_____

_____

_____

_____

_____

_____

Optional:

Your name: _____ Date: _____

May Brooks/Cole quote you either in promotion for *Health Counseling* or in future publishing ventures?

Yes: _____ No: _____

Sincerely,

Judith A. Lewis
Len Sperry
Jon Carlson

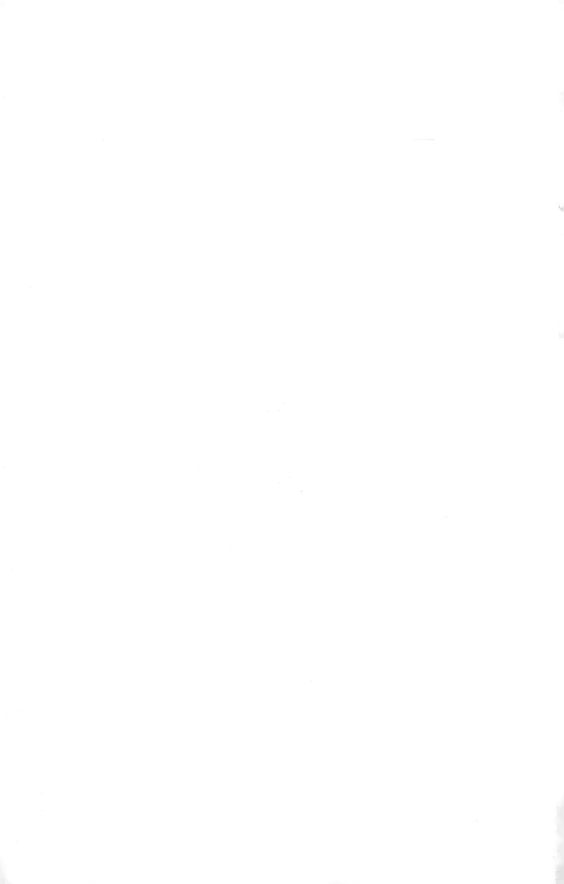